MILK

MILK

Its Remarkable Contribution to Human Health and Well-Being

Stuart Patton

Transaction Publishers
New Brunswick (U.S.A.) and London (U.K.)

Library of Congress Catalog Number: 2003070276
ISBN: 0-7658-0210-4 (cloth); 1-4128-0511-2 (paper)
Printed in the United States of America

Library of Congress Cataloging-in-Publication Data

Patton, Stuart.
    Milk : its remarkable contribution to human health and well-being / Stuart Patton.
        p. cm.
    Includes bibliographical references and index.
    ISBN 0-7658-0210-4 (alk. paper)
    1. Milk—Health aspects. I. Title.

QP144.M54P386   2004
613.2'6—dc22   2003070276

Dedicated to the memory of:

Donald Victor Josephson, 1911- 2001.

Don was of the third generation in a Swedish family that owned and operated a dairy farm near Stillwater, MN. He became a very successful university educator in dairy science serving as teacher, researcher, administrator, consultant to industry and a superb mentor of young people passing through the university. It was my lasting good fortune to gain his support, come under his inspiring influence and become one of his professional colleagues.

And to:

All my teachers, colleagues, especially my graduate students, and of course, my wife, Colleen. They made my career a fact and a joy.

Contents

Preface

Early in the last century, researchers were amassing the basic facts of human nutrition which led to the statement, "Milk is the most nearly perfect food." Milk was shown to contain more of the known vitamins, minerals, and other essential nutrients in significant quantities than any other single food. This was not to say that milk is perfect but that it is very nutritious, and the contention was not based on opinion; it arose from actual analytical data for nutrients in milk. In recent years, criticism of milk has become a popular fetish. There is a book claiming milk is poison; there are assertions that milk either causes or contributes to every major disease one ever heard of; there are anti-milk web sites; and the news media regularly carry negative implications and opinions about milk. In an attempt to set things straight, nutrition experts at the University of California Berkeley devoted part of their Wellness Letter to debunking wild and unjustified claims against milk. Virtually none of the criticism arises from research scientists, the bulk of it comes from political/cultural action groups. I never thought of milk as being very political/cultural, but these people will say anything to get attention and further their causes. Their actvism shows no concern whatsoever for the livelihoods and interests millions of Americans have in the dairy industry.

What is one to think of all this? It comes at a time when life scientists are generating a great outpouring of new facts, products, speculations and questions. I recently tried to find a newly advertised diet supplement in a local super market. Such stores used to carry a few kinds of vitamins and minerals in individual or one-a-day pills. This store had 30 to 40 feet of aisle, floor to eye-level, devoted to vitamins, minerals and bioactive supplements of all kinds. It was not very long ago that doctors were telling us, if we ate a balanced diet, we didn't need any supplements. They are changing their tune. And whose tune does one follow? Estrogen supplements were supposed to help older women avoid heart disease, but recent studies involving thousands of women do not support the earlier findings. How good are epidemiological studies anyway? They can be very good but they also are complicated and often confounded. The tone of the current times is nicely captured in a letter-to-the-editor of my paper this morning. This lady says in essence, how can one keep up with all these scientific claims especially when they contradict other highly reputable studies?

In light of this growing complexity and confusion, it seemed a good time for me to write a book providing an overview of milk. In one way or another, milk is important to all of us. It deserves to be understood and we should not accommodate its misrepresentation by activists. Evidence is indicating that it is an even better basic food for most people than had been assumed. See if you don't agree.

Acknowledgments

My efforts to produce the manuscript for this book were aided by a number of wonderfully willing people. First of all, there were my wife, Colleen, and various members of our family who would promptly proofread, give feedback and other help on request. There was Stacie Bird, a staff photographer at Penn State, whose assistance in preparing some of the photographic figures was indispensable. There also were professional colleagues who helped locate photographs, obscure information and other essential details. In that connection, I am very grateful to the following:

Thomas Anderson, Dale Bauman, Craig Baumrucker, Andrew Benson, Allen Duthie, Terry Etherton, Harry Farrell, John Fuquay, Arlyn Heinrich, Leif Jensen, Robert Jensen, Thomas Keenan, Philip Keeney, Ronald Kensinger, Manfred Kroger, Ian Mather, Lois Mc Bean, Thomas Palchak, Donald Palmquist, Tammy Perkins, Donald Puppione, Robert Roberts, Floyd Schanbacher, Lawrence Specht, Bridget Stemberger, Caroyln Summerbell, Marvin Thompson, Marc Tosiano, Gabriella Varga, and Ulrich Welsch. Of course, they do not bear responsibility for the text.

In addition, my sincere thanks goes to a cheering section which not only included my family and professional associates but also many friends and acquaintances. Such support is no minor matter during the up and down times that can occur during the writing of a book.

At the point of a completed manuscript, Irving Horowitz of Transaction Publishers, deftly headed the project toward publication. My sincere thanks to him and to Bernard Siegan who brought my need to Prof. Horowitz's attention. There are others to whom I'm grateful for their efforts to educate me about the book publishing business, in particular, Judy Jospehson, a successful author who gave very helpful orientation and encouragement. Last and by no means least, I thank Laurence Mintz and his assistants at Transaction Publishers for editorial refinement of the manucript.

1

Origins of Milk as Food

Milk is an important factor in the life of virtually every human being, whether it is one's initial nourishment following birth, the milk a woman makes in her breast, or the cow's milk and its products that form an important part of one's diet throughout life. Cow's milk contains more of the essential vitamins and minerals required by the human than any other single food. Breastfeeding is one of the most important occupations in which a woman can be involved. We need to know about milk. Science is constantly generating new information about it. The news media carry regular reports concerning it. Many of these are judgmental and provocative, a standard practice in the news business in order to arouse reader interest. However, as with all things that bear importantly on human health from cradle to grave, we need to have the best quality information possible. With respect to milk, that is one thing this book attempts to provide.

The Beginning—Evolution of Milk

Milk secretion has to be one of the most remarkable phenomena in nature. It is the means by which all the mammals were set apart from the rest of the animal kingdom. One is bound to wonder why and how milk came to be. According to the fossil records, mammals have existed for about 150 million years, but they tell us nothing about the emergence of lactation. Attempting to arrive at an understanding of this matter leads us to evolutionary theory. While it is the center of vehement debate at this time, such an approach to biology is highly useful in understanding the origin of milk. In fact, milk may supply one of the better lines of evidence that evolution did indeed occur.

A mammal is defined as a warm-blooded animal the female of which produces milk for the nourishment of her young. Structural and functional similarities suggest that mammary glands, in which milk is made, evolved from sweat glands. Considering that both are on the surface of the body and both elaborate liquids as their primary function, the explanation makes sense. A related fact is that piranha, a type of fish native to South America, feed their young by means of a secretion of mucus on the sides of their bodies—nursing of a sort. In a similar way, the female duckbill platypus, an egg-laying mammal of Australia, releases milk onto its abdomen where it is licked up by the young. This animal seems to have been stabilized midway in the evolution of a bird to a mammal.

So what would be the value of internal gestation of an embryo and nursing versus egg laying and bringing the nestlings food? Once in the world, all newborn are fairly helpless and at risk to predators, so there may not be much advantage one way or the other in that regard. But with eggs versus gestation in the womb, there is a clear-cut survival factor in favor of gestation. Eggs can be stolen and eaten. They are subject to the vagaries of the elements. Their desertion leads to almost certain death. In the womb, the developing fetus has the metabolism, size, and cunning of the mother taking care of it while maturation goes on. However, once born, the mother could continue to protect her young but a need to nourish them would be essential. Thus, it was very natural that lactation co-evolved with gestation to meet this early need. Compared to craw feeding, as in some birds, or bringing home food for the helpless young, milk has a number of advantages:

- Nutritionally, milk is tailor-made for the young of each species.

- It tends to be uniform and consistent in its composition and properties.

- It presents no problems of chewing and swallowing.

- It passes along specific disease inhibitors, such as antibodies, from mother to young.

- It is available to the young even when the mother is having difficulty finding food.

Considering the fragility of newborn life, all of these factors could make quite a difference in numbers of surviving young, and when we realize that millions of years may have been involved in natural selection of lactation for the nourishment of young, only very minor advantages could have been adequate to promote and develop that unique function. The mere fact that lactating mothers undergo appropriations from their own body stores to make milk during periods of inadequate food supply is a remarkable type of insurance for life of the newborn. That's not to say that a starving mother is going to make an adequate supply of milk, but lactation definitely accommodates short-term fluctuations in the mother's food supply.

It is a point worth some thought that gestation-lactation was not just a process that evolved to favor survival of the young. It also had to be developed in such a way as to not harm the mother. Most are aware that gestation-lactation can be a severe drain on the human female, but most mothers accomplish those demanding tasks with good health throughout and some over and over again. So it is highly plausible that natural selection has strengthened the woman for that job, including the extra nutritional and physiological stress with which she must contend.

If we think about lactation as a physiological process, and milk as its product, one could conclude, "Milk is milk. The species doesn't make much difference." This viewpoint is supported by the appearance of lactating tissue under the microscope. From species to species, the cell structure has much in common. Another line of evidence is that animal mothers are often enlisted or volunteer to nurse young across species—a practice sometimes featured by zoos to show that "the lion can lie down with the lamb" and be beneficial to the young in question. Indeed, all mammals have common nutritional needs at the organ and tissue levels. As discussed elsewhere (chapter 5), cow's milk is very beneficial food for the human. Nonetheless, one can appreciate that during past millions of years, there must have been specialized evolution of the milk for each species to favor maximum survival of the young. The merits of evolved changes in milk would be confirmed through maturation of the young to reproductive age. Failure to reach that goal would eliminate milk with detrimental characteristics. For a successful nursing mother (see figure 1.1).

Figure 1.1

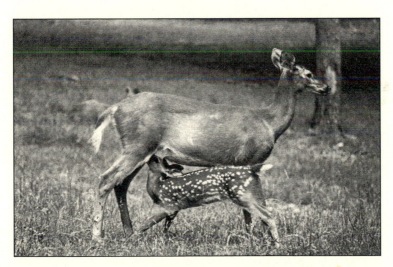

A whitetail deer providing milk for her fawn. It is one of the 12,000 known species of mammals, animals that produce milk for the nourishment of their young. Deer's milk contains 6 percent fat, 8 percent protein and 4.5 percent lactose. It is about twice as rich as cow's milk in fat and protein and about the same in lactose content. Photo courtesy of Don Wagner and Stacie Bird, The Pennsylvania State University.

While each species solves many subtle challenges to its survival, a few examples will illustrate how milk seems to fit into the designed-by-selection process. Across the spectrum of mammals, the fat content of milk varies from a few percent to as much as half of the milk. The marine mammals—whales, porpoises, seals, and sea lions—are the principal producers of the heavy cream. For example, milk of the gray whale is 53 percent fat, that of the northern elephant seal, 29 percent. Nearly all of the marine mammals have milk fat content of 25 to 50 percent. Why all that fat? These species need fat for fuel to produce energy, for flotation, for insulation in a cold, wet world, and as a source of water, via metabolism, in a salty world. The transfer of fat off of the mother's back onto the young by way of the milk is virtually a direct process—blubber to blubber. Observing the nursing of baby elephant seals on the beach from day to day is almost like watching a football being inflated. They need to achieve a condition promptly in which they can swim and fish just like their parents. Since fat is a main source of energy for the marine mammals and carbohydrate is minimal in the marine food chain, the milk of these species contain little or no carbohydrate (lactose).

Milk of humans and cattle illustrate differences in the needs of their young (see also, p. 42). Cow's milk is rich in high-quality protein, calcium, and phosphorus, the essential raw materials for making bone and muscle. The calf will reach a body mass of about 1,000 pounds in two years. The human, who is slower growing and will never reach such a weight, has milk that is much more dilute in those body building components.

Since milk is the means by which the newborn mammal survives and grows, mothers that do not produce milk of the proper quality in sufficient quantity produce no progeny or progeny with defects lethal to their development and ability to reproduce. Thus, these mothers contribute no individuals to the reproducing population; and as evolution has progressed, there has been a constant refining of milk's nutritional quality for each species. This is not to say that other factors had no effect on survival of mammalian species, only that the newborn mammal cannot even begin to develop without its mother's milk. So during the 150 million years or so of mammalian evolution, milk has undergone a constant and exceptionally long-term process of perfecting. While it is true that the milk of each species accommodates the special needs of its young, there is a common denominator in the cell biology of mammalian tissues and organs. Most of the factors that aid growth and maintenance of mammalian cells are required by all mammals. So it is not surprising that milk of many species other than the human have been utilized by mankind, and that mothers of one species can effectively nurse young of another.

Milk Supports Growth *and* Maintenance

There is a period following birth during which the newborn mammal is surviving on milk as its exclusive food. Eventually, there is a progressive adaption from milk to suitable food available in the environment; but in the early postnatal period, which in the human normally last at least several months, there is a lot of growth and development. For example, during the first six months of life, the human brain on average doubles in size. This brain growth, supported by milk alone, is impressive enough, but just as remarkable, at the same time, milk is having a similar effect on growth and development all over the body. So milk assures survival and health. While this capacity of milk as a single food to support life is strong evidence of its nutritive value, there is a distinction to be made. The accomplishment is not simply growth. It also involves maintenance of cells, tissues, organs, and bones that are already there. Actually cells and tissues are turning over throughout all of life. As a result, milk can make a valuable contribution to the diet *at any age*.

Human Food

Before considering the emergence of cow's milk as human food, it is worth asking what kind of background humankind has with respect to its food? These days we are subject to all kinds of food fads, advertising pressures, and health promotions to eat this and don't eat that. But the important basic question is what has been appropriate food for us from biological and evolutional standpoints? According to archeological evidence, an ancestor of ours named Lucy was pretty much down from the trees and walking upright on the ground about 3.5 million years ago. It is estimated from her skeletal remains that she was about 3.5 feet tall and weighed approximately sixty-five pounds. From other remains, it has been deduced that males of the time were about a foot taller and forty pounds heavier. Lucy's remains were discovered in Ethiopia in 1974. During the past year or two, bones of another pre-human of about the same age as Lucy were found in Kenya. Because of the skull shape, this find is being referred to as Flat-face which suggests that ancestor may be more closely related to us than is Lucy. But it is pretty exciting to realize that human-like beings were walking upright about 3.5 million years ago.

What did Lucy, Flat-face, and those who came after them for several million years eat to survive; and what kind of a digestive/metabolic system did they pass on to us? They surely were not like carnivores who could run down or ambush prey, attack with claws and teeth, tearing flesh off the bone. Nor were they like herbivores that could survive exclusively by munching vegetation. Actually, it appears that early humans were sorely challenged to find food and spent most of their days roaming around searching for it. In order to exist, humans had to be omnivorous, that is, eating all kinds of both plant and animal materials. Consider for example, the effects of season and geographic location. These would greatly alter what was available. It seems likely that the menu included: fruits, nuts, seeds, grasses, leaves, roots, bugs, worms, birds and their eggs, fish, and small animals.

Considering the spectrum of human foods throughout the world today, the foregoing list still covers the situation pretty well. Today, bugs and worms would not be appreciated except in a few locations, but as a people broadly considered, we are not squeamish when we need something to eat. Rats and dogs are acceptable in areas of the Far East. Certain fat worms that live in dead tree trunks are a delicacy in New Zealand. The point is we humans have a biological background of benefiting from a very wide variety of foods. Admittedly there must have been a big learning process in all this. Not everything is good for us. Some plants are horribly poisonous, and one would need to know which. An example from the animal side, Eskimos know not to eat the liver of polar bears. The organ contains a tremendous concentration of vitamin A and is thus very toxic. In addition to finding out what would agree with us, we also had to learn how to hunt and fish, how to preserve food, and eventually how to grow food.

Why didn't primitive humans eat only plant materials, as in the modern practice of vegetarianism—a diet exclusively comprised of fruits, vegetables, and grains? Because that is not the way we evolved. It was not natural to our forbears nor good for them to eat only vegetation. There is rather convincing evidence why that would not have worked, namely vitamin B12. That essential nutrient only occurs in animal matter and we cannot live without it. Vitamin B12 is of very broad importance in the growth and maintenance of the human body. Two of its classic deficiency symptoms are pernicious anemia, a failure to produce red blood cells, and painful degeneration of the nervous system as a result of failure to produce myelin for the sheath of nerve cells. A lack of B12 also renders the vitamin known as folic acid non-functional. So inadequate B12 intake also produces folate deficiency. In people with normal B12 absorption, these various deficiency symptoms have been reported only in strict vegetarians. Synthetic vitamin B12 became available about twenty years ago. So vegetarians who eat no animal products can now remain healthy by using a B12 supplement and a carefully balanced diet. But the human is not naturally a strict vegetarian. For some concerns about vegetarian diet practices, see chapter 6 in Miller et al. (suggested references).

The Human and Milk of Cattle

It is not surprising that man came to understand the milk of livestock as a valuable human food. In all probability, primitive humans evaluated the taste of milk from mammary glands of animals killed in the hunt and found it quite acceptable. No doubt, the idea passed through their minds at some point to use such milk for needy human infants, that is, ones not having lactating mothers. The observable fact that milk is the sole and unique food of growing mammalian young, including the human, was probably not wasted on them. Coupling these observations that milk is palatable and life-sustaining may well have led to its use as a basic human food. One cannot know precisely when milk was adopted as a food by primitive man. Archeological evidence from the Middle East indicates that livestock (cattle, goats, sheep, camels) was being milked at least eight to ten thousand years ago. Cave paintings in France dating to 30,000 years ago depict robust horned animals looking very much like current domestic cattle. So man knew, used, and admired ruminant animals in that epoch. Humanity has had a unique relationship with livestock, particularly cattle. The cow is sometimes called "the foster mother of the human race." This term is based not only on the use of bovine milk as human food but also on the worldwide use of formulas based on cow's milk to feed human infants. Another aspect that promoted the man/livestock relationship was lack of competition between them for food. Grasses, favored by ruminants, have little value or use as food by man.

Milk is mentioned prominently in the Old Testament in circumstances that are estimated to have occurred over 3,000 years ago:

> Then he (Abraham) took curds and milk and the calf that he had prepared, and set it before them, and he stood by them under the tree while they ate. (Genesis 18.8)

> —and he brought us into this place and gave us this land, a land flowing with milk and honey. (Deuteronomy 26.9; also 26.15)

It is an interesting implication of this latter quotation that abundance of milk and honey apparently is the ancient writer's definition of a fine place. A time scale relating some important events to man's adoption of milk as human food is presented in figure 1.2.

In addition to their meat, hides and wool, the milk of livestock became important to man. In respect to human nutrition, cow's milk frequently is described as "the most nearly perfect food." This is not to say that it has no limitations, but that it can supply more of the known essentials in significant amounts than any other single food. One is led to believe early human populations that utilized milk (or milk products) as a lifelong food had advantages, discussed following, over those that did not. In the meantime, production of milk and milk products has spread all over the world.

Lactose Digestion Capability (LDC)

An early limitation on mankind's extensive use of milk from livestock as food involved the problem of digesting lactose, a sugar which for all practical purposes exists only in milk. It occurs at a level of about 7 percent in human milk and 5 percent in the milk of cattle. Lactose is not used as such by the human but must first be broken down in the intestine into its component sugars, glucose and galactose, which serve energy and other needs in the body. The human infant is born with a capacity to express on its intestinal mucosa the

Figure 1.2

0 -	- The present -
-	
2,000 -	- The birth of Christ -
-	
4,000 -	
-	
6,000 -	- Milk adopted as human food -
-	
8,000 -	
-	
10,000 -	- Livestock domesticated in the Near East -
30,000 -	- Cave paintings of wild cattle in France -
4,000,000 -	- Man's progenitors walking upright in Africa -
150,000,000 -	- Evolutionary emergence of mammals -

Time frame in years (left) of some past events in relation to our adoption of milk from livestock as human food.

enzyme,[1] lactase, which can accomplish this hydrolysis of lactose. An enzyme is a protein that promotes a precise (chemical) change in the structure of a substance. Because single units of the enzyme can repeat their effects over and over again, enzymes are said to be catalysts. In certain of us, as explained as follows, there is progressive loss of the enzymatic activity that cleaves lactose such that by about eighteen months of age it has virtually disappeared; and if substantial quantities of cow milk, or milk products containing lactose (e.g., ice cream) are later introduced into the diet, especially in adulthood, a high level of intestinal discomfort involving gas and/or diarrhea might result in some individuals. This is due to fermentation of undigested lactose by bacteria in the lower digestive tract and bowel. As a matter of evolution, it is plausible that a weaned mammal might be programmed to lose its intestinal lactase activity since it never again would encounter lactose in its food.

Existing in cow's or goat's milk at about 5 percent concentration, lactose usually exceeds the content of milk fat (3-5 percent) and milk protein (3-4 percent). Historically, under a widening practice of milk drinking, it would not have been surprising if an individual showed up with a genetic mutation to enable metabolic use of that lactose. This individual would not only benefit generally from the milk as food, but he/she would derive additional energy and improved calcium absorption from the digested lactose.

Geographic distribution of older child/adult LDC

Not all human infants lose their lactose digesting capability (LDC). Child/adult LDC is associated with populations in certain areas around the Red Sea, where livestock tending is believed to have originated, along regions of the Mediterranean Sea, in Europe, parts of Central Africa and as far east as India. The circumstances of the Fulani people are relevant. Though dark-skinned, they have Caucasian racial features and are thought to have migrated from the Middle East through North Africa to Senegal (West Africa). The livestock-tending portion of their population is mainly LDC-positive, whereas the sedentary Fulani are much less so. The Tutsis of Rwanda (Central Africa), who also tend cattle and drink milk, seem unique in that only 7 percent of them are reported to lack LDC. One wonders if milk consumption over the centuries or millennia was a factor in the tallness of these people. The Hutus who live in the same area as the Tutsis have much less LDC than the latter. LDC is lacking in Native Americans and Asians among others. Interestingly, the Japanese may be acquiring this trait in parallel with their growing dairy industry. Some data on the incidence of low LDC in a few ethnic populations throughout the world are presented in figure 1.3.

Figure 1.3

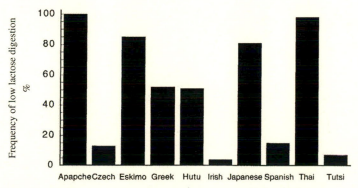

Frequency of low lactose digestion capability in some ethnic populations.
From data collated by Holden and Mace (see suggested references).

Genetic aspects of child/adult (LDC)

Protracted drinking of milk, that is, cultural induction, appears to be the plausible and remarkable explanation for the origin of child/adult LDC.[1] This human trait is associated with areas, pastoral populations, and ancestors involved in dairying. A single, inheritable, dominant gene is involved. This gene is in addition to the gene for lactose hydrolysis (lactase) which we all have in infancy; so somehow it seems to be a regulator of lactase production in the intestine.

Thus far, the geographical data are consistent with a gene mutation involving older child/adult LDC that appeared six or eight thousand years ago among livestock owning people in the Middle East. Migration of them, and perhaps their livestock-associated life style, could account for the spread of LDC into Africa, Europe, as far east as India, and eventually to other areas including the Americas, Australia, and New Zealand. However, emergence of the gene at multiple locations is also a possibility. For example, both the Tutsies of Central Africa and the Irish have a remarkably high incidence (>90 percent) of LDC (see figure 1.3). It is hard to rationalize these two populations in terms of common inheritance in that they are of different races and both have been notably non-migratory. However, dairying is common to them both.

Since the gene controlling child/adult LDC is dominant and may be induced or selected by milk drinking, it may take very few generations for it to establish itself where it has not existed, such as in Oriental, Native American, and most African populations. It seems likely that many African-Americans are lactose tolerant since they are extensively crossbred with Euro-Americans. Eventually there may well be little or no incompetence in digesting lactose. Further research regarding how and when LDC becomes heritable, and how well inheritance of the ability is retained after milk drinking is abandoned, should produce very interesting results. For further discussion of genetics and evolution in relation to LDC, see notes to chapter 1.

Remedies for Lactose Intolerance

It is notable that those who are lactose-intolerant have no serious limitation concerning milk consumption today. Milk with lactose predigested is increasingly available, as are tablets containing the enzyme lactase, which can be added to milk to hydrolyze its lactose. Lactase provided by the bacteria in fermented milk, such as yogurt, also benefits the lactose intolerant. Cheeses, in which lactose is usually greatly reduced, if not completely absent, pose no lactose problem. Short of some limiting allergy, almost anyone anywhere in the world can consume a glass of milk or two incrementally over a day's time with no discomfort. It is also important to understand that not everyone lacking LDC experiences discomfort when drinking milk. On the contrary, there are milk "regulars" who have no idea of their inability to digest lactose. The state of LDC with respect to milk consumption throughout the modern world has been reported and reviewed in depth, see chapter 8 in Miller et al. (suggested references).

Benefits of LDC

Thus, among the ancient, livestock-tending people there appeared a genetic mutation enabling the digestion of milk sugar by older children and adults. This would have conveyed two advantages, that is, milk would become a much better source of energy, and discomfort of occasional or frequent intestinal distress from lactose intolerance would be eliminated, thereby encouraging milk consumption. A practical consequence of acquiring LDC was that some peoples of the ancient past benefited from milk in their diet and the impact of this sound nutrition may have aided them in the human struggle for good health, long life, and so on. For example, from an extremely primitive beginning, Europeans developed an increasingly productive dairy husbandry which has been passed on to the United States and other parts of the world where it has evolved to monumental proportions. By the late 1900s, dairying, that is, the production, distribution, and sale of milk and milk products, had become the seventh largest industry in the U. S., and that did not include its substantial contribution to the meat industry which was ranked fourth largest.

At one point a few years ago, I was seeking an attention-getting title for a paper I was writing about milk. In the growing avalanche of communications that the reading public deals with every day, that's not easy to do. "The Rise of Western Culture or How Milk Conquered the World" came to mind. It's an overstatement, and the world is far from conquered. Compared to many other areas of the world, America is like a wonderland. Most Americans live the good life. They grow up with great expectations and learn early in their lives to have the wants. Much of what benefits them in that life often gets taken for granted. Lots of good food, including milk, is such an assumed benefit. To many people, milk has become like a public utility, resembling such things as water, electricity, gas, and so on. It's needed by many and it's there—anywhere you go in the United States, you can get good milk. Things weren't always like that, and in the case of milk, it took great, concerted effort and ingeniousness to reach that point. One of the objectives of this book is to deepen the public understanding and appreciation of milk, because, like anything else, we could lose it. There are many activists working hard to eliminate the dairy industry. Of course, milk and milk products as we know them today didn't just happen. An outline of how the industry evolved from a few dairy animals imported by early American settlers to the current huge enterprise is presented in the ensuing section.

Evolution of an Industry

The primary breeds of dairy cattle imported into America arose from wild stock in Europe that was first domesticated there about 8,500 years ago. Thus

Europeans have had a relatively long history of breeding and using cattle for milk, meat, leather, and as beasts of burden, among other things. They viewed ownership of cattle as a major aspect of wealth. In Ireland, domestic cattle were a central part of the culture and it is not surprising that the Irish have a very high incidence (>90 percent) of lactose digestion capability (see figure 1.3). They have been drinking milk for thousands of years. As a consequence of this prior European background, early settlers of the American colonies brought a few dairy animals with them plus the practical knowledge of milk and of the required animal husbandry. One might ask why bother bringing these large animals onto small boats with enough feed to keep them alive during dangerous crossings that would often take several months? Clearly, it was considered worth the expense, effort, and risk. It was common knowledge among those pioneers that milk was a good food and that it could also be converted into butter and cheese. It is also worth noting that they were not being subjected to high-pressure advertising or activist political groups about the merits or limitations of milk. They simply recognized the need for food to survive and that milk was useful for the purpose. In those times, a cow or two were part of the operation of most families and to the extent that they had more milk than needed, it was shared or bartered with neighbors. No doubt a few enterprising individuals specialized in the "dairy business." They bred cattle, expanded the number of cows in their care and the amount of milk produced. They, or others performing vendor service, supplied the milk to local families in the early settlements.

So from a spare beginning of a few animals imported into the American settlements during the early 1600s, a giant industry arose. Milk production is now approaching 200 billion pounds a year. Presently there is one cow for every four or five Americans. The growth of dairying in America is a remarkable story that parallels industrialization of the country. It is of interest to know why milk succeeded despite its limitations and the many growing pains of the dairy industry.

Keeping Quality of Fresh Milk

Anyone with even limited knowledge of fresh, unpasteurized milk knows that it can spoil rather quickly. However, there are certain properties of the milk and methods of handling it that can inhibit deterioration for hours and, in some instances, days. We should not assume that the early settlers were ignorant of these facts. Thousands of years before application of scientific experimentation, people were making trial and error observations. That is, by observing many times one way of doing something as compared with another or others, the superiority of a particular procedure might become evident, and where this was a matter of getting sick from drinking spoiled milk, the teaching process may have been very effective. For example, it certainly would not have taken very long for one to deduce that milk keeps better in winter cold as compared to summer heat. All one would need to establish that point would be to taste and smell the milk to perceive the difference; and if one got sick a few times from drinking milk with a strong odor or flavor, the point would be reinforced.

What else did our early American forbears do to avoid spoilage of milk and sickness that might ensue from drinking such? This would be the era from the 1600s to the mid-1800s. Milk exhibits a bacteriostatic period for some hours after it is removed from the udder.[2] Depending on what kind of bacteria enter the milk before and during milking, the extent of natural antibiotic activity in the milk, and the temperature at which the milk is held following milking, bacterial multiplication may be held in check for two to ten hours or more. Milk is often close to complete freedom from bacteria (sterile) at the time of milking, and it may actually experience a drop in bacterial numbers during the first few hours post-milking. Milk is known to have a number of natural antibiotic activities that are imparted to it within the mammary gland during its synthesis.[3,4] For example, the protein lysozyme, which occurs in tears as well as milk and other body fluids, destroys bacteria and thus, protects the eye against infection. Lysozyme is quite active in human milk but less so in cow's milk because of its comparatively low concentration there.

Another natural tendency that would have been helpful to the early American dairyman would have been the desire to keep milk clean just as one would want any food to be clean. It has been shown in the development of medically certified raw milk, which is available in quite a few markets today, that efforts to get milk from the cow's udder into the bottle with little or no bacterial contamination of any kind can result in a milk which is almost bacteria-free and of excellent keeping quality. Such practices prior to milking as washing the udder with disinfectant, stripping out a small amount of fore milk from each teat and sterilizing the milking machine, or in the old days, having the milker wash his/her hands, promote clean milk of low bacterial count. Stripping the teats tends to wash out bacteria that may have entered the teat canal from outside the udder.

One simple means of demonstrating the initial quality of fresh milk and its resistance to spoilage is the methylene blue test. Methylene blue is a dye which is blue in the presence of oxygen and is colorless in its absence. The milking process tends to saturate milk with oxygen of the air and the growth of bacteria in milk will tend to deplete this oxygen. So addition of the dye to fresh milk produces a blue color. The test consists of incubating the milk with the dye under standardized conditions. The length of time required for the sample to become decolorized is a good indicator of its bacterial quality. This is based on the fact that most common bacteria require oxygen to live and if there was heavy initial contamination of the milk the oxygen would be used up quickly leading to decolorization of the blue dye. Milk samples that decolorize within an hour or two are of relatively poor bacterial quality; those which resist the change for ten or more hours are considered to be of excellent quality. Another procedure used to assess the initial bacterial quality of milk is known as the direct microscopic count in which the number of bacteria in a standardized quantity of a milk sample are determined by observation through a microscope.

Of course, colonial Americans didn't have the methylene blue test or microscopes available but such tests make clear that fresh, cleanly produced milk tends to resist spoilage. A further consideration is that the normal generation time of most bacteria is about twenty minutes at room temperature (70° F). Since spoiled milk has a bacterial count in the millions, almost any milk produced under reasonably clean conditions is going to take several hours to spoil.

Other very simple, extremely sensitive criteria of food quality used not only by early Americans but also by anyone today are taste and odor. Milk because of its bland odor and flavor when fresh and properly produced is very easily screened for spoilage. No doubt humanity applied such tests with increasing effectiveness down through the ages because they helped to determine what practices preserved food and keep people from getting sick. For further consideration of flavor in milk and milk products, see chapter 8.

Small was Good Public Health

With many local families in early America producing milk primarily for themselves, transportation and keeping quality of milk were not a problem. Within a few hours of its expression from the udder, the milk could be delivered and consumption of it could begin. As mentioned, it was common knowledge that cold winter weather preserved foods and the heat of summer quickly spoiled them. Just when and how this knowledge was applied to milk is not clear. Spring houses probably became common on American farms very early in the country's history; and it was the practice to use such facilities to cool fresh milk. While those structures could be very simple and superficial, the eastern countryside of the United States is dotted with these small free-standing spring houses. They were often built of the limestone ever close to the surface in many parts of the northeast and make very picturesque outbuildings near the farmhouse. They provided protection of a small pool of spring water at or near the point at which it emerged from the ground. In more recent years the holding pools were constructed of concrete and the water was pumped from a nearby source either under or above ground. Spring water in the northeastern United States runs about 50° to 55° F. the year around. While this is above the operating temperature of a modern refrigerator (34° to 40° F.), it is well below the optimum growth temperature for most bacteria. Thus, cooling cans of fresh milk in spring water greatly enhanced keeping quality of the milk.

Use of mechanical refrigeration did not begin to spread widely in the United States until the late 1920s. Up to that time, ice cut from ponds and lakes in the winter was stored in buildings for use as needed all year around. Cabinets called iceboxes, which were about the same size as a modern refrigerator, were used in the home to preserve perishable foods such as milk. These cabinets would accommodate large chunks of ice, delivered as needed, in an upper compartment which cooled food held below.

Up until 1900, most of the United States population was living in rural areas, residing on farms and in small towns (see figure 1.4). This enabled distribution of milk to most of the people without milk spoilage and public health problems. However, as pointed out by Du Puis,[5] supplying growing populations of cities with adequate quality and quantity of milk became very challenging. She has documented this extensively as it applied to New York City. Basically the dilemma was how to transport enough milk over relatively long distances, that is, up to hundreds of miles, to supply closely living people by the thousands and later millions, with a food commodity that could easily spoil and become contaminated with bacteria capable of generating epidemic sickness. Such innovations as milk plant mechanization, pasteurization, mechanical refrigeration, tank trucks for hauling milk, and foresighted regulatory laws, including farm inspection, eventually brought this problem under control. However, not before a lot of cost was experienced in terms of maladjusted milk supply and human sickness. Indeed the success of milk as a food commodity in America involved many interacting factors as discussed following.

Figure 1.4

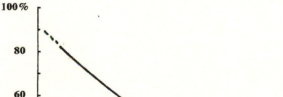
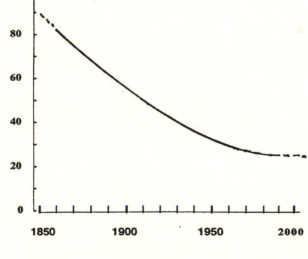

Trend over time in the rural population of the United States as a percentage of the total population. Adapted from U. S. census data.

Milk Succeeded

The Human Side of the Equation

In her carefully and extensively documented analysis of why milk succeeded as a food in America, Du Puis details the economic, sociological, political and religious factors involved and the interplay of numerous interest groups in the advancement of the industry. In her humanistic focus on this situation, she points to a central image that was being fostered of milk as "nature's perfect food." This was being toned down to the more realistic "nature's *most nearly* perfect food" as nutrition science began to enlighten the world in the late 1800s. It soon became clear that no food contains every nutrient required by humans and all of them in the right amount. Nonetheless, there was a sustained image in the evolving American culture that saw milk as divinely inspired and specially designed to support human well-being. Children's need for milk was unquestioned. In bringing out some of the more subtle factors involved, Du Puis points to the fact that men became supportive of "liberating" women from breast feeding which tended to make cow's milk more indispensable for infant feeding.

With this image of milk as a great and much-needed food, social, political, regional, and city planners and uplifters became engaged in the knotty problem of how to get good, clean milk produced, transported, and distributed to the ever-growing population. The deadly public health conditions that prevailed in the young cities of America during the late 1700s and early 1800s, particularly during the summers, are almost unimaginable in light of today's standards. There was no understanding of sanitation in the modern sense. The elevated summer temperatures promoted typhoid and yellow fever, malaria, food poisoning, and many other sicknesses to epidemic proportions. It is evident from the biography of John Adams,[6] who was to become our second president, that people would leave such places as Philadelphia and New York in the summer to save their lives. Supplying milk under such conditions often produced disastrous consequences. This was a completely different situation from the simple matter of a farmer supplying his family and his neighbors, in some instances, with fresh milk each day. So it is little wonder that many human interest groups labored for most of the nineteenth century to solve the problems of milk supply to urban centers. Pasteurization, which was widely adopted toward the end of the century, arrived none too soon, although like all innovation it was seriously questioned at the time. In brief, pasteurization is heat treatment sufficient to kill all disease-causing bacteria and nearly all of the other bacteria in milk. It has a barely discernible but not unpleasant effect on the flavor of milk. So far as rendering milk safe from a public health standpoint, it was a godsend.

Other factions in addition to the planners were vitally interested in the success of the struggling dairy industry. Farmer/producers, processors, and marketers of milk and milk products had a strong vested interest because it provided them a living. Politicians could not avoid getting involved since happy producers and consumers of milk were and still are important issues of constituents. In a sense, the picture is ever changing, yet, never changing. Always there are many humanistic factors in food production, distribution, and consumption; and while the details change the principles do not. The dynamic roles of supply, demand, distribution, and price are everlasting.

Another human factor contributing to the success of the young dairy industry was the American genius for innovation and invention. Processes, machines, and equipment of all kinds were devised for handling and packaging huge volumes of milk. While this was by no means an exclusively American success story in that some of the key inventions and concepts came from Europe; for the most part, it was this country doing what it is exceptionally good at. For further consideration of milk processing including pasteurization see chapter 7.

A Triumph of Facts

The conquest of the Western world by milk has not been brought about simply by humanistic motivations. It is also a triumph of facts, mostly scientific and technical. There are some basic properties and characteristics of milk separate and apart from relativistic human concerns, that made for its large-scale success:

Milk, of and by itself, is a life sustaining food. It promotes the growth and maintenance of every organ and tissue in the body. This is not something that required proof from modern science. Anyone who has ever observed breast feeding of babies, the nursing of kittens and puppies by their mothers, or calves by cows readily understands it. Humanity has known it for thousands of years.

Milk has proven to be a food rich in essential nutrients. As basic facts of nutrition were being brought to light by scientific research during the last two centuries, it was established beyond question that cow's milk is a rich source of *essential* nutrients required by the human including vitamins, minerals, and amino acids. This simply provided a more detailed understanding of what was already known by the colonial culture of America (see above) and added to an already strong demand for milk.

Retail milk evolved to be a very uniform and sanitary food. It is a principle of economics that repeat sales are based on the customers' knowing the good character and quality of an item will not have changed if they come back to repurchase it. Milk has been so perfected that it can be obtained in acceptable quality anywhere from coast to coast in the United States. This is a tremendous testimonial to many years of research on quality control of milk by personnel at land-grant universities and in government laboratories. It also is an indication that milk is quite uniform as synthesized in the udder and will remain so if properly handled.

Milk tastes good to most people. An industry is not going to achieve mammoth proportions on the basis of a food that tastes bad. Milk is slightly sweet with a faint characteristic flavor. It is found refreshing when served cold, as is usually the case. Actually milk is pretty bland and there is not much to which one can object. Of course there are those that don't care for it, but they are a minority. For further consideration of milk flavor, see chapter 8.

The physical and chemical properties of milk lend it to transportation and processing in massive volumes. Milk is easily pumped, agitated, heated, homogenized, cooled, and packaged. Invention of the cream separator made it easy to remove or adjust the fat content of milk. This is a rather unique situation; a first-class food that can be extensively and satisfactorily manipulated in the customer's interest. These attributes enabled tank truck shipment of milk and processing of it in huge, highly efficient plants. Thus, the milk that was supplied by the neighbor's cow in colonial days could become the product of a remarkable nationwide industry.

Much of the United States is ecologically suited to the pasturing of cattle. Considering that our forebears from Europe were used to raising and maintaining dairy animals on pasture, America offered vast lands to do more of the same, especially in the east and midwest. This like the rest of the industry required development, but a great potential for growth was there.

It is true that milk "boosterism," public relations, sales promotions, lobbying, and politics contributed to the success of milk as a food in America. However, it can be argued also that separate and apart from such manipulative efforts, there were known facts and conducive conditions, such as those listed above, that may have inevitably produced such success. Sometimes despite all the pushing and shoving, the facts win and humanity benefits. At least in part, that seems to have been the case regarding the growth of the milk industry in America. But the pushing and shoving goes on, and it was ever so. What is needed now is a source of information on milk that not only can assist people in the understanding of this remarkable food, but one that will provide an update covering new research findings and what they mean. This is such a book.

* * *

In summary, when one ponders what factors benefited survival of the primitive human, good nutrition has to be a crucial consideration. Physical strength and good health (disease resistance) through the reproductive years could not have been achieved in any other way. Nothing chronically weakens a human like mal- or undernutrition. The relatively recent increase in stature of Europeans and Japanese suggests that most, if not all, of the human population has evolved under marginal conditions of nutrition. It is true that, within the past hundred years in many areas of the world, food quality and quantity have improved, sanitation is much better, some toxic elements in the environment are being controlled (e.g., lead), antibiotics and many other beneficial drugs have been developed, and medical practice is much more sophisticated and effective. But these are mainly recent innovations. If one were to ask what might have had a real impact on human well-being in the last 10,000 years, a different and better food for children and adults such as milk could have been very effective for those to whom it was available. Not only milk, but, as discussed, the acquisition of lactose (milk sugar) digestion capability by certain populations could have been of great and selective value not only with regard to survival but also human vigor and productivity. In more recent years, millions, young and old, have also experienced a sense of the good life in consumption of milk and its products (ice cream, cheese, butter, yogurt, etc.). It would be nice if the benefits of this outstanding achievement could reach everyone the world over.

Suggested References

Tattersall, I. *Becoming Human.* Harcourt Brace, Orlando, FL. 1998. pp. 258.

Miller, G. D.; Jarvis, J. K.; and McBean, L. D. *Handbook of Dairy Foods and Nutrition.* 2nd ed., Boca Raton, FL: CRC Press, 1999. pp. 443.

Holden, C.; and Mace, R. Phylogenetic analysis of the evolution of lactose digestion in adults. *Human Biology* 69:605-28, 1997.

Flatz, G. Genetics of lactose digestion in humans. *Advances in Human Genetics* 16:1-77, 1987.

Du Puis, E. M. *Nature's Perfect Food.* New York University Press, New York. 2002. pp. 310.

Notes

1.   Holden, C. and Mace, R. *Human Biology* 69:605-28, 1997.

Genetics and evolution of lactose digestion capability (LDC). A gene that distinguishes between those who are LDC-competent and those who are not has been detected and sequenced (Enattah, N. S. et al. Nature Genetics 30:233-7. 2002.) but the protein for which it codes has not yet been identified. Thus we do not know whether this protein is simply a marker or a true regulator of lactase activity (expression). The revelation of this gene's sequence does provide the basis for a new test for LDC. However, existing tests, especially the analysis of breath for hydrogen following ingestion of milk or lactose, have been relatively satisfactory.

One of the great current frontiers of research is the question of how genes are turned off and on. It seems that a man need only think about a woman and it may elevate his testosterone production and speed up the rate at which his beard is growing. There are many interesting research questions yet to be answered about LDC. For example, can one acquire LDC capability sometime during a lifetime as a result of continuing milk drinking or does it have an absolute dependency on a mutated gene, such as that reported by Ennattah et al., of one individual which spreads to succeeding generations? Is it possible that the ancient milk drinkers, probably at multiple sites, by sheer coincidence happened to carry the LDC gene? Could the LDC gene and milk drinking have been associated with survival in ancient peoples? How is the original LDC we all have in infancy turned off in those who lose it? Is there a use-it-or-lose-it character to LDC in adult life?

The fact that older children and adult humans acquired gene(s) enabling digestion of lactose presents an interesting challenge to the understanding of evolution., that is, how plant and animal life changed over time and became what they are today. We do not know how long it takes for a population of milk-drinking people to become LDC, nor do we know exactly what the mechanism is. The well-known Darwinian Theory of Evolution that change comes about due to random mutations (sudden changes in genes) and to natural selection is now considered inadequate and too simplistic to explain the astoundingly complex facts about life. In essence, Darwin proposed that if a mutation produced individuals that are better adapted to survive, then the characteristics of this "new breed" would become part of the heritable character of that animal or plant. Over very long periods of time, thousands or even millions of years, according to Darwinian theory, great changes, even the development of new species might occur. Darwin (1809-1882) himself was very conservative in his claims about this explanation. He didn't necessarily feel that it could account for the origin of life or even explain all evolutionary change; and he did his best to refine and upgrade his hypothesis during his years after introducing it. Prior to Darwin's Theory, there were others who offered explanations of how changes occurred in the appearance, behavior and survival of living things. One was a very accomplished French biologist by the name of Jean Baptiste de Lamarck (1744-1829). He wondered, for example, how the giraffe acquired its great long neck and speculated that from constantly reaching up to eat the leaves of trees, the animal acquired the long neck and passed it on to the young. At about the same time, a rabbi by the name of Rav David Luria, studying the Torah and the observable facts of life, came to a similar conclusion, that is, acquired characteristics are heritable. Without going into detail, this idea of inheritance was rejected and Lamarck, who was rather famous at the time, ended his life in poverty and reputational ruin.

Lamarck, Luria, and others of their persuasion appear to have been discredited prematurely. The writer can remember in his earliest biology class being told—"So they chopped off the tail of this laboratory rat; and after it healed, they bred the rat: and its offspring had tails of normal length." So much for the explanation that acquired characteristics are heritable. But as is often the case with science, the investigators of the day broad-jumped to a premature conclusion.

Since that time there have been many experimental observations that effects of environment can modify progeny of exposed individuals. LDC certainly seems to be a case in point. Others have involved the shape of a songbird's beak the inheritance of which proved quickly responsive to the nature of the weather and available food (see *The Beak of the Finch: A Story of Evolution in Our Time* by Jonathan Weiner); the imprinted headflicking behavior of rats which was immediately passed on to some of their young, and a change in the way moths construct their cocoons that proved immediately heritable (cited by Gordon R. Taylor in "*The Great Evolution Mystery*"); and even the adaptation of bacteria to the fermentation of lactose, which, as an initial step, requires the same cleavage of the molecule as does LDC in the human (in "*Not by Chance*" by Lee Spetner).

So, yes, blunt traumatic acts, such as losing a limb or chopping off a tail, do not create heritable characteristics. But changes produced by repeated stimulation over prolonged periods of time, such as the constant drinking of milk for years by an LDC incompetent individual, especially into the reproductive years, may lead to a change that can be inherited.

The reader may wonder why spend so much time on how the human acquired LDC? By way of explanation, it seems important enough simply from the standpoint of trying to understand how cows' milk became such a valuable human food, but as a general principle, the concept of rendering acquired characteristics heritable is even more important. Let us consider the case of constant overeating with resultant obesity. This could thoroughly engrain behavioral and metabolic changes in the way food is handled by the body. Obesity is said to be reaching epidemic proportions in the United States with 50 to 60 percent of the population considered overweight. Admittedly this is a complicated problem with many contributing factors, such as high availability of food and growing human inactivity; but one solid contributor is whether ones parents were obese. If one of them was, ones chances of being fat are 50 percent; if both were obese, it is 90 percent. So it is concluded that inheritance is a big factor in incidence of obesity. But it would be important to know whether this inherited fate comes inevitably from a long, long chain of overweight forebears, or can it be acquired in the short-term? Has it become widely inherited just since our food supply became so abundant and we quit doing so much physical work? From an evolutionary standpoint, those changes are very recent. Another interesting question along the lines of inherited obesity, can one rigorous and dedicated diet control person break the chain? Seemingly, there are many human attributes that need to be rethought and researched with respect to inheritance of acquired characteristics.

In recent years, the emphasis has been on how important genes are in determining ones character—physical, mental, and emotional. However, it is becoming evident that something turns genes on and off—a principal area where environment can have an effect. Clearly there must be some kind of environmental factor involved in LDC, otherwise it would not be traceable to ancestral dairy farming/milk drinking. For those interested, there is a book on the gene vs. environment issue: Moore, D. S. *The Dependent Gene: The Fallacy of Nature vs. Nurture* (W. H. Freeman, New York, 2002. pp. 400).

2.   Jones, E. D. and Burrows, W. *Textbook of Bacteriology. 14th ed. (revised).* W. B. Saunders Co. Philadelphia. 1946. pp. 234-5.
3.   Reiter, B. *Journal of Dairy Research* 45:131-47. 1978.
4.   O'Toole, D. K. *Advances in Applied Microbiology* 40: 45-94. 1995.
5.   Du Puis, E. M. *Nature's Perfect Food.* New York University Press, New York. 2002. pp. 310.
6.   Mc Cullough, D. *John Adams.* Simon and Schuster, New York. 2001. pp. 446-7.

2

Milk Secretion and Composition

Milk is one of the most unusual products in nature. In chapter 1 we considered its biological evolution and the perfecting of it for survival by each species. In this chapter we focus on the production, secretion and composition of milk. Engagement of the whole female body in lactation as well as activities of the lactating cell are considered. This process is designed in such a way that the mother can pour nutrients out of her body continuously for months, and in some cases even years, without detriment to herself. In fact, the normal course of events is for it to occur over and over again.

The Mammary Gland

Conception in the female mammal brings about a sequence of hormone-triggered changes. A rise at that time in circulating estrogen and progesterone induces an extensive development of the ducts and alveoli that will accomplish the synthesis and secretion of milk. So at the same time the young are developing, the mammary glands are being prepared for their functioning.

Organization of the Tissue

The mammary epithilial cells which produce milk are arranged to form hollow spheres known as alveoli. The substances needed to make milk are supplied by the blood to the outer surface of the alveolus where they are taken up by the individual cells, made into milk, and the milk is exported from the cell into the hollow interior of the alveolus known as the lumen. All of the alveoli are connected in a branching pipeline system of ducts. The structure is often likened to a clump of grapes in which the grapes are like alveoli and the stems are ducts. The little ducts are connected to bigger ones that eventually terminate on the surface of the mother's body. This is a remarkable system. The product of every single milk-synthesizing cell can flow continuously to a point where it is accessible to the nursing young, that is, to a nipple or teat.

The number of nipples (teats) vary from two to fourteen among mammalian species. The goat has two, the cow four, and many others, such as the dog, cat, pig, mouse, rat have a row on each side. The total number of teats in these species ranges from eight in the cat to as many as fourteen in the pig. In a rough way, the number of teats seems to have co-evolved with the number of young at delivery. The human, almost always giving birth to a single offspring, has two. The species with rows of teats often have ten or twelve young at a time. However, there is an indication from whence we humans came. Many of us, both female and male, bear marks about five or six inches below our nipples where another pair may have existed many millions of years ago. Ordinarily it is just a brown spot on the skin. In very rare instances, women may have vestigial glands complete with nipples in their armpits. Along with the normal breasts, these may even produce milk and considerable discomfort as lactation commences. However, such extra glands will become inactive fairly promptly if they are not nursed or pumped to remove milk. According to Dr. Judy Hopkinson of Baylor College of Medicine, extra mammary tissue is estimated to occur in 2 to 6 percent of women. It is most common under the armpits but can occur in the form of nipples, areolae or breast tissue from the groin upward and even on the back and buttocks.

The fact that the male human has non-functioning breasts is of interest. This is due to regulation by the male (y) chromosome but due more specifically to the different pattern of hormones it dictates during development as compared to that for the female. By treating the young male with female hormones, especially estrogen, it is possible not only to induce breasts, but also to suppress male genitalia and promote development of those for the female. Further, the biomedical literature makes clear that persistent suckling of the nipple can induce lactation in the human, including men, as well as in experimental animals.

The basic structural unit of lactation is the alveolus, a scheme of which is shown in figure 2.1 (left). Note that there is arterial circulation, bringing essentials such as oxygen, glucose and fatty acids for the cells, as well as a venous system for taking away waste products. Figure 2.2 shows what alveoli of lactating tissue from a cow actually look like under the microscope. There is great similarity in the structure of alveoli from lactating tissue of the various mammals. In fact, with the exception of fat cell deposits, the tissue itself has a structural resemblance from species to species. In distinction to other species, ruminants (cattle, goats, sheep, etc.), because of their low fat diets, tend to have little fat in their lactating tissue. A further factor is that in most species, such as the human for example, fat present in the tissue during pregnancy is gradually utilized during lactation.

The scheme of the alveolus (figure 2.1, left) also shows the location of myoepithelial cells, which are a type of muscle cell. They are wrapped around the outside of the alveolus. Suckling by the young prompts the release of a hormone, oxytocin, from the pituitary gland in the center of the head. This hormone, which reaches the mammary gland by way of the circulation, causes contraction of the myoepithelial cells. This serves the purpose of squeezing the

Figure 2.1

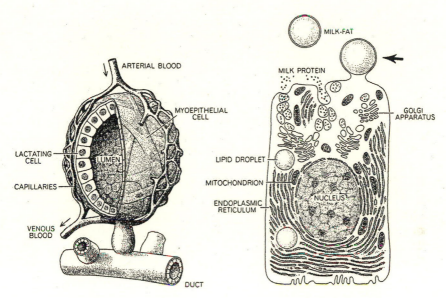

Structural scheme of an alveolus from lactating mammary tissue. Note that the lactating cells are arranged as a sphere the center of which forms an expandable lumen in which the milk they secret can accumulate. The lumens of all the alveoli in the gland are interconnected by a system of ducts (lower) that drain to the nipple (see also Fig. 3.1, p. 58). (right) Scheme of a single lactating cell enlarged from alveolus (left) and showing principal structural elements. The two major secretory mechanisms are: 1. by means of membrane-bound secretory vesicles containing the skim milk phase, see path of milk proteins, that empty their contents through the outer (plasma) membrane into the alveolar lumen; and 2. lipid droplets forming and growing in size as they move to and are enveloped by plasma membrane (arrow) which ultimately expels them into the lumen.

alveoli and expelling milk from their lumens into the ducts. Massage and manipulation of the bovine udder, as takes place in both hand and machine milking, also accomplishes the release of oxytocin. The resulting effect is known as 'let down' and it is commonly experienced by women as a change in tension within the breast. Simply the crying of her baby may induce milk let down in the mother. Without let down, the amount of milk the baby can obtain is quite limited.

Sometimes in work with experimental animals that do not lend themselves to milking, one resorts to injection of oxytocin, with or without anesthesia, as an aid to obtaining a milk sample. The effect of oxytocin can be dramatic. The writer vividly remembers such an effort with a mother pig. Under such conditions, pigs are totally uncooperative. So the help of an experienced veterinar-

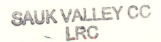

Figure 2.2

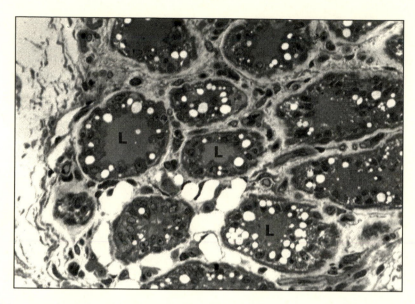

Mammary tissue from a lactating cow showing numerous more or less spherical alveoli with central lumens (L) into which milk is secreted. Note that most alveolar cells contain fat droplets (roundish white spots) of various sizes but that lumens are relatively small and mostly free of milk fat globules suggesting that the animal had been milked recently. Magnification 160X. Photo courtesy of Bridget Stemberger and Stacie Bird, the Pennsylvania State University.

ian who knew just how to do it was solicited. First he thoroughly restrained the pig and then he injected her with oxytocin. Next he produced a large oblong roasting pan and held it under her double row of teats. Within a matter of some seconds, milk began to stream out of all the teats into the pan. This only lasted a minute or so but it produced a good-sized milk sample. I was truly impressed and used the technique on a number of occasions to collect milk from anesthetized rats. Of course, one doesn't use a collecting pan with such an animal. After the injection, drops of milk can be massaged to the nipple and collected with a syringe or eye-dropper.

The alveoli, ducts, and blood vessels, including capillaries of the mammary gland, are retained in a structural network of adipose and connective tissues. In fact, these latter are the dominant components of the non-lactating gland. The function of connective tissue as a structured support system seems straightforward. On the other hand, adipose (fatty) tissue appears to have more sophisticated functions. In addition to serving as a storage reserve of fat that can be transformed into milk fat, adipose tissue seems to supply factors and structure needed for development of functional alveoli. A current speculation is that all of the major cell types of the mammary gland, including epithelial, myoepithelial, adipocyte and fibroblast may arise from a common forebear known as a stem cell.

The Lactating Cell

To properly appreciate milk and the mammary gland, it is necessary to have some understanding of the cell that makes milk. This will necessarily introduce some technical words that may be new to the reader, but definition of these terms follow and it is hoped that a clear impression of this remarkable unit will be conveyed. The lactating cell, the one that secretes milk, belongs to a cell classification known as epithelial. These cells line the inner and outer surfaces of the body including the skin, intestines, other organs, and respiratory passages. It appears that lactation evolved in these cells from their related function in sweat glands of the skin.

In most respects, the lactating mammary epithelial cell is a typical animal cell. It has a nucleus, which houses genetic material; mitochondria, which produce energy substances needed for life of the cell; membrane systems required in the structural/functional activities of the cell; cytoplasm, which is the aqueous medium that carries essential dissolved and suspended materials to all parts of the cell; and an outer covering, known as the plasma membrane. It is not only part of the cell's membrane system, it physically defines the dimensions of the cell and regulates what enters and leaves the cell. In a secretory cell, this outer membrane, which facilitates entry of raw materials and secretion of finished products, is of great importance. It will be discussed further, but explanation of the many complex and fascinating aspects of basic cell biology should be sought elsewhere, such as in the text by Alberts et al., listed in the suggested references. Our objective here is to focus on distinctive features of lactation at the cellular level.

Membranes

Cell membranes are too small to be seen in detail even with the aid of an electron microscope (e.m.). They have a very thin, sheet-like structure. The production of milk in the lactating cell is made possible by a system of such membranes made of lipid and protein molecules. One of the useful classifications of lipids (fatty molecules) is according to their affinity for water. There are polar or water-loving lipids and there are non-polar or water-repelling lipids. The latter, because of their water rejection and self-attraction, form into oil droplets or layers of oil on water. The polar lipids, having a partial affinity for water as well as for each other, self-assemble into a bi-layer, that is, a very thin sheet only two molecules thick. When very well resolved in the e.m., one can see that in cross section a cell membrane looks like a line that is a little lighter in the middle than along its two edges. This is interpreted to show that the double layer of lipid molecules is oriented with the water loving ends to the outside. Certain proteins, because of their properties, embed in or attach to the outer surface of the lipid bi-layer. The resulting membranes have large surface area which facilitates physical and chemical interactions required in the life processes of the cell. As already mentioned, cell membranes compartmentalize structure and regulate movement of molecules, for example, the nuclear membrane confines the cell's principal genetic material to the nucleus. That membrane has pores which allow particular substances to move in and out of the nucleus. Other major membranes of the lactating cell are the endoplasmic reticulum, which synthesizes proteins and lipids; the Golgi apparatus membranes, which produce the lactose of milk and process and package proteins for secretion or transfer within the cell; lysosomes, which breakdown and recycle obsolescent, redundant or foreign proteins, lipids and carbohydrates; and mitochodria, which generate the chemical energy needed to keep the cell alive and functioning. A scheme of the lactating cell showing the major membrane systems is in figure 2.1 (right).

Regarding cell structure, the term, vesicle, is used to define a more or less spherical, membrane-bound particle. In a sense, vesicles are liquid-containing bubbles. Figure 2.3 is a photomicrograph showing a number of secretory visicles in a lactating cell. Vesecles of the type shown contain the skim milk phase of milk. In addition to the secretory vesicles released from the Golgi apparatus, there are many other vesicles carrying specific products and docking instructions for various locations in the lactating cell. For example, immunoglobulins, disease-fighting antibodies, from the mother's circulation attach to the basal plasma membrane and are enclosed in a vesicle that forms by invagination of that membrane. This vesicle then moves the full length of the cell, fuses with the cell's plasma membrane bordering the alveolar lumen and empties the immune globulin into the accumulating milk.[1] This is an elegant mechanism! Like all of milk secretion, it provides a way for the mother to send not only nutrients, but substances to defend against diseases and biochemical messages to her young.

Secretion of Milk by the Lactating Cell

There are two major mechanisms for the secretion of milk, one for the fat and the other for the skim milk. Micro droplets of fat which form in the endoplasmic reticulum at the base of the cell fuse with each other and larger droplets as they move to the apical (secretory) membrane. This membrane progressively envelopes the maturing fat droplet, and when the process is complete, the membrane-encased droplet, known from this point onward as a milk fat globule, detaches itself from the cell which places it in the accumulated milk of the alveolar lumen. At the same time, the milk proteins, lactose, salts and what will be aqueous phase of the milk, is packaged into spherical, membrane-bound

Figure 2.3

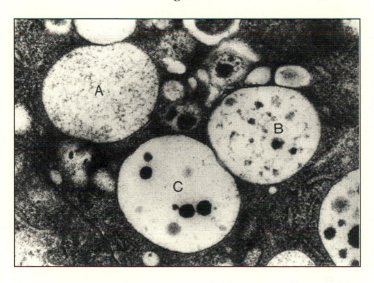

Photomicrograph showing three secretory vesicles (A, B, and C) within a lactating cell of cow mammary tissue. These vesicles show casein micelles in various stages of development with loose strands of protein evident in A, partial aggregation of the strands in B, and formed (rounded) micelles in C. Magnification 19,000 X. Photo from Beery, K. E. et al. Journal of Dairy Science 54:911-12. 1971 with permission.

vesicles which will also convey their contents to and empty them through the plasma membrane into the alveolar lumen. These mechanisms and the membranes involved in them can be visualized in figures 2.1 (right), 2.4 and 2.5. In addition, figure 2.4 suggests the rather exquisite nature of cell membranes. Figure 2.5 is a micrograph of a fairly typical lactating cell.

Membrane Flow

The observations of D. J. Morré and T. W. Keenan at Purdue University led them to propose that various membranes of the cell are derived and renewed by a process of flow and simultaneous transformation from their original site of synthesis in the endoplasmic reticulum.[2] The mechanisms of milk secretion are well explained by and expand on this concept. As shown in figure 2.1 (right), when secretory vesicles containing skim milk move from the Golgi complex and empty their contents, some of the vesicle membranes thereby become plasma membrane as a result of fusion, see also figure 2.4. A portion of the plasma membrane, in turn, is removed when a fat droplet is enveloped by it in the process of being secreted from the cell. So milk secretion is producing a constant flow of membrane from endoplasmic reticulum to the Golgi complex then

Figure 2.4

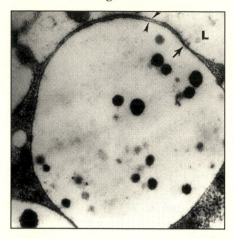

Photomicrograph showing part of a secretory vesicle in a lactating bovine mammary cell. The vesicle is at the point (arrow) of fusing with and rupturing the cell's plasma membrane with the result that the vesicle's contents will be emptied (secreted) into the alveolar lumen (L). Note at the top of the photo, the vesicle membrane (lower arrowhead) is in close parallel array with the cell's plasma membrane (upper arrowhead). Magnification 22,700X. Photo from Beery, K. E. et al. Journal of Dairy Science 54:911-12. 1971 with permission.

to secretory vesicles, followed by addition to plasma membrane and finally, to removal from the cell by fat droplet secretion. While evidence by electron microscopy indicates some variations in certain aspects of this membrane flow, the essence of it is precisely as described. Compensating somewhat for this flow in one direction is endocytosis of plasma membrane by envagination and internalization back into the cell.[3]

During the past century, one of the most intriguing research areas in all of biology has concerned the structural and functional nature of membranes. The fact that milk fat globule secretion provides a continuous sampling of plasma membrane under highly physiological conditions has provided an excellent circumstance for membrane research. As a consequence, that membrane is very extensively characterized and continues to offer further research opportunities as the knowledge and tools of science grow more sophisticated.[4,5]

Whole Body Metabolism and Lactation

The mammary glands are isolated appendages maintained by the blood circulatory system which functions whether the gland is dormant or lactating. In the case of breast cancer, the tumor cells, just like other cells of the body, require oxygen, nourishment and removal of waste products.

Figure 2.5

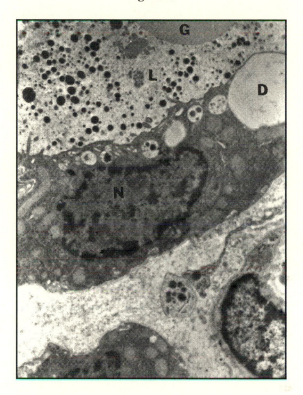

Photomicrograph of lactating rat mammary tissue showing fat droplet (D) emerging in the process of secretion from the cell into the alveolar lumen (L). Note how the outer membrane of the cell is enveloping the droplet. This mechanism will eventually place the droplet outside the cell. The relatively flattened condition of the alveolar cell, with nucleus (N), and an abundance of secretory products in the lumen indicate that the animal had not been nursed for some time. The dark particles in the lumen are casein micelles. The edge of a secreted fat globule (G) is evident at the top of the micrograph. Magnification: 6,500X. Photo courtesy of Bridget Stemberger and Stacie Bird, the Pennsylvania State University.

Lactation increases the demands on the circulation. During gestation, as the mammary glands are preparing to make milk, there is a large increase in the numbers of capillaries, the very smallest blood vessels which maintain our cells. Beyond greater tissue needs for oxygen and removal of CO_2, there will be the need to bring large quantities of precursor molecules into the gland for the synthesis of the major milk constituents, that is, fat, protein, and lactose. The supply of these precursors must be generated in addition to other normal whole body requirements. For the nine months of gestation, the human mother is not only maintaining herself, she is also growing baby and developing milk making tissue; and after the baby is delivered, she will be producing milk. As a consequence of these demands, she must take in more food than normal and it needs more than ever to be food of good nutritional quality. These requirements hold not only for the human but mammals in general. For economic reasons, efficient, profitable conversion of feed into milk has been studied in great depth with the cow. Some of the special considerations in that context are covered in chapter 6.

The digestion of food is the process for breaking down the fat, protein and carbohydrate we eat into their simple components, that is, fatty acids, amino acids, and simple sugars. These products are then absorbed into the circulation and supply the cells all over the body with these needed substances. This process also provides the lactating mammal, either directly or via some additional processing at other sites such as the liver or adipose tissue, with the precursor molecules for milk synthesis. Food is not the only immediate source of precursors for milk synthesis. Under dietary stress, the mother will, if necessary, meet the demand for metabolites with which to make milk from her own body stores. Her body proteins will be used as a source of amino acids, fatty acids will be removed from her adipose tissue, calcium taken from her bones, etc. Of course, this is an unhealthy condition that can injure both her and her offspring if pressed too far. In the case of the human infant, both physical and mental development can be permanently damaged by insufficient nourishment; that is, too little food or food of poor nutritional quality.

In the advanced industrial nations, where there is plenty of food and high quality health services, a pregnant woman is dealing with some cross currents, usually manageable ones. On the one hand, there are the developmental needs of her baby pre- and postpartum. On the other hand, the obstetrician doesn't want the baby (fetus) to get too big or it will be a problem to deliver which could be bad for all concerned. Then there is Mom herself who, in our culture at least, is very sensitive about her appearance and the possibility of getting too heavy. She knows that putting on some weight is inevitable but she doesn't want to get any bigger or more out of shape than necessary. For the most part, natural selection via evolution has taken care of this by bringing down to modern times women who have metabolic systems to deal with the situation. However, there are always exceptions, and obesity is currently a growing problem at all ages in our culture. As humans, we just don't labor physically and move enough anymore. Fortunately, this is a made-to-order problem for today's nutritionist/dietician. Rather than go off on far-out diets at such a crucial time, it is much better to consult one of these professionals for an appropriate nutrition program, and above all, to get regular exercise.

Milk

Major Components and Their Synthesis

The major nutritional components of milk from a quantitative standpoint are classified as the same three basic macronutrients as occur in other foods: carbohydrate, protein and fat (lipid). While it is not necessary to deal in depth here with the chemistry of these three, some definition of them will aid in the understanding of milk in that it will help make clear how the carbohydrate, protein and lipid of milk are unique.

Carbohydrate. It is so named because this class of substances is comprised of the element, carbon, which has, so to speak, been hydrated, that is, treated with water. Actually, the combination of the carbon with the elements of water, two atoms of hydrogen and one of oxygen, is somewhat more complicated than that; but if carbohydrates are heated to a suitable high temperature, the principal decomposition products are carbon (charcoal) and water.

There are many carbohydrates and as food; they are used by humans and other living things primarily as a source of energy. They drive energy requiring reactions and changes within cells, and they enable the expansion and contraction of muscles which makes us animated living beings. Some typical carbohydrates are the ones we are familiar with in our foods including starch, such as occur in cereals and potatoes, sucrose, glucose, fructose, cellulose and lactose. Sucrose is the common sugar we use to sweeten things. It is a white crystalline solid, and like salt, a very pure material. In fact, crystallization is a process of purification because only the specific molecules of a substance will tend to form crystals and the crystals will be very characteristic of the substance; for example, salt crystallizes in the form of cubes and lactose, the sugar of milk, crystallizes in the shape of hatchet heads.

Sucrose, obtained commercially from sugar cane or sugar beets, is comprised of two simpler (smaller molecule) sugars: fructose and glucose. These latter are released from sucrose in the human gut by the digestive enzyme, sucrase. They also are sweet tasting and are found widely distributed in foods. Fructose is particularly common in fruits and is also known as fruit sugar. Cellulose is a widely distributed structural carbohydrate in plants. We cannot digest it, so it is one of the basic components of fiber which passes through us pretty much unchanged. Cellulose is readily utilized by ruminants, including the cow, which enlists the help of bacteria in their rumens. That distinction is one reason why cattle do not necessarily have to be in competition with humanity for food. Digestion of cellulose in the cow is discussed in chapter 6.

Lactose, also known as milk sugar, is produced from blood glucose. Two units of glucose are taken up from the circulation by the lactating tissue and converted to one of lactose. One of the glucose units is used as such and the other is converted in the lactating cell into a closely related sugar called galactose. These two units are then linked together to make lactose. There are traces (< 0.1 percent) of glucose and galactose in both human and cows' milk. Lactose averages about 5 percent in bovine milk and 7 percent in human milk. This is sufficient to make human milk slightly sweeter than cow's milk. However, lactose is only about one-fifth as sweet as sucrose.

Protein. All living systems contain an array of proteins which are composed of amino acids, compounds containing the elements carbon, hydrogen, oxygen, nitrogen and in two instances, sulfur. Proteins are made by connecting these amino acids to each other in long chains which can fold in various ways to provide proteins of different shapes and reactivities. There are twenty naturally occurring amino acids, nine of which are classified essential, meaning that we *must* have them, but can't make them, and are dependent on our food to supply them. The other nine are known as non-essential and we are able to make them as needed. Proteins vary greatly in their size and amino acid composition.

The specific sequence of amino acids in a protein is known as its primary structure. This sequence for each protein is determined by its gene (DNA) and the RNA template that is produced from that gene. Because of many factors involved, including the eighteen different amino acid building blocks, proteins vary greatly in size, primary structure and amino acid composition. Every species of plant and animal has its own unique set of proteins. The current estimate is that we contain about 70,000 proteins. To make the situation even more complex, carbohydrates, lipids, or phosphates may be connected to or associated with proteins to form glyco-, lipo-, and phosphoproteins, respectively.

Most of the milk proteins, including casein, alpha-lactalbumin and beta-lactoglobulin, are derived mainly from free amino acids or very short chains of them contained in the circulation. Some, including the immune globulins and serum albumin, are transported directly from the circulation across or around the mammary cell and into the milk. In the case of colostrum, the secretion of the mammary gland for the first few days postpartum, these globulins pass between the alveolar cells and are present at highly elevated levels. They are particularly important in protecting the newborn against infection. There are literally hundreds of proteins in both human and bovine milk. Many are present at levels of a few parts per million, especially the proteins known as enzymes which facilitate chemical reactions. Bovine milk proteins have been the subject of extensive reviews.[4,6]

One of the most important and characteristic proteins in milks of the various species is casein. Actually it is a family of phosphoproteins that self-assemble into small particles which then further assemble into units known as micelles. This unique process is evident in the photomicrograph of lactating tissue (figure 2.3). Casein micelles are relatively big on the cellular scale. For example, such a micelle in cows' milk is about 300 times bigger than serum albumin, another protein of average size co-present with casein in the medium. These micelles are what give skim milk its white appearance. They are on average about 0.000004 of an inch in diameter. Without them, it would be a clear, greenish-yellow fluid.

Casein is very important nutritionally. It is of excellent quality regarding content of essential amino acids, and it contains abundant calcium and phosphorus. The casein of cow's milk, which is 80 percent of the total milk protein, is recognized as the best dietary source of calcium in the United States' food supply. For further details on the milk proteins, see the handbook cited in the suggested references at the end of this chapter.

Fat

It is especially important these days that one have some fundamental understanding of fat. The image of this dietary component in the public's mind has become dreadful. It conjures up worries about obesity, diabetes and heart attacks. Along with the good cholesterol and bad cholesterol, concepts of good fats and bad fats have emerged. As with all progress in science, agonizing reappraisals have been going on and the bad image of fat is being rehabilitated on the basis of new knowledge. However, no one is questioning the not-too-much edict, which holds, not just for fat but food in general.

So what is fat? In common terms, it is readily recognized as the oily, greasy aspect of our food. Almost everyone knows what fat in the form of salad oil is and the difference between fat and lean tissues of meat, either before or after cooking. However, the fat in many foods is not readily evident. This is especially true of processed foods where many ingredients are finely blended and one cannot see the fat. This is true of cookies. A dead giveaway is when they leave a big grease spot, a spot that won't dry or go away, on a paper napkin. For those who must be concerned, searching food labels for fat content can be a help. The amount of fat in sauces or gravies is harder to judge because with good preparation, the fat is so thoroughly dispersed you cannot see it. A dilemma with fat is that, like sugar, it makes foods taste good (see also chapter 8) which invites us to eat more.

The main constituents of fats are fatty acids. They vary in size and structure and thereby determine whether the fat is a liquid or solid and whether it is relatively saturated (solid) or unsaturated (liquid). Further discussion of structure and properties of fats, is presented in the notes for this chapter, p. 53.

Another factor about fats in respect to milk is that enzymes, known as lipases, can release the fatty acids from their glycerol structure in which condition they become known as free fatty acids. Thus, the lipases are said to be fat-splitting enzymes. They are among those which digest our food; they also occur in cells throughout the body. The fatty acids can have one of two fates: degradation and use for energy or other purposes, or resynthesis into fat. Such resynthesis can be for storage in adipose deposits or, in the mammary gland, it can be for production of milk fat.

Milk fat, butterfat, or milk lipid, as it is known, is made using two sources of fatty acids: from the circulation (blood) and newly made in the mammary tissue. Those from the blood may originate from ingested food lipids or they may be mobilized from fat in adipose tissue. In that connection, making milk can remove fat from ones body but exercise and eating a proper diet are a better way to eliminate excess fat. Glycerol for fat synthesis is derived from glucose. Fatty acids and glycerol in the lactating cell come together in the presence of enzymes that will combine them to make triacylglycerols (fat). As is characteristic of fat-in-water systems, these newly synthesized molecules of fat seek each other and gather to form micro fat droplets which then fuse with each other and go on to form large droplets in the secretory region of the cell. Eventually, the enlarging droplets touch the outer membrane of the cell and are progressively enveloped by it. This process leads to the separation of the droplet from the cell and its release into previously secreted milk that has been accumulating in the lumen of the alveolus (figure 2.1). Overall, the synthesis and secretion of milk fat is a truly unusual process.

Compositional data for the principal fatty acids of human and bovine milk fats are in table 2.1. These data show rather profound differences between milk fats of the two species. That of the cow contains a set of unique short carbon chains (4:0 - 10:0) fatty acids and very little polyunsaturated fatty acids (18:2+3). Both of these differences are a result of the unusual digestive system of the cow. It has what is called a rumen as its first stomach. In essence, it is a large fermentation tank in which food is broken down and modified by microorganisms before it goes to the intestine to undergo the more typical digestive processes of most animals, including the human, which have no rumen. The abundant polyunsaturated lipids in the grasses, legumes, silages, and grains consumed by the cow are hydrogenated, that is saturated, in the rumen, which is the reason bovine milk fat is designated a saturated fat. Dominant among the fermentation products of the rumen are acetic and beta-hydroxybutyric acid. These two acids are absorbed directly from the rumen into the circulation and are carried to the mammary gland where they are used to make the short chain fatty acids of bovine milk fat. Lack of a rumen makes for much less radical digestive activity. This is shown in the data for human milk fat produced while the mother was on a corn oil diet. Feeding corn oil, which is rich in linoleic acid (18:2), produced a level of 43 percent 18:2 in the human milk fat. Digestion simply released the 18:2 from the corn oil making it possible for the breasts to pick it up and use it as such to help make milk fat. Both human and bovine milk fats contain many other fatty acids in addition to those shown in table 2.1, but all are at low levels (<1 percent). The rumen in relation to milk synthesis is discussed further in chapter 6.

Table 2.1
Fatty acid composition of human and bovine milk fat.[1]

Fatty acid[2]	Human		Cow	
	Fat-free diet	Corn oil diet	Summer	Winter
4:0	-	-	3.6	3.5
6:0	-	-	1.3	1.4
8:0	-	-	0.9	1.1
10:0	-	-	2.4	2.7
12:0	7.9	3.0	2.7	3.9
14:0	9.0	2.3	9.8	12.7
15:0	-	-	1.1	1.0
16:0	23.5	13.1	25.4	34.4
16:1	6.8	1.4	0.9	1.3
17:0	-	-	0.7	0.7
18:0	3.2	3.0	15.8	11.6
18:1	36.9	31.3	-	-
18:1 *cis*	-	-	24.3	19.9
18:1 *trans*	-	-	6.4	2.5
18:2+3	7.3	43.0	1.9	1.5

[1] Data are weight percent taken from studies of human (Insull, W. et al. Journal of Clinical Investigations 38:443. 1959) and bovine (Patton, S. et al. Journal of Dairy Science 43:1187. 1960) milks.
[2] Number of carbons in the chain colon number of double bonds. The cis and trans forms of 18:1 were only measured in the cow samples. The cis double bond was in the 9-position and the trans double bond in the 11-position.

Mysteries of the Blood to Milk Pathways

A scheme showing the involvement of blood components as precursors of the major milk constituents is presented in figure 2.6. The precise means by which these precursors move from within the extremities of the circulation, the capillaries, into the lactating cells is not known with certainty. To some extent, this may simply involve diffusion of these substances through pores from the rich source within the capillary to the depleted condition in the lactating cell. The critically involved gases, oxygen and CO_2, appear to move in and out of mammary cells by such a mechanism. There is evidence in the case of glucose that receptors on the basal surface of the lactating cell specifically bind and internalize it. In the case of fatty acids, there is morphological evidence of transport by a secretory mechanism out of the capillary to the base of the lactating cell.[8,9]

The microenvironment for these molecular events is shown in a remarkable photograph of lactating mammary tissue, figure 2.7, taken through the electron microscope. The large oval-shaped body containing two dark structures is a

Figure 2.6

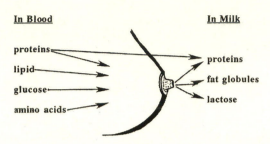

A scheme showing components taken up from the blood in the synthesis of major milk constituents by the mammary gland. The lipid, more commonly called fat, used from the blood is in the form of lipoproteins and the lipid in milk is in the form of fat globules. Some blood proteins pass unchanged through the tissue into the milk; however, most of the total milk protein is made in the gland. Among species variations, ruminants, such as the cow, also utilize fermentation products from the rumen (forestomach) by way of the blood in making milk; and marine mammals produce little or no lactose, the dominant carbohydrate of milk.

capillary endothelial cell shown in cross section. These cells, when aligned with each other, assume the form of a tube by folding back on themselves. This particular cell has closed on itself at the point where the two tips can be seen to touch each other (arrow). This results in the formation of a tube with a hollow central region called a lumen (L) which carries blood. By astounding good fortune, a red blood cell (RBC) was captured in the lumen by this particular photomicrograph. It is notable that the lumen is barely large enough to accommodate an RBC. The nucleus (N) of the endothelial cell is the sausage-shaped object at the immediate lower left of the RBC.

A further merit of figure 2.7 is that it shows the intimate association of the capillary with the base of two lactating cells (M1 and M2). An extensive array of what are thought to be secretory vesicles can be seen in the cytoplasm of the endothelial cell (arrowheads) next to the base of the two mammary cells. This structure is consistent with the forming and filling of the vesicles on the lumen surface followed by their migration and emptying out of the cell at the (outer) plasma membrane. In essence, this would represent a means of bathing mammary cells in blood plasma constituents which they can import as needed. In any event, something of this nature must happen since it is known that milk precursor molecules, such as glucose and fatty acids, when radioactively labeled, can be detected as moving from blood to mammary cell to secreted milk component.

It is notable in figure 2.7 that the space below the cells does not appear to have any structure. This region presumably contains lymph, an interstitial fluid

Figure 2.7

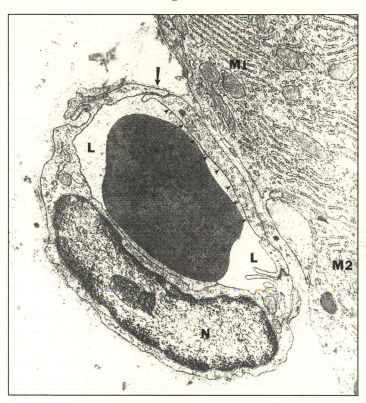

A photograph of lactating mammary tissue taken through an electron microscope. It shows a blood capillary at the base of two mammary cells, M1 and M2, and containing a red blood cell, the dark mass in the lumen (L). Magnification: 15,000x. For further description, see text. Photo courtesy of Bridget Stemberger, The Pennsylvania State University.

that normally drains back to the blood by way of a system of special vessels. It is in this interstitial space that colostrum is assembled and instead of returning to the blood, it will be the first substance secreted by the mammary gland upon birth of the young.

Milk as a Product of the Cell

Let us suppose that we have just obtained some milk from a cow. We can see that it is a white fluid, but beyond that, what do we have? If allowed to stand for twenty or thirty minutes, it will be noticed that a layer, known as cream, has formed. Depending on the breed of cow and what she has been eating, it may be noticed that the cream phase has a more yellowish-orange hue compared to the lower (skim) milk. The cream is a concentration of fat globules which are carriers of yellow plant pigments known as carotenoids. Yellow, orange, and red molecules of this pigment group contribute to the color of tomatoes, lemons, carrots and autumn leaves. Cows of the Guernsey breed tend to deposit carotenoids in the fat to a substantially greater degree than do Holsteins which make up 87 percent of the cows in America. You may have heard the term, "Golden Guernsey," in reference to the rich yellow color of milk from that breed. On the other hand, goats and some breeds of cattle transport no pigments into milk fat, with the result that, in their case it is white. Regarding cows' milk fat, it is known to be less yellow during the winter months when the cows are housed inside and are eating dry feeds. A noticeable increase in the pigmentation occurs when the cows are put out to pasture in the spring. Pasture plants, including grasses, clover and alfalfa, are good sources of beta-carotene, the principal yellow pigment of milk fat. It is converted to vitamin A in the human and thus is also known as provitamin A.

Milk fat, like any other fat, will float on water. Thus, in our sample of fresh milk, the fat globules rise to the top of the milk. This process is greatly hastened by the fact that the globules tend to clump and sweep others along with them as they rise. The part of the cream layer that is not fat globules, that is, between them, is identical in composition to the lower milk phase. After the cream layer has formed, the appearance of the milk is quite stable. The skim milk phase still remains white, but with a somewhat bluish cast, and nothing more seems to be rising or settling from it. The whiteness is due to particles of casein, the major milk protein. They are round, rather uniform in size and known as micelles. Fat globules are about thirty times bigger than casein micelles in mean diameter. Unlike fat globules, the micelles of casein in fresh milk repel each other. That coupled with their small size tend to keep them suspended in milk due to their repelling negative electrical charge.

If we remove the cream layer from our sample of milk and subject the resulting skim milk to high-speed centrifugation, that is, spinning it in a glass or plastic tube at many thousands of revolutions per minute, the casein micelles will be forced to the bottom of the tube where they will form a sediment or pellet. It will be noted that a clear greenish yellow liquid remains above the pellet. This liquid contains all the other milk constituents including the lactose, some of the milk proteins, the milk salts, water-soluble vitamins and many other trace substances. A similar liquid is obtained in the process of cheese making. In that case, the casein micelles are induced to aggregate in a process known as curd formation, discussed in chapter 7. The liquid that is left is known as whey and the proteins contained in it are known as the whey proteins; principally alpha-lactalbumin, beta-lactoglobulin and immune globulins totaling together about 0.6 percent of the milk. These whey proteins are the same ones contained in the clear whey-like liquid of our centrifugation experiment.

This liquid has a greenish yellow color arising from the water-soluble B vitamin, riboflavin or B_2 as it is known, of which cow's milk is an excellent source. This liquid is clear because all the components not in true solution have been removed either in the cream or the sedimented pellet. We may notice a very thin skin of cream on the surface of the liquid. This is due to the forced rising of extremely small fat globules. Though numerous, they are quantitatively insignificant with respect to the fat content of the milk. One other milk fraction distributed under these conditions is the cellular material which includes macrophages and other cell types of the body's immune system, bacteria, viruses, cell debris and tissue fragments. From a quantitative or mass standpoint, this fraction of milk is inconsequential and the particular components of it will either rise with the fat globules or sediment with the casein micelles depending on their numbers and affinities.

Cow's milk contains cells of the immune system which originate from the circulation, that is, macrophages, lymphocytes, and leukocytes. While the numbers of these cells in milk will go up when an infection, known as mastitis, occurs in the udder; some of them are always present and represent a perfectly normal condition in milk from healthy udders. In fact, they are around prowling the udder to gobble up and destroy bacteria in order to maintain health of the tissue. Further, cow's milk with inordinate numbers of these cells is not allowed to be used for human consumption. These are the same type of cells as occur in human milk and in our circulation. There is nothing the matter with them as such; it's that high concentrations may mean an infection is present. Bacteria associated with infection are more of a concern, of course, but if present in milk they would be destroyed by pasteurization.

Generally speaking, a fresh sample of human milk, treated in the manner we have described for the bovine sample, will compartmentalize in the same way. However, on formation of the cream layer, it will be noted that the lower phase is not white like bovine skim milk, but more of a watery-looking, slightly cloudy liquid. The cause of this difference is that human milk contains about one-tenth the amount of casein that cows' milk does and this makes for a lack of whiteness in human skim milk. Sometimes lactating mothers seeing this condition are concerned that their milk is too watery and not healthful, that is, not concentrated enough for their babies - not true, perfectly normal. Mean composition data for human and bovine milks with respect to their major components and nutrients is given in table 2.2. As can be seen in the table, there are a few notable differences between milks of the two species. Among these are the much greater levels of protein and minerals in cow's as compared to human milk. This is why cows' milk is especially beneficial food for the human from ages one to thirty years during which time tissues, organs, and bones are maturing. See also chapter 5.

It has been known for many years that cow's milk is an excellent source of riboflavin. However, not until adapting Table 2.2 for use in this chapter did I

Table 2. 2
Nutrient composition of human and bovine milks

Nutrient	Human[1]	Cow[1]	percentDV[2]
Water, (percent)	87.50	87.99	-
Food energy, kcal	70	61	(160)
Protein, g	1.03	3.29	17
Fat, g	4.38	3.34	13
Carbohydrate, total, g	6.89	4.66	4
Fiber, g	0	0	0
Ash, g	0.20	0.72	-
Minerals			
Calcium, mg	32	119	30
Iron, mg	0.03	0.05	0
Magnesium, mg	3	13	8
Phosphorus, mg	14	93	23
Potassium, mg	51	152	12
Sodium, mg	17	49	5
Zinc, mg	0.17	0.38	6
Vitamins			
Ascorbic Acid, mg	5.00	0.94	4
Thiamin, mg	0.014	0.038	6
Riboflavin, mg	0.036	0.162	24
Niacin, mg	0.177	0.084	11
Pantothenic Acid, mg	0.223	0.314	8
Vitamin B_6, mg	0.011	0.042	5
Folate, mcg	5	5	3
Vitamin B_{12}, mcg	0.045	0.357	15
Vitamin A, IU	241	126	6
Vitamin D	-[3]	-[3]	25[4]
Other (fat soluble)	-[3]	-[3]	-[3]
Cholesterol, mg	14	14	12

Abreviations and Conversions: percentDV (daily value) -the percentage of the suggested daily intake of an essential nutrient recommended for an "average" person, g-gram, mg-milligram, mcg-microgram; 1,000,000mcg=1000mg=1g; lb-pound, 453.6g=1 lb, IU-international unit.

[1]Amount in 100 g. [2]Daily Values supplied by a glass of cows' milk (1/4 quart). [3]Small, variable amounts of Vitamins D, E and K are also present. [4]By fortification.

Adapted from: *Newer Knowledge of Milk and Other Fluid Dairy Products,* National Dairy Council, 1993, p. 47. With permission.

realize that cows' milk contains about 4.5 times as much of this B vitamin as does human milk. This fits well with the greater protein and mineral content of cow's milk because riboflavin also is a potent growth factor. They are all involved in quickly making the calf a large, relatively mature animal in only a year or so from birth. While the human on average is gaining about fifteen pounds during its first year of life, a Holstein calf puts on about 600 pounds. Note also in table 2.2 that some of the other B vitamins, including thiamin (B_1), B_6 and B_{12}, are comparatively elevated in cows' milk. Vitamin B_{12} is also profoundly involved in growth.

Interestingly, cow's milk is not nearly as good a source of thiamine (B_1) as it is of riboflavin (B_2), but the bovine has no problem with this because a bacterium in its first stomach, the rumen, makes this vitamin. Thus, cattle have no need for an outside source of thiamin and the calf has its own rumen supply going a few weeks after birth. The rumen synthesis of this vitamin was revealed by ingenious research at Penn State about seventy years ago. S. I. Bechdel, a dairy scientist, R. A. Dutcher a vitamin biochemist. M. H. Knutsen, a microbiologist, and J. Shigley, a veterinarian teamed up to create a cow with a permanent hole, known as a fistula, in her side so that the contents of her rumen could be sampled at will. She was known as Penn State Jessie (figure 2.8).

Figure 2.8

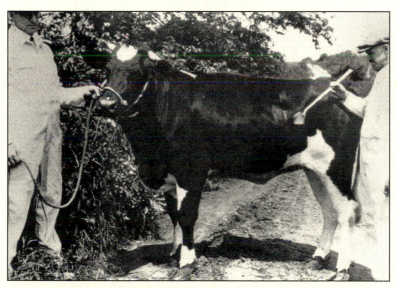

Penn State Jessie, the famous Holstein cow with a hole in her side. Shown with her is Prof. S. I. Bechdel (left) and Dr. J. Shigley, the veterinarian who performed the surgery. The hole, known as a fistula, allowed researchers to sample Jessie's stomach (rumen) contents and to discover that bacteria were synthesizing vitamin B_1 therein.

They kept a rubber stopper in the hole when she wasn't being sampled. This research was still going on some years later when I was a freshman working in the barns. I was entranced by all of this which had led to the identification of the bacterium that was generating the thiamin.[10] It was given the genus name, *Thiaminbacillus.* What an impressive example of teamwork in research! What a contribution to the understanding of animal nutrition!

Factors Influencing Milk Composition

Because of bovine milk's economic importance and nutritive value to the human, factors influencing its composition and yield have been extensively studied. Much is known about the effects of such variables as feed, breed, season, stage of lactation, frequency of milking, length of dry period, numbers of lactations (age), and so on. For the most part, fluid milk sold for beverage purposes in the U. S. does not exhibit wide variations in composition and nutritive properties excepting, of course, where the amount of fat is purposely reduced (2 percent, 1 percent and non-fat milks) and where supplementation with vitamins A and D or milk solids are optional to the customer.

There is some confusion about the fat content of milk sold to consumers. Whole milk contains about 3.25 percent fat. That means the other 97 percent or so of the milk, also known as skim milk, fat-free milk or non-fat milk, has essentially no fat in it. Three or 4 percent is not much fat. It means that there are about two teaspoonfuls of fat in a glass of whole milk. Considering the water content of milk (87 percent), it is not particularly fattening on a calorie to volume basis because one will feel full long before very many calories have been consumed. Of course, it will be even less calorific when the milk fat is reduced or totally removed. Another point is that 2 percent-fat milk has about half the fat removed, not 98 percent of it.

Regarding the composition of cow's milk, health needs of particular individual consumers may render one or another milk component problematical. The one most seriously debated in this regard is milk fat. In distinction to the negative image many have with respect to it, especially with reference to obesity and heart disease, there are clear indications from current research that milk fat prevents those conditions (see chapter 5). As to human milk, it is widely considered quite adequate and preferable for the normal infant up to four to six months of age, assuming of course, that the mother is well nourished. Breast-feeding beyond that period is considered very desirable, but supplements of both other foods and micronutrients are normal practice by that time. Human milk is also subject to variations in composition and yield but these are not usually of such magnitude as to interfere with well being of the normal infant.

One interesting variation concerning the amount of fat in both bovine and human milks is the increase in fat content as a milking or nursing progresses.

The first milk suckled from the breast at a nursing may be as low in fat as a fraction of 1 percent, and as high as 12 percent in the last milk obtainable by the baby at that nursing. The same is true in the milking of a cow. The reason for this is not known but back pressure of accumulated milk in suppressing fat droplet secretion is one possibility. As the milk is withdrawn, pressure within alveoli should fall and droplet secretion increase. There also may be some relative drag on the movement of fat globules to the nipple or teat because of their size, affinity for cell surfaces and tendency to form clumps.

A variable component of the pregnant woman's diet, which has received a good bit of publicity lately, is the B vitamin, folic acid. Inadequate levels of it in the expectant mother can lead to defects in the spine and brain of her fetus. A government requirement in 1998 that flour and other grains be fortified with folic acid has more than doubled the levels in blood of women in the child-bearing age range, fifteen to forty-four. In the three years since this program was initiated, the incidence of these dreadful birth defects has fallen 19 percent.

Green Milk? No and Yes

Perhaps you have been asked by some young person, "Why do brown cows eat green grass and give white milk?" The answer to this not entirely naive question involves some interesting phenomena. The question describes a situation which is quite true for the cow, although some breeds, especially the Guernsey, when on green feeds, tend to have noticeably golden yellow milk and this is, as previously explained, from the yellow plant pigment, carotene, which comes through into the milk fat at higher than usual concentrations in the case of the Guernsey. This is the natural yellow pigment of butter produced from all the Western breeds of cows: and we actually do not know, at the cellular/molecular level, how it gets from the circulation into the milk fat. But the much more noticeable green pigment, chlorophyll of grasses and leaves, which cows consume in abundance, does not reach their milk. It appears to be destroyed mainly in the cow's first stomach, also known as the rumen. The abundant fat globules and casein micelles in the milk do not preferentially absorb any wavelengths of light in the visible spectrum, so being solid particles, white light is reflected back for us to see.

On the other hand, human milk is a different story, and green human milk happens especially at garden harvesting time. Dr. Judy Hopkinson of Baylor Medical College collected many samples of donated human milk at one point in her career. She observed that at the time of year when fresh green vegetables are widely available, the samples often had a definite green caste. On checking with the donors, there was a good correlation between consumption of green vegetables and production of green milk - except for one lady whose milk was consistently green but who said she never ate vegetables. The explanation was that she was taking chlorophyll pills daily. So Dr. Hopkinson's observations are quite supportive that chlorophyll, the common green pigment of plants, is the source of the green tint which occurs in some human milk. Of course, there may be a lot more green human milk than we think because the close connection between producers and consumers precludes observation.

Actually chlorophyll is quite insoluble. One cannot extract it from leaves or grass with water. But when we consume chlorophyll-containing foods, our digestive enzymes split the chlorophyll into phytol, a fatty substance that accounts for about one-third of the molecule and chlorophyllin, the green component. This latter, on being freed from the phytol becomes water soluble. So it is reasonable, based on Dr. Hopkinson's observations, when we eat green vegetables, a certain amount of the green chlorophyllin is released and passes from our intestine into our circulation. How it is metabolized, in addition to passing into milk, and whether it benefits one in any way is not presently known. There seems to be room for some research here. How does chlorophyllin get across the mammary gland? Does it get into all our cells? Is it beneficial? The orange pigment in carrots, known as carotene or provitamin A, is good for us, but in excess, it can turn one orange.

Environmental Contaminants

Analytical Capabilities

Instruments and methods for analyzing body tissues and fluids such as blood, urine and milk are becoming ever more sensitive. It is possible to detect 200 compounds at concentrations as low as a few parts per billion in a teaspoon of blood. As this highly sensitive methodology is applied increasingly to detect interactions of environment on humans, animals and plants, we should become much more fully informed as to what kinds and amounts of environmental substances are present in and on us, which ones pose health risks and at what concentrations. After that, we have to determine, as individuals, at what levels we will have peace of mind. The whole thing is both reassuring and yet annoying. With more sensitive means of analysis, we find that things are present we didn't even know were there or worry about at all. But then, if no reliable data are available about toxic thresholds of the now-measured substances, how much and intense should our worry be? Unfortunately, the human tendency is to react negatively to the detection of a toxin at any level. On the other hand, maybe we should take solace in finding that a toxin exists at a reassuringly low level.

That highly sensitive analysis can be informative is revealed by recent results from a few strands of Mozart's hair, a sample having been collected at the time of his death. Wolfgang Amadeus Mozart (1756-91) the musical genius, only lived to be thirty-five years old. His death has been attributed to typhoid fever but the hair analysis indicates he must have been suffering greatly from lead poisoning, a widespread environmental problem in Europe at the time. The moral of this story is that we are much better off than was Mozart about lead poisoning.

Environmental Awareness

There are concerns today that the air, our food, industrial activities, consumer products and life styles are exposing us to deadly toxic substances. At the same time, we are living on average close to eighty years and enjoying pretty good health. There is no question that we come in contact with potential hazards during our lives, in fact, unavoidably so. We must breathe air; our skin is touched by many things; and we must take food into our bodies. All human foods are exposed to the environment and, as a result, pick up things that are not strictly part of the animal or vegetable material making up the food. For example, non-essential substances can be taken up by the wheat plant through its roots; foreign substances can settle on the plant from the air, including dust, smog particles, and pesticides. The harvested grain will be contaminated with these things. Yet other matter can become included with the grain during harvesting, storage and further processing, such as, insects and their eggs, rodent hairs and rodent droppings. The grain will absorb molecules of a fumigant used to kill insects and their eggs. The amounts of these things in grains are kept to a minimum by law; and while the idea of them in the grain may not be aesthetically pleasing, they are relatively harmless. In fact, humankind has been eating foods naturally contaminated in various ways since time immemorial.

Consider wood smoke, which is comprised of a tremendous inventory of organic chemicals. Primitive humans slept around fires, cooked food over fires, and dealt with the many intimate consequences of forest fires. They breathed smoke, ate smoked food and absorbed smoke through their skin. No doubt they smelled smoky, and through natural selection, any humans that couldn't take smoke were eliminated from the gene pool. Similarly, sunlight, dust, bacteria, parasites, poisonous soils, toxic plants and weather extremes are environmental factors that have been shaping human hardiness. So over the many years involved in human evolution, we have been well prepared to deal with our environment. Our bodies have many detoxification and elimination systems for getting rid of harmful substances. This is fortunate because we simply cannot avoid contact with the environment and neither can the plants and animals we use as food. The main requirement is that contaminants, especially those known to be toxic, not be allowed to reach levels in our food that would be unhealthy.

Toxic Elements

There is a group of toxic substances that is in a special class. It is the elemental poisons, particularly lead, arsenic, and mercury, that can build up to lethal levels in the body. Such elements cannot be broken down so there is no ability of our bodies to detoxify them by degradation. While a single dose of them that is large enough can kill, they also have the insidious ability to accumulate from repeated low doses, such as in drinking water, and thus to make one sick and eventually to cause death, see Mozart above. Fortunately, effective state and federal regulations have greatly minimized the environmental threats of these poisons. They are not a problem in milk and milk products.

Because it is currently such a potent environmental issue, a few comments about arsenic in (drinking) water supplies seem appropriate. It is a classic cost/benefit problem. The question is how much will human health benefit at what cost in improvements required of offending water companies throughout the country? There seems to be an impression that a zero level of arsenic in water would be ideal though impractical. No doubt people in certain areas of the country where natural water content of arsenic is high, such as New Mexico, would have to support costly renovation of their water processing facilities. So the next question is whether the acceptable upper limit should be reduced from the present 50 parts per billion of water to 20 or 10 ppb? There could be a lot of difference in lives/health saving vs. dollar costs between those latter two figures. Unfortunately, defining the values accurately is not easy but it should be done. In all of the big vaccination programs for childhood diseases, there are dollar costs *and always a few fatalities.* The U. S. public has agreed to accommodate that drawback in order to protect the rest of the children. So decisions can be reached on these difficult issues.

Another part of the arsenic—drinking water problem is the human variable. There are not a lot of good basic data on how humans handle various levels of arsenic. An arsenic level that apparently would kill some people would not bother some others. There also seems to be some feeling that people can adjust to ingested arsenic. Further, there are indications in experimental animals (goat and rat) that arsenic may even be an essential nutrient at very low levels. In humans, elevated levels of arsenic in the 150 to 200 ppb range are known to cause bladder and lung cancer, but the element has also been reported as a cancer inhibitor. Hopefully, research will develop more precise information on what is a safe upper limit for arsenic in drinking water and whether arsenic can have health benefits for us and under what circumstances. At the moment, the decision has been reached by the United States government to lower the maximum level to 10 ppb to be reached by 2006.

Neither human nor bovine milks are considered to be important sources of human exposure to arsenic or lead. Actually, there are data indicating that the cow tends to screen fed arsenic away from the mammary gland and milk. Regarding mercury, which is a well-known toxin to the nervous system, concern has been expressed recently by pediatricians that high levels of the element in seafoods may be transferred from a breast-feeding mother to her infant. For a literature review of trace elements in human and cows' milk, see Casey and coauthors, in the suggested reference, *Handbook of Milk Composition* (pages 622-674) at the end of this chapter.

Bacteria

Some things by their very name may conjure up harm. The word, bacteria, also known as microorganisms or microbes, is an example. Some bacteria cause disease, and thus are known as pathogens, while others do not; and some are highly desirable, such as those inhabiting a healthy human intestinal tract and those used to make cheese, buttermilk and sauerkraut. Bacteria are virtually everywhere and it is impossible to eat without consuming them along with the food and drink. Cooking foods, pasteurizing milk, refrigerating foods during storage, and washing ones hands before eating are all practices designed to minimize contamination with and growth of bacteria. The pasteurization of milk discussed in chapter 7, has been set at a level of heat treatment that will destroy all pathogenic bacteria and most of the non-pathogens as well.

Food Contamination, Summary of Some Principles

So, as most of us are aware, our food always has a history, and the main concern is to regulate it in a healthful way. One relevant concept, not always appreciated, is that poisonous contaminants, and even natural toxic constituents of foods, must achieve a certain level in a food before they can make people sick. There is, so to speak, a threshold level that must be exceeded. Up to the threshold level, our bodies can handle toxic substances; above that level, our detoxifying and eliminating capabilities are swamped sooner or later and we are in trouble. It may be an ideal to keep all man-made pesticides, note that many plants make their own, out of our food, but it is unnecessary and impractical to do so as long as the amount of our intake is at a harmless level.

A related general principle is that there are no perfect solutions to the food contaminant problem—only more or less desirable ways of doing things on a cost/benefit basis, that is, what will we have to pay for the reputed improvement? For example, a local supermarket offered the option recently of regularly grown bananas at $0.39/lb. versus organically grown bananas at $0.74/lb. In the minds of some, organic cultivation has advantages. It is supposed to avoid commercial fertilizers, insecticides and weed killers, which are known to be harmless to humans when properly used, but they aren't always properly used. Are these changes worth that increase in the cost of bananas? Remember, organically grown foods also have a history and are exposed to contaminants, too, especially when manures are used as fertilizer. In addition, some 'natural' insecticides approved for organic farming, such as rotenone and pyrethrum, are not without toxic effects.

Contamination of Milk

As a food and processed food raw material, milk implicates another factor in the contamination chain, the mammal that made it. Following is a presentation of this issue as it relates to human and bovine milk.

The Mammal Mother Screens Contaminants Away from Her Milk

In evaluating milk as a food, an important attribute is often overlooked. The making of milk from ingested food by the mammal mother involves a physiological selection process. Only particular molecules from the food are used, ones that will be good for the newborn. Others that do not fit the blueprint or that aren't needed are left out. In addition, some toxic molecules that come into the mother's body on or in her food are subject to detoxification and/or elimination in her urine and feces. In essence the lactating mammal screens out much, if not all, undesirable contamination during the making of the milk. This is in distinction to many other kinds of food materials which, either because of their composition or environmental exposure, may contain substances harmful to human health. This is not to say that milk, either human or bovine, is always free of all substances detrimental to the human, but as compared to many other foods, milk has undergone *a purification.*

Possible Contaminants—Human Milk

Despite all the filtration and detoxification mechanisms that exist in the human, some undesirable substances that the mother consumes may get into her milk and thus into her baby. For the most part, this is because the processes of deflecting and detoxifying the substances in question are not 100 percent efficient. For example, if a mother is consuming alcoholic drinks, her body will be burning and eliminating the molecules of alcohol, but if her alcohol consumption is excessive, a small amount of it may get into her milk. The likelihood is that this will do no harm to her baby as a one time or occasional thing. However, habitual and excessive drinking by a breast-feeding mother can harm her baby and should be avoided. The problem can be much more serious during pregnancy when the fetus in the womb is directly exposed to alcohol in the expectant mother's blood. This can produce fetal alcohol syndrome which stunts growth and causes memory and learning problems in the baby. About one in every 1,000 babies born in the U. S. suffers from this disorder.

In the interest of maximizing a baby's health and lifelong well being, a mother is well advised, while pregnant or during nursing, to avoid alcohol, recreational drugs and smoking. There are also other substances, such as antibiotics, allergens, prescription drugs, toxins, and carcinogens that may in some instances be a hazard to infants by way of the mother's milk. Generally such substances do not achieve toxic levels in the milk. Each mother and her baby are a unique circumstance and in instances where there appears to be a problem, a pediatrician or nutritionist should be consulted.

It is of interest that the human not only stores fat in adipose tissue, substances that are soluble in the fat are also stored with it. One such substance is the yellow plant pigment, beta-carotene, a fat-soluble precursor of vitamin A. It is contained in carrots and green vegetables. Surgery on the human reveals this fact because the adipose (fatty) tissue invariably has a yellowish color due to carotenoids. There are other fat soluble substances from human environmental activities that are stored in our fat, such as DDT, the famous insecticide which is so effective against malaria, and PCBs (polychlorinated biphenyls) used in paper-sizings and many other industrial applications. The concentrations of these types of fat-soluble substances from the environment can build up in our tissues over time, and in the case of a nursing mother, they can be released throughout a lactation into her milk and baby. In the case of one woman employed to work with PCBs, it was noted that the highest levels of PCBs in her milk were immediately after delivery from which point there was a progressive decline during her lactation.[11] This experience serves as a model as to how some environmental contaminants behave with respect to lactation. PCBs are mentioned as examples here. Whether or not they pose an environmental contamination problem continues to be debated.

Contaminants—Cow's Milk

For a number of reasons, cows' milk involves a different set of advantages and disadvantages compared to human milk regarding contaminants. The cow consumes different foods, doesn't smoke or indulge in recreational drugs. Further the bovine digestive apparatus is uniquely different from that of the human. And whereas human milk is usually distributed directly and immediately to the consumer, cows milk has a number of opportunities for contamination before it is consumed.

In consuming pasture grasses, hay, corn and other silages, and grain mixtures, the cow is fed almost exclusively on crude plant materials. The first stop of these inside the cow is the rumen, a large fermentation chamber. As explained in chapter 6, the rumen microorganisms bring about many unique chemical changes in these materials before they reach the true stomach. While the human and other monogastric mammals have such a stomach, they have no rumen. Its fermentation reactions probably destroy some plant-born toxic substances but may even generate others, although there is no evidence that such actions, if they exist, are of any significance to the healthfulness of cow's milk.

The most important and consistent type of contaminant of cow's milk after it leaves the udder are bacteria. As produced in a healthy animal, cows' milk is close to bacteria-free (sterile) as it leaves the udder. If the teats and the milking machine have been sanitized before milking, the withdrawn milk will continue uncontaminated. Milk is an excellent growth medium for most bacteria, especially at body temperature which is 97°F for the human and about 100°F for the cow. Unless fresh milk is cooled, the few microorganisms it contains will begin to multiply producing a new generation in roughly fifteen minutes. At that rate, the bacterial counts can be in the millions rather quickly. So the industrial practice is to cool the milk immediately after milking. Milk is known to be bacteriostatic for a period of time immediately following milking.[12,13] This is at most only a few hours during which the bacteria are prevented from multiplying by natural (not fed) antibiotics in the milk. However the length of this period is variable and undependable. The type of activity, although much weaker, is like that in our tears which keep our eyes from becoming infected by bacteria that are ever present on our skin and in the environment. Sweat also contains inhibitors of bacterial growth.[14]

The various other steps in processing and distribution of cow's milk, as explained in chapter 7, are all designed to keep milk clean and free of contaminants until it reaches the consumer. Actually the dairy industry is very experienced and successful in achieving those objectives, not only with milk but with dairy products in general. Because of the human element involved, the industry doesn't have a perfect record, of course. But the rare exceptions prove the rule. One of these occurred in a Japanese milk plant recently. After the day's processing of milk, someone forgot to dismantle and clean a valve assembly, and perhaps the lines leading to it. This allowed residual milk in the equipment to warm up and for bacteria to proliferate therein. The bacteria, apparently of a highly toxigenic strain, were swept into milk that was being processed the next day. The net result, 20,000 people were rendered sick. Yes, this was bad, but the miracle is that it practically never happens. Everyday untold millions obtain commercially processed milk of excellent quality.

* * *

In summary, milk is a product of the mammalian mother involving not only the mammary glands but also her total body metabolism. The raw materials for making milk are brought to the lactating cells by the blood. In one of the great miracles of cell biology, milk components are made, assembled, packaged, and secreted by the lactating tissue. The milk of each species of mammal is of such a nutritional quality that it *alone* can support the life and development of the newborn for a substantial period. Obviously a substance which can do that is a remarkable food. Maternal metabolism tends to deflect many toxic contaminants from the mother's milk, but in the case of both human and bovine milks, it is important that measures be taken to protect and preserve their healthfulness.

Suggested References

Alberts, B., Bray, D., Johnson, A., Lewis, J., Raff, M., Roberts, K. and Walters, P. *Essential Biology of the Cell.* Garland Publishing Inc., New York, 1998. pp. 630.

Hamosh, M. and Goldman, A. S. (eds.) *Human Lactation 2. Maternal and Environmental Factors.* Plenum, New York, 1986. pp. 657.

Jensen, R. G. (ed.). *Handbook of Milk Composition.* Academic Press, San Diego. 1995. pp. 919.

Jensen, R. G. The composition of bovine milk lipids:January 1995 to December 2000. *Journal of Dairy Science* 85:295-350. 2002.

Mather, I. H. and Keenan, T. W. Origin and secretion of milk lipids. *Journal of Mammary Gland Biology and Neoplasia* 3:259-273.1998.

Mather, I. H. A review and proposed nomenclature for major proteins of the milk-fat globule membrane. *Journal of Dairy Science* 83:203-47. 2000.

Morré, D. J. and Keenan, T. W. Membrane flow revisited. *Bioscience* 47:489-498. 1997.

Mulder, H. and Walstra, P. *The Milk Fat Globule.* Centre for Agricultural Publishing and Documentation. Wageningen, The Netherlands, 1974. pp. 296.

Newburg, D. S. ed. *Bioactive components of human milk.* Kluwer Academic/Plenum, New York. 2001. pp.592.

Notes

1.   Mostov, K. and Cordone, M. *Bioessays* 17:129-38. 1995.
2.   Morré, D. J. and Keenan, T. W. *Biosciences* 47:489-98. 1997.
3.   Welsch, U. et al. *Cell and Tissue Research* 235: 433-8. 1984.
4.   Mather, I. H. *Journal of Dairy Science* 82: 203-47. 2000.
5.   Keenan, T. W. *Journal of Mammary Gland Biology and Neoplasia* 6: 365-71. 2001.
6.   Eigel, W. N. et al. *Journal of Dairy Science* 67:1599-1631. 1984

Structure and properties of fats. At the more basic chemical level, fats are related in structure to the hydrocarbons, such as gasoline and petroleum. Like them, fats can be burned and used as fuel or as a source of light. All such substances are insoluble in water and float on it. That is why droplets of fat can be seen separated on our foods. The structural basis of these substances is long chains of carbon atoms (-C-C-C-C-C-) with hydrogen atoms attached, two hydrogens per carbon (-CH_2-CH_2-CH_2-CH_2-) When there is only one hydrogen per carbon, it creates an extra bond between the carbons (-CH_2-CH=CH-CH_2-). This double bonded condition is called "unsaturated," and if a fat contains many of these double bonds, it is said to be polyunsaturated. Most of us have been coached to think that polyunsaturated fats are better for us than saturated fats. It is not quite that simple, but we need to be aware of what unsaturation is. Polyunsaturated fats are more liquid and tend to oxidize, that is, deteriorate on exposure to air, more readily than more saturated fats. These two types of fats may have different health consequences, discussed in chapters 5 and 6.

Fatty acids are the basic components of fats. These contain the aforementioned hydrocarbon chains; and the acid refers to a carboxylic acid group attached to one end of those chains. This group contains the element, oxygen, in addition to carbon and hydrogen. (-CH$_2$-CH$_2$-COOH). The other basic component of fat is glycerol which has the structure:

$$H-C-C-C-H \quad \text{or} \quad CH_2OH-CHOH-CH_2OH$$

```
        H H H
     H-C-C-C-H    or    CH OH-CHOH-CH OH
        O O O             2          2
        H H H
```

It can be seen that glycerol is hydrocarbon-like but that it has a different group known as an hydroxyl group (-OH) attached to each of its three carbons. These are the sites at which the fat synthesizing cell attaches fatty acids. So the basic molecule of a fat is a combination of one glycerol and three fatty acids. It is known as a triacylglycerol or triglyceride. Since fatty acids can vary in their chain length and unsaturation, fats are quite varied in their composition and properties. Mostly the fatty acids contain even numbers of carbons from 14 to 22, and double bonds (unsaturation) in a limited number of positions. However, there are some few fatty acids with odd numbers of carbons and others with branching of their carbon chains. In addition, depending on variations in bonding, shapes of the fatty acids and triacylglycerols can exist in more than one form. The upshot of all this is that fats can be very complex from a compositional standpoint. There are literally thousands of different triacylglycerols (triglycerides) in milk fat.[7]

7.   Jensen, R. G. *Journal of Dairy Science* 85:295-350. 2002.
8.   Schoefl, G. I. and French, J. E. *Proceedings of the Royal Society B* 169: 153-65. 1968.
9.   Scow, R. O. et al. *Lipids* 7: 497-505. 1972.
10. Bechdel, S. I. et al. *Journal of Biological Chemistry* 80: 231-8. 1928.
11. Yakushiji, T. et al. *Archives of Environmental Contamination and Toxicology.* 7:493-504. 1978.
12. Reiter, B. *J. Dairy Research* 45:131-47. 1978.
13. O'Toole, D. K. *Advances in Applied Microbiology.* 40: 45-94. 1995.
14. Nizet, V. et al. *Nature* 414:454-7. 2001.

3

The Breasts and Lactation

Most of the time, those two protruding mounds of flesh on a woman's chest don't appear to be doing much. However, they are very potent life-promoting structures, and among the most important objects in the world. Despite the fact that our culture has changed drastically from its simple biological beginning when humankind roamed around in search of food for the greater part of the day, the breasts continue in their basic primitive purposes. They supply a life-sustaining fluid for the human infant that surpasses all others, and they have a well-known power for getting the attention of the male. From the standpoint of biology, it is interesting how closely associated these quite different but fundamentally important activities are.

It would be a disaster if U. S. culture became indifferent to the breast. It is a tremendous driving force in our entertainment, art, advertising, clothing, and news media industries. It is of great importance in cosmetic surgery. There is so much money and vested interests tied up in breast appreciation, it is hard to imagine a world without it. On that particular issue, there doesn't seem to be much interest in gender equality.

Gender Definition and Sex

As a result of increased and cyclic hormonal activity in the human female during puberty, the breast areas enlarge and protrude. While there is at this time some slight development of the alveolar and ductal systems that may eventually make and enable flow of milk, the primary change is a growth of adipose tissue. This growth is unique to the human. In other mammals, it only occurs during pregnancy. Such early localized fat deposition does not appear essential for subsequent lactation. Women with relatively small breasts go on to a normal development and differentiation of the tissue during pregnancy and accomplish lactation and nursing of their babies very well. The implication is that adolescent breast enlargement is primarily for mate attraction and sexual activity.

Some people have commented to us that they think women's breasts are getting larger. We know of no studies on this matter. The fact that our culture is endorsing greater breast display via skimpier and tighter clothing and more emphatic bras could be misleading. Early in the last century, when women wore more and looser clothes and bras that flattened, the breasts may have been just as big but relatively concealed. Even today with bra padding and surgical breast augmentation, the true situation may be obscured. On the other hand, there are a number of reasons why an increase may have occurred. According to the latest USDA figures, over half the U.S. population is overweight. Since breasts are primarily adipose tissue, this uptrend in weight may be reflected in increased breast size. A further dietary factor may simply be good nutrition. Not only do we have an excellent food supply, we are being made increasingly aware of good nutrition practices. This may well contribute to overall body development, breasts included. Another possible factor is the increasing use of progesterone-type birth control pills. It is well known that this hormone is involved in breast development, and it is the feeling of some planned-parenthood professionals that these agents when used regularly by teenage girls promote greater breast size. Finally, if size of breasts has direct connections with reproductive success, there may be genetic selection going on for larger breasts.

Fat On, Fat Off?

To facilitate delivery of the baby and health of the mother, obstetricians recommend that weight gain during pregnancy be restricted to the twenty-four to thirty-five pounds recommended by the U. S. Institute of Medicine. A further consideration is that gaining too much can cause problems and failures in breast-feeding. The average, adequately nourished woman puts on about ten pounds of fat, not weight but fat as such, during a pregnancy. Some weight tends to be lost following delivery whether or not breast-feeding is elected. However, the net effect of these processes on any given individual is quite uncertain. In the unique circumstance of pregnancy, many women wonder, from the standpoint of figure and weight control, how can I come out of all this looking good? There is still a lot we would like to know about the body's deposition and mobilization of fat. We do know gender differences exist in that most men preferentially put it on their stomach area. They develop "pot bellies" so to speak. Women, normally and desirably, carry some extra fat in their breasts, hips, and back sides—generating the well-known curves. Not only can fat become too much of a good thing in those locations, but build-up can occur also in the arms, legs and on the abdomen. There are remarkable individual differences in which only single sites are affected. This and gender differences suggest that there are regulatory phenomena we still do not understand. For example, why do some women have everything but their hips under control, or why are others trim but large breasted? Perhaps knowledge from the new genetics will give us answers and suggest means of control.

Exercise is an important factor in weight control and health. It is not necessary to discontinue exercise programs during pregnancy. However, exercise at that time should be done regularly and not strenuously. Pregnant women are more sensitive to injury from intense activity, and their babies' development can be disrupted by intermittent exercise. For further information, visit the American College of Obstetricians and Gynecologists web site: www.acog.org.

It would be nice to know precisely where that average ten pounds of fat is gained during pregnancy and where it is lost following delivery and lactation. Does it come off of the same place it went on, or from some other location? Pregnancy and lactation may offer women opportunities to manage weight and figure, but it would be helpful to have more basic information about the processes involved. We do know from experimental animals that fat deposits in the mammary gland are used during lactation, presumably for milk synthesis. But we need to know more, especially about the woman.

Lactation is also a consideration in total body and breast image. About the latter, see the following section in this chapter on breast conformation. As mentioned there is a tendency toward weight loss during lactation but this will vary with a woman's individual circumstances. To support lactation and her own well being, a mother needs additional food. So, as major factors influencing her body weight during and at the close of lactation, there is her initial weight condition, the calories she needs for her own sustenance, the additional calories needed to support lactation and the amount of exercise she gets. Nutritionists recommend additional food intake to the extent of 600 to 800 calories per day to support lactation. Since the health of both mother and baby are at stake, a calorie-adequate, well balanced diet is of prime importance. Problems in this area should be taken up with a nutritionist or pediatrician.

Lactation

The factors which build the human mammary gland into a prolific milk producer are complex and the subject of continuing research. The newly formed, teenage breast has initial structure consisting of a rudimentary duct system, a few alveolar nodules and an extensive matrix of adipose (fatty) and connective tissues. Upon conception, a rise in circulating factors stimulating development of alveoli and the duct system occurs, and in time, the structural-functional essentials for lactation are in place (figure 3.1). From the study of simplified systems, such as cells and tissue slices, it is evident that the two hormones, estrogen and progesterone, are essential to the development of what will be the lactating gland. However, the high level of progesterone, essential at this phase, actually inhibits lactation. When the placenta is expelled on birth of the baby, a major source of progesterone is eliminated and within a few days, lactation begins in earnest. The commonly used phrase is, "my milk came in." It is a very recognizable sensation in which the breasts take on a full feeling. From then on, the baby will be able to get something more than colostrum.

Figure 3.1

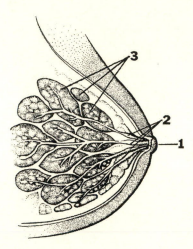

Structural scheme of the lactating breast: 1. nipple, 2. major ducts, 3. lobules of alveoli. Milk synthesized within individual alveoli passes through a system of smaller ducts into larger ducts which terminate in the nipple. Adipose and connective tissue provide the supporting matrix for blood vessels and the foregoing structures involved in milk synthesis and secretion. The non-lactating breast is comprised mainly of the adipose—connective tissue matrix. (Reproduced* with permission, Elsevier Science).
*From: Patton, S. and Jensen, R. G. Biomedical Aspects of Lactaion. Copyright Pergamon Press 1976.

Colostrum

The circumstances of the breast at the time of delivery are of considerable interest and concern to the expectant mother. The fluid that is available from the breast then and shortly after the baby is delivered is called colostrum. Compared to milk, it is yellowish and somewhat viscous. The color arises from carotene, a yellow plant pigment, which comes originally from the mother's diet. It tends to associate with fat and wherever fat is stored in the human, carotenoids are found. Carotene is converted to vitamin A in the human, but beyond that, it is not known whether the high level of carotene in colostrum serves other purposes in the infant. Colostrum is also a rich source of immune globulins which function as antibodies against diseases in the newborn.

During pregnancy, the developing cell structure for making milk is fairly open and bathed with lymph, the clear portion of blood, which is constantly entering the fine structure of breast tissue and draining back into the circulation. It is this lymph and what has accumulated in it that makes up colostrum at the time of delivery (see figure 3.2.)

Figure 3.2

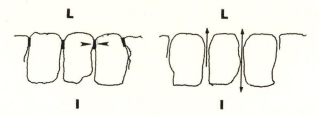

A scheme showing the structural configuration of the mammary epithelial cells before and after lactation (right) and during lactation (left). At the outset of lactation, tight junctions form between the cells (arrowheads). They create a barrier that prevent secreted milk constituents, which accumulate in the lumens(L), of the alveoli from diffusing back into the interstitial area (I), and ultimately from there into the circulation. They also suppress entry of interstitial substances from getting into lumens and being secreted with the milk. In the non-lactating state (right), there is no barrier structure formed by attaching the cells to one another. So fluid, and whatever it contains, can move back and forth between the cells (arrows). This latter condition prevails during the formation of colostrum (gestation) and throughout the resting, i. e., non-lactating, state of the breasts. So potentially, epithelial cells of any non-lactating breast may be producing bioactive substances that enter the general body metabolism.

Exactly how colostrum is created is not known. Presumably there is selective retention of immune globulins from the circulation because they are at an exceptional concentration of 5 to 10 percent in the first colostrum withdrawn at the time of delivery. It is not very useful to give volume and compositional data on colostrum without specifying the time in relation to delivery of the sample collection. The following scheme describes changes in the breast secretion as a function of time after delivery.

Days Postpartum	Character of the Secretion
0 to 2	Primarily a lymph-like, transcellular fluid* containing in addition a minor amount of material secreted by epithelial cells over an indeterminate period of time.
1 to 3	Transcellular fluid is diminishing due to closing of junctions between epithelial cells from which significant milk secretion is beginning to arise.

| 2 to 4 | Milk secretion begins in earnest. Material of transcellular origin is reduced, not only through closing of tight junctions, but also by dilution in the expanding milk flow. Mother reports that, "My milk came in." |
| 4 to 6 | Although further and gradual changes in milk composition will be occurring, the secretion product arises almost exclusively from the lactating cells and approximates normal milk in composition. |

* Fluid which is able to enter secretory ducts by passing around cells.

So the composition of a woman's colostrum is changing day by day, and in fact, hour by hour. My colleagues and I analyzed samples from five women during the 0- to 6-day post-delivery period.[1] From their protein patterns, samples collected during days 0-1 were seen to be pure colostrum. However, for two of the five, no sample could be expressed during that two-day period. All yielded a sample at the forty-two-hour collection and the pooled sample for the five women appeared to be relatively pure colostrum although a trace of beta-casein, a major protein of mature milk, was detected. Subsequent samples collected at sixty-five and eighty-eight hours postpartum showed large amount of this protein and the secretion had gone from a watery, yellow appearance to the characteristic whiteness indicating that milk secretion had begun. The average protein and fat contents of the pure colostrum for the five women averaged 7.3 and 1.4 percent, respectively; typical values for mature milk are 1.0 percent protein and 4.0 percent fat. According to our results, the very high protein content of clostrum is due almost exclusively to immune globulins.

To our knowledge, no one has ever investigated the quantity of colostrum produced by women. In order to do this, one would want to collect the total secretion from a group of women for a period of about six days postpartum using a marker, such as beta-casein, to define the amount of contaminating milk. Since women have a distinct sense of when lactation has begun by the filling of their breasts, one assumes that the amount of colostrum is comparatively small. This is confirmed by the fact that samples collected by our group using a breast pump on mornings of the first few days postpartum averaged about a tablespoonful. For comparison, milk yields of well-nourished women in full lactation average between a pint and a quart per day.

In contrast to the calf, which needs colostrum to survive, the human can get along without it. This is because there is active transfer of antibodies across the placenta during pregnancy in the human but not in the cow. So the human newborn starts off with significant resistance to infection. Most authorities advise that babies receive the colostrum. Although, there is no problem of survival without it, possible functions of colostrum in the infant deserve additional research. For example, there are indications that carotene may function in the immune system and that lactoferrin, a protein at elevated levels in colostrum, inhibits the growth of pathogenic bacteria and viruses. The fact that colostrum does not appear essential, is produced for only a few days, and in limited quantity has tended to minimize its significance so far as pediatricians are concerned. Allowing the baby to nurse for colostrum poses a problem if the mother does not intend to breastfeed. Suckling at that time encourages full lactation to begin and that is more easily suppressed if never encouraged. So it is the common practice in this situation for formula to be the baby's nourishment from the outset.

Pregnancy makes a woman realize that, to some extent, her body is no longer her own. It is mobilized to support development of the fetus within her. While not as demanding and all pervasive, the same is true of lactation. At that time, the body has, in addition to its own maintenance, a special metabolic focus on moving precursors of milk to the mammary gland by way of the circulation. For example, during lactation, dietary and adipose fat tend to move to the mammary gland for use as milk fat rather than to move to or remain in storage as adipose fat throughout the body. A mother's synthesis of milk establishes requirements of her diet in addition to those needed for her own well being. One simple, beneficial measure is for her to drink several glasses of milk a day. This supplies precursors, electrolytes and fluid volume needed for making her own milk. Whole body metabolism in relation to milk synthesis is also discussed in chapter 2 and dealt with more extensively in selected references at the end of that chapter.

Milk synthesized and secreted by alveoli in the human mammary gland collects through a system of ducts leading to fifteen or twenty larger ducts that terminate in the nipple (figures 3.1 and 3.3). Unlike the gland in the cow or goat, there is no large terminal cistern in which milk can accumulate, and one cannot simply squeeze the breast to express milk. However, by using a stripping action toward the nipple with the fingers and thumb, it is possible to remove milk a little at a time. If the idea is to set aside milk for the baby regularly, a breast pump is more convenient and efficient.

The modern mother can be caught in a dilemma. During the period 1900 to 1960, the popularity of breastfeeding lost ground to the use of formula. Ironically, this was at a time when most women were still based in the home, a rather ideal place for breastfeeding. The view was that formula feeding was modern, less confining and just as healthful as the breast. In 1965 it was estimated that only 26.5 percent of mothers leaving the hospital were nursing their babies. By 1980, the figure had increased to 50 percent because of growing evidence that human milk is superior to formula. Then another decline set in. This latest

Figure 3.3

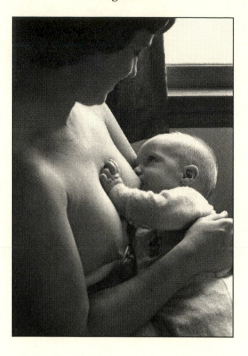

Made-for-each-other lunch partners. Development and functioning of the breasts are dependent on the action of various hormones including estrogen and progesterone from the ovaries and placenta, insulin from the pancreas, hydorcortisone from the adrenal glands and prolactin from the pituitary. Photo courtesy of Robert S. Beese, the Pennsylavania State University.

reversal is probably linked to the huge increase of women in the workforce, which made breastfeeding impractical for many. Currently in the United States, only 24 percent of homes involve traditional families of husband, wife and at least one child eighteen or under. The decline in marriages and the rise in numbers of children born out of wedlock have increased the responsibilities and stress on women. Lactation proceeds best under relaxed, peaceful conditions. Nursing mothers risk "drying up" when they are under constant strain. However, some manage to work things out. We know of one young mother who was working days and going to law school at night. She carried an electric breast pump with her and periodically pumped her breasts to maintain the flow of milk and keep up the supply for her baby. The corporate world seems to be recognizing the need for and benefits from enlightened policies regarding mothers. There also has been a great expansion in home-based employment possibilities. So it is becoming feasible for a woman to deliver and nurse a baby and work it in with her job situation. Currently, 64 percent of mothers leaving the hospital are nursing but this figure falls to 29 percent by the end of six months. According to the U. S. Surgeon General's office, at least several billion dollars would be saved in medical expenses due to childhood diseases by increasing levels of breast-feeding to 75 percent leaving the hospital and 50 percent at six months.

Non-Influence of Implants

In 1999, there were 167,318 cases of breast augmentation surgery in the United States About 3,000 of those cases were patients under eighteen years of age. Between 1993 and 1998, the incidence of cosmetic surgery, such as breast enlargement and liposuction, tripled. How breasts look seems to be growing in importance. One unique worry of these modern women is, will my implants or other surgery interfere with lactation and breastfeeding? The opinion of medical authorities and the experience of mothers is that normally there is no problem. An important objective of implant surgery is to avoid interfering with the lactation/nursing potential of the glands. Of course, in unusual implant installations, loss of some or all capacity to make and deliver milk may occur. For example, there are cases of radical mastectomies (total removal of the glands) to forestall breast cancer. In these unusual circumstances, women are usually well aware of their limitations.

Merits of Human Milk

As previously mentioned, milk was perfected as a food for the young during millions of years of evolution. Thus, human milk is as ideal for the initial nourishment of the infant as nature can make it. Formulas can approximate mother's milk and babies can survive and even thrive quite well on them, but no formula will have all the components in the same proportions as in human milk. Biological systems are exceptionally complex, and as a matter of fact, we don't know how many significant components of milk remain to be identified. This is why cow's milk will not be reproduced by some combination of vegetable components, and why soymilk, which has nutritive value in its own right, will never be a complete substitute for mammalian milks.

Because human milk is such an excellent food for the human infant, it is important that the lactating mother try to keep it that way by avoiding noxious substances like cigarettes, alcohol and drugs that can harm her baby via her milk. Fortunately, most women are very conscientious about this matter.

Breastfeeding, How Long?

While most mothers enjoy nursing their babies, there are limitations. Nursing is not always convenient from the standpoints of time and place; sometimes one would prefer to wear a different kind of top; and at some point, it would be nice to get on with life unencumbered. The consensus of pediatricians seems to be that six months is ideal, a year although a lot to ask is even better, three months is an indispensable minimum, and something is better than nothing.

Help

Breastfeeding is something of an art and the rewards from mastering it are considered great by most nursing mothers. Each baby presents a somewhat different challenge. Nature has worked out most of the kinks in the process, and that is a main reason why we are here. But things do come up and moms are good at worrying. Two of the most common are: "I don't think I have enough milk" and "My milk doesn't seem to be of the right quality." In most instances, these are needless concerns. Nature goes to extremes to make milk of the proper quality, sometimes even at high cost to the mother. The building blocks for making milk not only come from the mother's food, they also can be extracted from the bone, muscle, and fat of her body. In order to minimize body break-down, mothers need to realize that making milk and ensuring the baby's health, as well as her own, depends on her eating an adequate diet. The inclusion of cow's milk in her diet is a good practice in that it supplies fluid and precursors to the mother for making her own milk. Another distress call is, "my milk won't let down." This mechanism, which depends on the hormone, oxytocin, from the pituitary gland, is discussed in chapter 2. In the absence of "let down," milk simply is not available at the nipple. It is held back in the alveoli and smaller ducts. Normally, all that is required for "let down" to occur is preliminary suckling by the baby in a pleasant ambience for breastfeeding. With many mothers, just the cry or the sight of the baby will induce let down. Mothers get where they know the conducive conditions. Stress and emotional tension in the mother's life can be counter-productive.

The baby's lack of vigor or interest in sucking is sometimes a problem at the outset of breast-feeding. Normally, a strong response is instinctive, and that is why the world is full of people. Usually, it is just an initial sluggishness which will eventually be overcome by natural hunger and repeated presentation of the breast. When the initial sucking is weak and ineffectual, offering sweetened water (two teaspoons per cup) in a bottle with nipple may be worth a try to encourage sucking power. Sweetness is highly appreciated by infants, and al-though human milk is slightly sweet, sweetened water may be more effective in getting the baby's attention directed to the sucking task. Some hospitals make it a practice to start newly delivered babies on glucose in water from a bottle. This is usually before the mother's milk has come in. Glucose like ordinary sugar is also sweet and this practice also may help to get the baby adjusted to sucking with vigor. In the interim between delivery and nursing, the glucose water helps clear congestion, prevents dehydration and supplies some energy to the baby. Note that allowing the baby to consume a lot of sugar/water should be avoided. Actually, after a baby has gotten used to the breast, he/she may be pretty emphatic about rejecting a bottle. So this is one of the possible bumps in the road mom may encounter when she wants a night off or to phase out breastfeeding.

It is beyond the scope of this book to deal with all the many maternal and pediatric considerations involved in care of infants. Mothers are very effective in networking about such things. From having been dependent a long number of years on breastfeeding women for research samples of milk, we learned how wonderfully cooperative they are when it is understood that the findings might be helpful to other mothers and babies. It is one of the purest evidences of goodness in the world. There is at this writing a National Registry for Lactation Research on the Internet with 360 breastfeeding women enrolled. They are willing to donate samples and cooperate in research on lactation. For mothers needing help, local La Leche League chapters, professional support individuals and organizations, hospital staffs, and pediatricians are good sources. There also are excellent reference books on human lactation and infant care, a few of which are listed at the end of this and other chapters.

In these times, the Internet is a very helpful source of information. While many websites come, go and change, it is likely that at least some of those providing information on breast-feeding will continue indefinitely. Following is a list of current sites, courtesy of Dr. Judy Hopkinson of the USDA Children's Nutrition Research Center at Baylor College of Medicine:

http://www.breastfeeding.com	A wealth of information and articles.
http://www.nmaa.asn.au/bfinfo/faq.htm	Information site of Nursing Mothers of Australia.
http://www.aap.org/family/brstguid.htm	American Academy of Pediatrics site.
http:www.waba.org.br/	This is breastfeeding information site with many relevant links.
http://www.bflrc.com/newman/articles.htm	This site provides access to handouts.

ttp:www.linkagesproject.org/	Handouts in English, Spanish, and French. Linkage project and resource.
http://public.bcm.tmc.edu/cnrc/	USDA Children's Nutrition Research Center. Features article, questions and answers on breastfeeding from lactation scientists.
http://www.lalecheleague.org/bf.html	La Leche League information

Induced Lactation

In the current U. S. culture, a woman can find herself in many non-traditional circumstances. One of them is to be non-lactating but wanting to breastfeed a baby, perhaps an adopted baby or that of a relative or friend. She may simply want to be helpful or perhaps not to miss the classic experience of her gender. While it is not a common practice, lactation can be induced in a woman by administering a suitable program of hormones, estrogen and progesterone, for a period of about a week or ten days. Any of a number of drugs stimulating production and release of prolactin, the indispensable hormone for lactation, may also be recommended. Breast pumping or suckling by the baby then will initiate the flow of milk which will be maintained as long as milk continues to be periodically removed from the breast. Women interested in such a program should consult a pediatrician. Sucking alone, if repeated and persistent, can cause milk to become available, but the yields are usually below those of natural (postpartum) or hormone-induced lactation.

Breast or Bottle

There are many things to be considered when a woman decides whether or not to breastfeed. Unfortunately many new mothers are intimidated by the prospect of it. They have never done it and some think they might fail at it. There is a lot required. At the very outset it becomes tempting to say, "I'll pass." It is important that these new moms receive adequate information and support to assist them with their decisions. The considerations can be broken down into those involving the feeding activity and those relating to human milk and formula.

Breastfeeding vs. Formula Feeding

There is no question that breast feeding an infant provides a very unique experience for both mother and baby. The bonding that occurs is considered to be of very great value to both parties. It would be a pretty peculiar baby that would prefer to suck on a bottle rather than to nurse its mother; and mothers have a very natural proclivity for holding and nursing their babies. Mothers speak of the great peace they feel during this time and the relief they often experience from rather hectic daily activities (figure 3.3). There are some definite practical advantages to breastfeeding. The breast is ready to go; the milk is clean and at the right temperature. There is little or no expense involved. Formula has to be bought, made up, if in concentrated form, and adjusted for temperature. Formula feeding is more expensive than the breast. On the other hand, formula liberates mom in a very real sense. Anyone willing and able can make formula and feed the baby. Whether breastfeeding can be accommodated in a contemporary mother's life is something each new mother has to decide. Lactating breasts do indeed tie one to her baby, but women can be remarkably ingenious in working these things out for some period of time.

Some of the other considerations in the breast-vs.-bottle issue concern benefits that may accrue regarding health of the mother. It appears well established that women who have gone through gestations and lactations, especially in early adulthood, experience a reduced incidence of breast cancer. It is not uncommon for a woman's body fat to be reduced by lactation. Lactation seems to aid in promptly restoring a woman's body to the normal nonpregnant condition. It is also known to be an inhibitor of conception, but as such, is not a particularly reliable means of birth control. For example, fully lactating women have been known to conceive as early as ten weeks postpartum, and in the longer term, as many as 50 percent of women may become pregnant while still lactating.

Human Milk vs. Formula

Generally speaking, human milk is the gold standard for infant feeding and formula manufacturers try to produce products that measure up to it. Something which enabled human infants to get started in life for many thousands of generations is not liable to be full of serious imperfections. Mothers giving defective milk would have been weeded out of the human race by natural selection. So in that general sense, the nutritional content of human milk is superior to any formula. More specifically, human milk contains antibodies and related factors that suppress infections of the ear, respiratory tract and gut. The latter (diarrheal) disorders kill millions of infants and children throughout the world every year. According to the American Council on Science and Health, suppression of infections is the main advantage of breast over formula. In addition, human milk produces fewer allergic reactions in infants compared to formulas based on soy protein or cow's milk. In infant feeding, the most important allergens are proteins and the most common allergy symptom is eczema. Human proteins are less problematical than animal or plant proteins; and because of the close genetic relationship between mother and her baby, mother's milk proteins are least likely to cause allergies. However, allergens from the mother's diet are known on rare occasions to reach her milk and affect her baby. Breastfed babies have fewer problems with constipation; in fact, their stools tend to be loose. One clear advantage of formula feeding is that the amount the baby is consuming can be accurately determined. Most breastfeeding mothers know whether their babies nursed adequately but they don't know exactly how much milk they took, and on some occasions this can be worrisome.

Provided the mother is well nourished, human milk is a completely adequate food for the first four to six months of a baby's life, and all that a baby requires. After that, it is common practice to start introducing other foods. Supplemental iron, vitamin D and fluoride may also be needed at about that time. Since each mother/baby is a unique situation, it is a good time to check with the pediatrician regarding an extended nutrition program.

There are some concerns that may arise with respect to preparing formula. If it is a dried or concentrated preparation, sanitary quality and possible environmental contaminants of the diluting water can be a problem, especially in developing countries. Related to this is the matter of spoiled formula. If the intent is to make up formula and use it over a period of time, it needs to be refrigerated until used. A few hours at 90°F, or even less, not only can spoil formula but even make it toxic. Some sense of sanitation on the part of the person preparing formula for the feeding(s) is imperative. It is a basic requirement that utensils, containers and water (if needed) be clean. Formula should be used promptly following warming for the baby. Such warming sets the stage for growth of contaminating bacteria. Thus, it is safest to dispose of any unconsumed residual formula.

Some years ago certain makers of infant formula, in the interest of developing new markets for their products, were making a strong effort to sell mothers in third world countries. Product use under the conditions often involved every no-no in the book, that is, an uneducated user, contaminated water, no refrigeration, a hot climate and poor sanitation. Not only is breastfeeding vastly superior under such conditions, but the whole sales campaign was soured by the public relations nightmare of infant sickness and death caused by "the greedy corporations."

Infant Feeding and Future Health

Regarding health of babies, it needs to be recognized at the outset that a lot has been going on in them before they ever see the light of day. Obviously, the nine months *in utero* influences the map of a lifetime. Even earlier, the mother, as she comes up to conception is defining the health potentialities of the situation, as does her post-conception nutrition and life style. It is something of a mystery why so many people are now living into their eighties, nineties, and beyond. However, the mothers of those people were born at a time when the knowledge of nutrition, the supply of good food, and the understanding of disease were making progress as never before. Very likely, healthy mothers not only make healthy babies but also babies with good potential for long life.

The normal expectation is that effects of infant feeding, either with breast or formula, will be more or less immediate and that when the practice is phased out, its influence on the infant will end. From recent research, we are beginning to get hints that this is not necessarily so. A British study suggests that formula fed infants become at higher risk of high blood pressure as adults than those who were breastfed. In the following section on the brain, evidence is discussed that breastfeeding may favorably influence subsequent development of human intelligence when compared to formula feeding. In other studies with mice regarding incidence of diabetes and obesity, there are indications that the mother's genes somehow acting in concert with her milk help promote or suppress the disorders when her offspring become adults. These kinds of observations are another indication of the remarkable significance of milk as a food.

The concept of functional foods has existed for several decades. These are foods that have beneficial effects over and beyond their basic nutritional contribution of protein, fat, carbohydrate, vitamins and minerals. For example, a functional aspect of breast milk is that it tends to establish a healthy population of bacteria in the infant gut. Any health-promoting effect of a food beyond its classical nutrient makeup would be in the functional category. That what a newborn is fed may have a directing effect on its development as a child and adolescent, and its health as an adult is a new and exciting hypothesis. For further information on bioactive components of human milk, see the suggested reference of that title at the end of the chapter.

As a field of research, long-term health effects of breast or formula feeding is in its infancy and much additional work will be required before a good-sized body of useful information has been acquired. However, what little we know to date seems to clearly indicate that future effects occur at least in some individuals. One would expect that the effects of having been breastfed would be beneficial. The primary evolutionary thrust of milk as a food is to assure survival and vigor of the newborn into its reproductive years. But in terms of infant formula, this does not mean that breast milk is in every instance perfect, or that nature can never be improved upon. Further, there have been millions of formula-fed babies that grew up to be very normal healthy adults. The challenging question now is whether they would have been even better if breastfed. Health in later life always seems to be at risk and somewhat of a mystery. Perhaps research in this area will help to clarify the matter.

The Brain, DHA, and Formula.

Some ten or twelve years ago, it was reported[2] that preterm babies (those born approximately five to twelve weeks early); who had been fed human milk as compared to formula subsequently developed to score slightly better on IQ tests. This created a lot of interest and discussion. It is hard to think of things that might be of greater concern than factors influencing intelligence. The particular study was confounded by the fact that mothers of the babies receiving human milk may have been brighter than those of the formula fed babies. This raises the possibility that the breastfed babies, on average, simply inherited a greater intelligence potential than the babies fed formula in which case what was fed might not have been the factor determining the experimental result. We found it exasperating that the actual details of what was in the formula were not revealed. So one could not know precisely what differences existed between the two groups of infants regarding intake of dietary components. Still, the study, as well as others to follow, was clearly suggestive, but they did not allow us to say with certainty whether or not feeding human milk, as compared to formula, has an effect on intelligence.

A recent study[3] evaluating duration of breastfeeding in relation to adult intelligence shows a clear-cut association between the two. The longer individuals were breast fed, up to nine months, the higher their adjusted mean scores were on two different intelligence tests. Beyond nine months, there was no additional benefit. The study involved both sexes and corrected for a wide range of possible confounding factors. The tests were administered at mean ages of 27.2 years for one sample (973 men and women) and 18.7 years for the second sample (2,280 men). The results, along with earlier findings, seems to firmly establish that breast feeding as compared to other means of nourishment during the first nine months of life, leads to somewhat better performance on intelligence tests even into adulthood. Of course, this heightens interest in the possibility that a component(s) of human milk is responsible for this difference, and in identifying the substance(s) so that it can be added to infant formula. Most exciting of all, it could establish for the first time, the relationship between something that is eaten and one's intelligence.

Studies on mental ability in infants helped to focus attention on two fatty acids present in human milk that are involved in development of the nervous and visual systems. These are docosahexaenoic acid (DHA) and arachidonic acid (AA). Both are present in substantially higher amounts in human milk as compared to cow's milk. Some European countries are now allowing DHA and AA to be added to infant formulas. In a recent move, the U. S. Food and Drug Administration has approved addition of the two fatty acids to infant formula. Growing recognition that DHA and AA are more important in human health than had been appreciated emphasizes the value of keeping up with research findings about them. For this purpose, reviews are noted here that cover the subject in terms of pregnancy,[4] human milk, infant formula and infant development[5,6] and in general human health and development.[7] Another report of interest is that lower DHA consumption is associated with higher rates of postpartum depression.[8]

There are some considerations in a more general sense about brain development and milk feeding. Man's brain is his best survival weapon. He does not have fangs or claws and he can't fly or even run very fast. He seems to have lost much of his ability to climb trees. But he is a fantastic sleuth and problem solver. The human brain doubles in size during the first six months of life. It is said that over half of our genes are concerned with brain growth, repair and function. Obviously, adequate nutrition is of great importance in brain development. Both breast- and formula feeding must sustain this process very well. However, there is abundant evidence that inadequate quantity and quality of food in infancy can irreversibly damage mental development. Provided that the lactating mother is healthy and well fed, it appears that human milk is the best designed "brain food" for her infant.

Pieces of Mom

A rather interesting difference between human and cow's milk concerns the occurrence of pieces of lactating cell on milk fat globules of the human but not on those of the cow.[9,10] Literally, mom is secreting bits of herself in her milk. Because these pieces are shaped like a new moon, they are called crescents and are known to contain all the different parts of the cell except the nucleus. These crescents occur because the plasma membrane of the lactating cell does not tightly adhere to some fat droplets when they are being secreted. Instead, the membrane encompasses some of the cells cytoplasm along with the fat droplet. For description of how milk fat globules are secreted, see chapter 2. The nucleus is not included simply because it is too large and well anchored in the cell. In the milk of some women, there can be as many fat globules with these crescents of cytoplasm as there are without. The average proportion seems to be about 7 percent of globules with crescents. It is not known what, if any, significance the crescent material may have for the infant. Crescents occupy much less than 1 percent of the milk volume. However, large quantity is not always an indication of nutritional significance, witness the vitamins. The crescents can be viewed as a concentrate of substances and structures that keep the lactating cell alive and functioning. Thus, they may serve similar purposes in the nursing infant. It is also possible that crescents have something to do with absorption and digestion of milk fat. We have noted that the globules with crescents have a tendency to fuse together (figure 3.4). Possibly such globules may fuse with and become part of cells in the infant's intestinal mucosa. This might provide a shortcut for transport of milk fat into the infant's circulation. In any event, one wonders why crescents occur? Constantly losing parts of the milk producing cells of the breast would not appear useful unless it was serving some purpose in the infant.

Figure 3.4

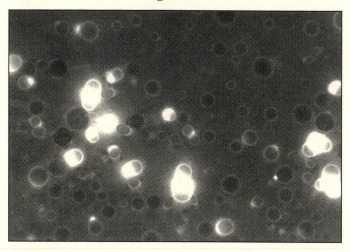

Photograph of human milk stained to show milk fat globules containing crescents of cytoplasm from the lactating mother's mammary cells. Note tendency of globules with crescents to fuse or clump (at right). Staining was accomplished with the dye, acridine orange; photo was taken through a microscope at a magnification of X650. Data of S. Patton and G. E. Huston. For details see Biochimica et Biophysica Acta 965:146-53. 1988.

There is other cellular material in milk; for example, sloughed mammary cells and parts thereof. Milk also contains other cells of various kinds, such as macrophages which spend their time searching the body, including the mammary glands, for bacteria, viruses and cell debris. This is all in the interest of host defense against disease and keeping tissues clean and orderly. These so-called phagocytes engulf and digest within themselves these enemies and tissue debris of the gland. Some of them are always present in the milk and when their numbers become unusually high there, one suspects infection, which, in the case of the mammary gland or breast, is known as mastitis. It should receive prompt medical attention and usually requires antibiotic treatment.

At one point in my research, I became interested in determining whether a particular component of human milk reached the lower intestine of the breastfed baby. The substance in question is known as a mucin, a protein with a lot of attached carbohydrate. It exists on the surface of cells in many tissues throughout the body including the mammary epithelial cell, and it is a component of the membrane on milk fat globules.[11] Dr. Horst Schroten and his colleagues in Germany had shown that this mucin binds a pathogenic form of the bacteria, *E. coli.*[12] The whole idea that components of milk are acting as decoys to sidetrack pathogens from binding to and infecting the intestinal mucosa excited me. I obtained fecal samples from a number of breastfed and formula-fed infants and analyzed them for the mucin. The results were gratifying in that none of the samples from the formula-fed babies was positive for the mucin, whereas most of the breastfed samples were.[13] So parts of milk passed all the way through the baby intact and thus could help protect the entire length of its digestive tract against infection. Evidence that human milk contains substances that are anti-infective is substantial and growing (see suggested references by Neville and Newberg at the end of the chapter). An area worthy of research is antibiotic activity of peptides resulting from the digestion of the milk proteins. It would certainly make sense for products of milk digestion to control the bacterial microflora of the gut, not only for preventing contagious diseases but also for suppressing diarrheal disorders.

An interesting sidelight to the foregoing research concerned the nature of the fecal samples. I had always heard that bowel movements from breastfed babies were relatively odorless. Having had seven children, I was familiar with diaper changing, but all had been formula-fed, so I could only attest that feces from formula are hardly pleasant smelling. The samples from my study bore out these observations. Formula generates a foul odor while human milk does not. Actually, the relatively mild odor connected with samples from the breastfed babies resembled that of buttermilk which is logical. Human milk fosters the growth of *Lactobacillus bifidus* in the infant intestinal tract. It is a lactose fermenting bacterium related to some of those used in buttermilk cultures. While this line of evidence about odor is not exactly high science, it does indicate the remarkable capacity of human milk to control microflora of the intestine.

Resting Breasts, Endocrine Function?

When the nursing mother weans her baby, i.e., stops nursing, the milk flow ceases. Then a marvelous natural program called involution takes over. Residual milk and most of the milk producing alveoli and milk-delivering duct cells are degraded and the products are recycled for use in other cells or disposed of. When this process is complete, the breasts are said to be inactive or in a resting state. Examination of breast tissue in this state under the microscope reveals evidence of residual secretory activity. What is being made and whether it has any significance to the metabolism and health of women has received virtually no attention. We suggest the matter is worthy of research. A gland producing secretions containing such substances as hormones and enzymes that are used elsewhere in the body is known as an endocrine gland. The pancreas which produces insulin is such a gland. The breast is not considered to be endocrine since its product, milk, is used outside the body. However, any residual secretory activity of the resting gland may release substances of use internally. It is pertinent that when lactation is full on and milk is being continuously removed from the breast, feed back of milk into the body is blocked structurally. All of the lactating cells are tightly joined to each other so that flow can only occur through the ducts to the nipples. However, after weaning, the tight junctions between these cells open and it is possible that anything they secrete diffuses back into the circulation and thus may be carried all over the body (figure 3.2).

Many bioactive substances are produced in lactating tissue and gain their way into milk.[14, 15 16] While it is true that after weaning, the major constituents and the volume (water) of milk may no longer be produced in significant amounts; some molecules of possible benefit to the mother may continue to be synthesized and released. Such molecules may not be a matter of life or death but they may be healthful nonetheless. For example, the milk protein, alpha-lactalbumin, for which there is evidence of anti-carcinogenicity,[16] comes to mind. Could this be a factor in the reduced incidence of breast cancer associated with lactation (see following section on breast cancer)? Another milk protein that could have many potential health consequences in the mother is lactoferrin (p. 120).

Conformation of the Breasts

The Initial Condition

As mentioned above, developed breasts of a teenage girl are largely adipose (fat) cells distributed in a connective tissue matrix. There also are a system of blood vessels that nourish the cells and some beginnings of a duct system for future handling of milk, but these vessels and ducts are minor aspects of the virgin breast. While there is a promise of function to come, initially the breasts seem to be primarily a structural display—smooth and firm. In our current society, both women and men are concerned about this situation and pleased when optimum size and shape of the breasts prevail both initially and for the long term. The hope seems to be that women may become pregnant, have and nurse babies, grow older, but that their breasts will remain well shaped and, where insufficient, increase somewhat in size.

Finding and maintaining what one considers an optimum breast size and conformation is challenging. It is by no means a problem just of too small. Many women are distraught with even modest-size breasts. They don't enjoy large masses of flesh that have to be strapped down all the time. This is basically the same old dilemma of obesity and exercise—the less one moves, the more weight one puts on and the more difficult and unpleasant it becomes to move. It appears that the best solution to this problem in our current culture, is for a woman to get ahead of the weight problem with diet and regular, continuing exercise *starting early in life* so that she can stay ahead of it.

Pregnancy and Lactation

With the onset of pregnancy, things begin to change in the breasts. In fact, their increased sensitivity is often the first symptom a woman has of her new condition. While both blood vessels and ducts will expand through branching and extension and many milk-producing structures (alveoli) will develop at the ends of the ducts during pregnancy, the adipose-connective tissue matrix remains relatively unchanged. Even though, the breasts increase in size, it is possible for some women to go through a pregnancy, suppress lactation following birth of their babies, and experience minimal change in their breasts. Cellular aspects that developed during pregnancy are for the most part selectively removed and the breasts are restored to more or less their original condition. As mentioned previously, it is easiest for a new mother to terminate lactation before it starts, and, preferably with medical care and advice, before she leaves the hospital following delivery.

Lactation has effects on breast structure, the principal one being utilization of the fat deposits of the virgin breast. Fat is quantitatively the primary component of the breast. So when lactation shuts down on weaning the baby, the original fat accumulation is largely if not completely gone. At the same time the milk-producing structures are dismantled by a process known as involution and there is no more milk in the breasts. The result is a slackness. It is as though the breasts have collapsed. Some of this change may be overcome by renewed deposition of fat in ensuing weeks and months following weaning. However, there is little chance the breast structure will be *exactly* as it was before. The new fat will not be deposited into the exact same co-developing structural matrix of fat cells and collagen fibers as in the virgin breast. One thing that seems to be working these days is the production and display of some cleavage irrespective of breast size. Lactation can help with the development of cleavage. Whatever the difference, use of the breasts to nourish babies is one of the most natural activities in the world. It has many merits for both mother and baby. If restoring or "improving" breast size and shape is crucial, one can always resort to a better bra; and there is always surgery.

Breast Cancer

Because of its complexity as a disease and the huge amount of information that has been amassed about it, breast cancer is beyond in-depth discussion here. However, total neglect of the subject would be an unjustified omission. Breast cancer is a serious concern in the lives of most women; and their pregnancies and lactations, or lack of them, have an important bearing on the matter.

What is Cancer?

From the time a human is conceived in the womb, cells of the embryo begin to multiply and differentiate into the many functional forms that make up the growing fetus. In addition, this process, which continues into the baby, child and adult, involves death and destruction of cells that are no longer needed as well as any abnormal cells, which if not killed, might go on to produce various forms of cancer. So all our lives our immune system is eliminating cells of the self that it identifies as abnormal or obsolescent, and thus unneeded. In time and as a matter of chance, one's immune system may be faced with an abnormal cell that is capable of evading all of its defense mechanisms and of multiplying out of control. This cell either forms a tumor, an abnormal cellular infiltration or, if it is a cell type of the blood, a leukemia—in any case, it is cancer.

What is Breast Cancer?

The epithelial cells of the breast are the structural units of the ducts and alveoli. These latter are involved in milk synthesis and secretion during lactation but they also exist in a resting state and reduced numbers before and between pregnancies and lactations. Epithelial cells are the principal ones involved in formation of breast cancers. By virtue of natural selection, life tends to be supported and protected through the reproductive years. That is the sick tend not to reproduce thereby leaving the healthy to perpetuate themselves. Thus, lethal forms of cancer have less tendency to develop in younger people. For example, breast cancer is primarily, but not exclusively, a disease of post-menopausal women. In the United States, more than three-fourths of all breast cancers occur in women fifty years or older. Since both environment and genetic are active, ever changing factors in the disease, there is earlier onset in about 20 to 25 percent of cases. In recent years, about 190,000 women in the U.S. are diagnosed annually as having breast cancer; and in 2002, roughly 40,000 were projected to die from it.

Risk Factors: Roles of Pregnancy and Lactation

There are a number of risk factors that increase ones chances of getting breast cancer including: being female, post-menopausal or obese, having a family history of, or an earlier occurrence of breast cancer or benign breast disease, late-in-life pregnancies or lack of a full-term pregnancy, early onset of menstruation and late onset of menopause, lack of physical activity, and exposure to radiations.[17] Consumption of alcohol and estrogen supplementation are recent additions to the list. A profile for the American woman with an elevated risk for breast cancer has emerged from many studies. She is well educated, middle class, has children late in life if at all, enjoys alcoholic drinks and may use hormone supplements. Some of the differences in breast cancer rates throughout the world may have their origin in the variations and complexities of such profile factors

Our particular interest here is in the roles of pregnancies and lactation. Simply stated, the more of both and the earlier the first full term pregnancy, the better. One can not do much about some of the big risk factors: being female, numbers of menstrual cycles, increasing age, family history or one's previous breast diseases. With regard to family history, genetic testing and counseling is

Figure 3.5

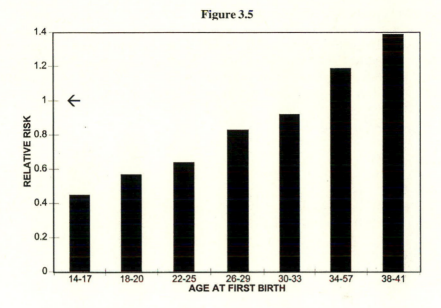

Trend in the relative risk of developing breast cancer as a function of age at first full-term pregnancy. as compared to the risk for women having experienced no full-term pregnancy (arrow) (Adapted from data of Mac Mahon et al. Bulletin of the World Health Organization. 43:209. 1970).

available. Pregnancies, lactations, weight control and exercise involve personal options that could help. Pregnancies and lactations have the benefit of eliminating populations of cells in the breast that may have picked up unfavorable mutations. Another possible benefit is that they spare the breasts from the monthly bombardment of hormones, particularly estrogen which is a well-known promoter of breast cancer. That is why later onset and earlier termination of menstrual cycles in life is thought to have a protective effect. Taking tamoxifen, a drug that blocks the estrogen receptor of cells, reduces the risk of breast cancer by about half for women in general.

It has been known for many years that an early full-term pregnancy is protective against breast cancer. The trend in risk as a function of age at first pregnancy is shown in figure 3.5. A theory regarding the beneficial effect of an early, full-term pregnancy involves the fate of stem cells in the breast. Such cells are flexible with respect to their further development into various final forms. For example, they might become duct, milk-synthesizing, or fat-storing cells, and they might be transformed at some point in later life into cancer cells. According to the theory, if these stem cells are driven into a normal mature state by an early pregnancy, this would reduce or eliminate the possibility of their later becoming cancerous. Another consideration is that the end of a pregnancy or lactation involves natural death of a lot of cells in the breasts and those cells will never be transformable to cancer. In the current public dilemma about stem cells for research, it has been brought out that fat cells, among others, have stem cell properties, meaning that they could be used to develop a variety of other tissues, organs, and *even possibly cancers.* Not only is this relevant to the breast, which is primarily comprised of fat cells, it also would correlate with obesity as a breast cancer risk factor.

Until recently, the picture regarding lactation in relation to breast cancer has been somewhat difficult to interpret. There have been many studies covering women in various areas of the world. A collaborative (meta) analysis[18] of data from forty-seven studies involving thirty countries and many thousands of women has now clearly shown the protective effect of breastfeeding—in fact, the longer the better. This epidemiological reanalysis indicates that the relative lack of breastfeeding among women in developed countries, including America, is a major factor in the greater incidence of breast cancer in those countries. It is heartening to have this kind of decisive answer to such an important question and coming from such a large amount of data.

Another factor associated with reduced incidence of breast cancer is consumption of milk and milk products. In that connection, we discuss in chapter 5 the capacity of a fatty acid of milk, conjugated linoleic acid (CLA), known more specifically as cis 9, trans 11octadecadienoic acid, to suppress mammary cancer in experimental animals. Moreover, recent studies[19, 20] of Scandinavian women have shown that reduction in incidence of breast cancer was proportionate to their consumption of milk. A related research question is why mammary tumors are rare in cows and much more common in some other species including the human. One may well suspect there is something protective about both cow's milk and all that lifelong lactation activity in its mammary glands. Since milk drinking and breastfeeding both appear to be protective against breast cancer,[18-20] it would seem worthwhile to study their combined effect on incidence of the disease in an appropriate population of women.

* * *

The female breasts provide a remarkable confluence of considerations about food, sex, and cancer. In the food realm, it is a matter of common sense that human milk is good for babies. Research reveals increasingly why this is true. In simple terms, breastfeeding makes for healthier babies but it also may have beneficial lifelong effects on them. Moreover, it is an activity that is much enjoyed by both parties. Hopefully, in this rather crazy breast-worshiping culture, the unique merits of those glands for making healthy babies will not be lost sight of. Full-term pregnancies, especially early ones, lactations, and regular milk drinking are associated with reduced incidence of breast cancer.

Suggested References

Hamosh, M. (Ed.) Human milk and infant development. *Biology of the Neonate* 74(2):79-192. 1998.

Hamosh, M. and Goldman, A. S. eds., *Human Lactation 2,** Plenum Press, New York. 1986. pp.231-239.

Howe, H. L. et al. Annual report to the nation on the status of cancer (1973 through 1998), featuring cancers with increasing trends. *Journal of the National Cancer Institute* 93(11): 824-842. 2001.

Meister, K. Should long-chain polyunsaturated fatty acids be added to infant formula? *A report of the American Council on Science and Health,* 1995 Broadway, New York, NY 10023. 2000. pp.19.

Meister, K. and Morgan, J. Risk factors for breast cancer. *A report of the American Council on Science and Health*, 1995 Broadway, New York, NY 10023. 2000. pp. 25.

Neifert, M. R. *Dr. Mom.* Signet, New York. 1987. pp. 529.

Neville, M. C. and Neifert, M. R. (Eds.) *Lactation.* Plenum, New York. 1983. pp. 466.

Newburg, D. S. (ed.) *Bioactive Components of Human Milk.* Kluwer Academic/Plenum, New York. 2001. pp. 592.

* This and other volumes in the series contain extensive information on human lactation.

Notes

1.   Patton, S., et al. Approaches to the study of colostrums—the onset of lactation. In: *Human Lactation 2,** M. Hamosh and A. S. Goldman, eds., Plenum Press, New York. 1986. pp. 231-239.

2.   Lucas, A. et al. *Lancet* 339:261-4. 1992.

3.   Mortensen, E. L. et al. *JAMA* 287:2365-71. 2002. Note: this paper is particularly useful because it reviews the literature in the 10 years since the Lucas (preceding note) et al. investigation.

4.   De Vriese, S. *Inform* 12: 1075-80. 2001.

5.   Hamosh, M. and Salem, N. *Biology of the Neonate* 74(2): 106-120. 1998.

6.   Meister, K. Should long-chain polyunsaturated fatty acids be added to infant formula? A report of the *American Council on Science and Health*, 1995 Broadway, New York, NY 10023. 2000. pp.19.

7.   Simonopoulos, A. P. *American Journal of Clinical Nutrition* 54: 438-63. 1991.

8.   Hibbeln, J. R. *Journal of Affective Disorders* 69: 15-29. 2002.

9.   Patton, S. and Huston, G. E. *Biochimica et Biophysica Acta* 965: 146-53. 1988.

10.   Huston, G. E. and Patton, S. *Journal of Dairy Science* 73: 2061-66. 1990

11.   Patton, et al. *Biochimica et Biophysica Acta* 1241:407-23.1995.

12.   Schroten, H. et al. *Infection Immunology* 60:2893-99.1992.

13.   Patton, S. *Journal of Pediatric Gastroenterology and Nutrition* 18:225-30. 1994.

14.   Campana, W. M.; and Baumrucker, C. R. Hormones and growth factors in bovine milk. In *Handbook of Milk Composition,* edited by R. G. Jensen. Academic, San Diego, CA, 1995.

15.   Newburg, D. S. ed. *Bioactive components of human milk.* Kluwer Academic/Plenum, New York. 2001. pp. 592.

16.   Sternhagen, L. G. and Allen, J. C. Ibid. pp. 115-120.
17.   Meister, K. and Morgan, J. Risk factors for breast cancer. *A report of the American Council on Science and Health*, 1995 Broadway, New York, NY 10023. 2000. pp. 25.
18.   Beral, V. et al. Breast cancer and breast feeding: collaborative analysis of individual data from forty-seven epidemiological studies in thirty countries, including 50,302 women with breast cancer and 96,973 women without the disease. *Lancet* 360:187-95. 2002.
19.   Knekt, et al. *British Journal of Cancer* 73:687-91. 1996.
20.   Hjartaker, A. et al. *International Journal of Cancer* 93:888-93. 2001.

4

Image of Cow's Milk: Roles of Media, Research, and Critics

Thus far we have examined the origin, composition, properties, synthesis and secretion of milk. We also reviewed those wondrous facts of life, the breasts, and how important they are both biologically and culturally. Next, let us consider the healthfulness of cow's milk. The value of human milk for the well-being of babies is not, and never has been seriously questioned. This was also true of cow's milk as a human food until about 1960. From that time on, milk has been receiving various criticisms, often amplified by the press, which thrives on reporting controversy, cultural clashes, and the destruction of icons. We live in an era in which nothing is sacred.

Before we can evaluate criticisms of milk and gain a valid understanding of its healthfulness, it is necessary to define the reliability of the various kinds of information available to us on human nutrition and health. Another area needing characterization is the forces and purposes of antagonism to milk. Who is attempting to discredit milk and why? To meet these needs, this chapter is divided into two parts: Kinds and Reliability of Health Information and Forces of Antagonism to Milk. Specific considerations regarding Healthfulness of Milk are taken up in the next chapter.

1. Reliability of Health Information

There is a realm of nutrition information that is comprised of facts. This information has been checked and tested many times by many people and found to be accurate. There is another level of understanding that is suggestive but not yet on solid ground. It leads to speculations and explanations that are neither true nor false until proven one way or the other. It involves ideas about how things *may* be. They can also be partly right or wrong. There is a good deal of confusion about the difference between association and cause and effect. Two things can be associated but they are not necessarily related by cause and effect. For example, there may be an association, that is, a correlation in incidence, between alcoholism and syphilis. This does not mean that alcoholism causes syphilis or vice versa. Heart disease is most common in English-speaking countries; however, speaking English doesn't cause heart disease. Milk drinking is associated with many things and for the benefit of maintaining our health, we must carefully evaluate the information we are receiving about it. Of course, anyone who wants to demean milk may claim that it is associated with some dreaded disease. The information may be incorrect in the first place but even if it were true, the intent is to have us conclude that milk *causes* the disease—not necessarily so!

Kinds of Knowledge about Nutrition

Common Experience

Until scientific effort began to characterize and identify the essential nutrients, vitamins, and minerals in foods, the only guidance humans had about healthfulness of a food was common experience. In evaluating such experience, if it comes only from one or a few individuals, scientists will say it is "anecdotal," which is a way of warning people that more and better evidence is needed before we can have confidence in the findings. With anecdotal evidence, there is too much possibility that the human subjects involved cannot, for various reasons, convey an accurate and representative result. So one needs consistent results from many observers for an answer to be reliable.

That is the way humankind arrived at what is good to eat and what isn't—an endless trial and error process which all of us continue to practice. If literally millions of people over thousands of years find by experience that a food is acceptable and healthful, this is at least as certain as the results of modern day scientific experimentation. It is by such long-term, collective wisdom that humanity knows cow's milk is a good food for humans. Thus, one would realize immediately that such scary statements as, "milk is poison," are preposterous. In this era, when it is common to read and hear these kinds of shocking messages, it pays, first of all, to make ones own calm evaluation, that is, in terms of the long-standing common knowledge, could this pronouncement possibly be true? Could the dairy industry have grown to its current immense size if milk were a deadly poison? The next step if one feels uncomfortable with his/her knowledge of the situation is to take it to the experts. Most announcements of the type mentioned are not made because of dedicated interest in the truth; their main purpose is to get attention for one reason or another. With regard to milk, there is no need for scary scenarios. Human experience and scientific research have supplied a tremendous amount of information about cow's milk, and we can specify rather precisely what its merits and limitations are.

The Hard and Soft Science of Nutrition

In thinking about the concept of food, diet and nutrition, it is essential to understand that nutrition has two scientific aspects, one concrete and certain and the other somewhat nebulous and not only uncertain, but involving a range of uncertainty. In the first instance, vitamins are essential for everyone—this is an incontestable fact; it is also absolutely true that one must maintain an adequate intake of them or ones health will deteriorate. The same thing is true of the essential minerals. For example, if one does not consume a sufficient amount of iron, either in one's food or as a supplement, anemia results. This is a condition of inadequate hemoglobin in one's red blood cells. Hemoglobin is the iron-containing protein that carries oxygen from the lungs to all the tissues and cells of the body. The symptoms of anemia include chronic fatigue, feelings of weakness, dizziness, and shortness of breath. Iron deficiency anemia is the leading nutritional inadequacy in the United States and throughout the world. Addressing this problem, Professor Paul Saltman, a nutrition biochemist at the University of California, San Diego, used to say, "If you can't afford red meat, at least cook with a rusty frying pan." In other words, red meat is a good source of iron but transfer of rust from an old-fashioned frying pan into one's food is another way to get it. While this was one of the unlimited successful ploys Paul, a truly outstanding teacher, had for getting and holding students' attention, the rusty frying pan is not a prescribed source of dietary iron. It does not lend itself to even crude quantitative control; and too much iron in the diet can be toxic.

Nonetheless, all of us need regular intake of iron, other essential minerals and vitamins, not only for good health but just to stay alive. These are hard scientific facts. However, when one raises the question, "How much iron do I need in my food or, as a supplement?" we are already into a softer aspect of nutrition science. The answer is that the requirements for essential nutrients vary among individuals. To determine each person's daily need for every nutrient would not be worth the trouble and expense. Nutritionists have solved this problem for us by determining the average person's needs. Of course, these values do not take into account all the individual variations due to such things as age, gender, body size, activity, life style, reproductive state (pregnant or lactating), and variations that exist between individuals because of genetic factors. Research has provided information on the range of requirements in the human population. From these data, the nutritionists derive optimum amounts plus an additional safety factor and these figures yield the so-called minimum daily requirements (MDRs), recommended daily allowances (RDAs), or daily values (DVs) —all of which mean more or less the same. These are encountered on food charts, in tables and on food labels in the form of percentages which tell one approximately how much of ones daily need, which is 100 percent for each of the various essential nutrients, that is being met by a serving of the particular food.

DVs are based on an imaginary average adult who would be consuming 2,000 calories per day. As mentioned, there will be variations. For example, a large male whose daily work is eight hours of hard physical labor would need more like 4,000 calories a day and commensurate increases in vitamins and minerals. Nonetheless, the DV is a very useful concept. It is a close enough fit for most of us that it can be used without correction. As an example, let us say one buys a can of applesauce, and on the label it indicates that one serving (about 1/3 cup) of that applesauce contains half the amount of vitamin C per day required by the average person. Thus, if one wants to completely satisfy the daily need for vitamin C using that particular applesauce, it will be necessary to consume two servings.

A Balanced Diet

The fact that one serving of a particular food provides only parts of one's daily needs for nutrients and calories introduces the concept of a balanced diet. In order to fulfill the daily requirements, allow for some choices and compensate for the nutritional limitations that each and every food has; selecting the right kinds and amounts of foods will be necessary. Otherwise, one may become deficient in one or even several essentials. For this reason, all of us need some basic understanding of nutrition. We will be selecting foods to eat all our lives and what we choose or don't choose can be very important to our health both short- and long-term. A balanced diet is one that supplies all of the nutrients one needs. Since most of the essential nutrients are not stored for long-term use in the body, a balanced diet is usually thought of in terms of a day's food, more particularly in our culture, breakfast, lunch, and dinner. The fact that no single food comes close to providing a balanced diet makes necessary and desirable the inclusion of a variety of foods in our daily intake. As discussed above, data have been produced on the nutrient contents of virtually every conceivable food so that we can know what a normal serving of any given item is contributing to our daily need (i.e., percent DV). The Nutrient Data Laboratory of the U. S. Department of Agriculture makes available extensive nutrition information on nearly 6,000 foods. This used to be available as USDA Handbook No. 8. While no longer available in paper, the entire database is accessible and can be downloaded wholly or in part from the Internet. The address is *http:// www.nal.usda.gov/fnic/foodcomp*.

Some Nutrition Guidelines

"Well," you say, "I can't be going around with a pack of nutrition tables covering all foods and a pocket calculator every day of my life. Is there anything I can do to make this process simpler?" The answer is yes. There are some practical steps that can help.

Consider taking a basic course in nutrition. All your life you are choosing foods and rejecting others. These choices are helping to determine how much energy you have, how healthy you are, how you look and feel, and so on. You might say it is one version of a "this-is-your-life" show; and it is certainly worth learning how to make good choices. The quality and variety of food in America is an incredible blessing, and it is very easy to select a healthy and enjoyable diet if you know what you are doing. So enroll for that course - and don't tell me you are too old or too busy to go to school. These days, people are going to school all their lives. Nutrition is taught very widely—at universities, community colleges, extension programs and night schools. The Internet also makes such courses accessible but my suggestion is to attend a live class if possible. With a subject such as nutrition, the on-site teacher/student interactions greatly enhance ones motivation and enliven the learning. Would you believe that as little as twenty-five years ago, nutrition was not included in educational requirements at most medical schools? So don't feel inferior, even some doctors aren't very far ahead of you on food and nutrition. If you want to keep up-to-date on nutrition via the Internet, try the Tufts University Nutrition Navigator at: <www.navigator.tufts.edu/index.html>. It provides review by experts of many other important sites providing nutrition data and information. About being too busy to take a short course on nutrition, you're not too busy to get sick; nutrition is about staying healthy, so a knowledge of it could save you a lot of time lost when you weren't feeling well or productive during your life.

Get a variety of foods into your diet. Any nutritionist will so advise. It is simply good insurance. There is no perfect food that has everything you need. Don't get into a rut. Certain foods prepared in a certain way can be very enjoyable and become habit forming. You can't make it on burgers, french fries, and soda forever. Mix it up with meat, poultry, fish, fruits, vegetables, grains, milk, and dairy products on a regular basis. Try to include five or six servings of different fruits and vegetables every day.

There is no such thing as junk food. All foods contribute to one's continuing need for nutrients, some better than others. The term came into being because some people insist on eating the same few foods over and over such that they were not getting a balanced diet. In an effort to discourage such eating, someone coined the "junk food" term and it caught on. However, there is absolutely nothing the matter with having a hamburger and french fries once in a while but not exclusively and constantly. Related to this is the emerging idea that restaurants have a responsibility to protect us from our ignorance about nutrition. I don't think we should count on that. It's too important to us. How about taking a course?

Consume at least a glass or two of milk a day. The reasons for this are presented throughout this book, but to put it simply, it is the best single food available from the standpoints of nutrition, refreshment, and convenience. When there isn't time or interest in preparing something and not time to sit down and eat a meal, a glass of milk is quick, and it makes a strong contribution to everyone's need for good quality food on a daily basis. Make it whole milk while you are at it. It tastes better and involves a very modest amount of fat that appears increasingly to have special benefits (see following, p. 117). Milk is an excellent insurance food for those times when you can't give your daily diet the care and attention it should have. Yes, tea, coffee, and soda are refreshing drinks, too, but they are not food. Yes, you can count the milk you put on your cereal but that's not enough.

Take a daily vitamin/mineral supplement (pill). For many years and even recently, one could hear, "If you eat a balanced diet, you don't need to take vitamin pills." There are a number of reasons why that is questionable advice. How many of us are carefully plotting each day to see that what we eat sums up to a balanced diet? Mom, who was something of a homegrown authority on such matters, is no longer spending much time preparing meals. Of course, there are exceptions, and I don't mean to insult the many women who continue to get family meals. But more and more, it is getting to be everyone is on his own about food. Another factor is the drive toward overweight avoidance. As a modern icon, the slim (well-nourished?) woman has been with us for some time. Now, however, 60 percent of us have been declared overweight. So the challenge is to eat less but still keep the diet balanced. Do we all have time to make a project out of that or would it be simpler to just take a multi-vitamin/mineral tablet to handle an important part of it? Another concern is our uniqueness as individuals. For various reasons such as genetics, life style, failing functions due to age, ravages of disease, etc., my actual requirements and balanced diet may not be quite like yours. Taking the daily tablet along with what we manage to design as a balanced diet is a simple insurance measure. However, vitamin/mineral supplements are not a substitute for good foods. In addition, the one-a-day pill is definitely not in the category where "one is good and more is better." Unhealthy overdoses of essential micronutrients can occur. For some people under certain conditions, this appears to be at a level not much above the recommended daily allowance.

Obtaining adequate vitamin D is somewhat challenging. Outside of milk, which is fortified with the vitamin at a level of 400 IU per quart, there are no good food sources. Regular exposure of the skin to sunlight is a suitable and very effective way to produce vitamin D in ones body, but the amount of sunlight varies seasonally and geographically. One also has to be concerned about skin cancer on overexposure to the sun. Again, a multi-vitamin supplement is good insurance.

The one-a-day supplement is really quite a technical achievement. Table 4.1 presents nutrition information of the type seen on labels for such supplements. The purpose of the table is to show that there are rather precise human requirements for a substantial number of micronutrients. One might wonder why the manufacturer sometimes includes less than the recommended DV in a tablet. This may be for reasons of cost, pill size or compatibility of ingredients. For example, calcium is not expensive but getting 100 percent of its DV, that is, 1,000 mg., into a tablet would make it too big for most people to swallow.

Table 4.1
Typical Nutrition Information for a Once-Daily-Type Tablet
Containing Vitamins and Minerals

Vitamins			Minerals		
Nutrient	*Amount*	*percent DV[1]*	*Nutrient*	*Amount*	*percent DV[1]*
Vitamin A	5000 I.U.	100	Calcium	200 mg	20
Vitamin C	60 mg	100	Phosphorus	48 mg	4
Vitamin D	400 I.U.	100	Iodine	150 mcg	100
Vitamin E	30 I.U.	100	Magnesium	100 mg	25
Vitamin K	10 mcg	12	Zinc	15 mg	100
Thiamin (B_1)	1.5 mg	100	Selenium	20 mcg	28
Riboflavin (B_2)	1.7 mg	100	Copper	2 mg	100
Niacin	20 mg	100	Manganese	2 mg	100
Vitamin B_6	2 mg	100	Chromium	120 mcg	100
Folic acid	400 mcg	100	Molybdenum	75 mcg	100
Vitamin B_{12}	6 mcg	100			
Biotin	30 mcg	10			
Pantothenic Acid	10 mg	100			

[1] percentDV (Daily Value) refers to the proportion of the daily requirement for an average adult supplied by the amount of the nutrient in one tablet.
Abbreviations: I U - international unit, mg - milligram, mcg - microgram

Sometimes more than 100 percent of the DV may be incorporated because recent research has suggested current recommendations are on the low side. Obviously, it is not a matter of life or death that every day we achieve those exact intakes shown in table 4.1. Some essential micronutrients, such as vitamin B_{12} can be stored in the body. Moreover, people can fast for days and apparently fully recover. However, for feeling good and energetically productive every day, the human health ideal is regular intake of the required kinds and amounts of nutrients.

Get some exercise. Yes, that's not food or diet, but it is inextricably involved in getting the good out of food and preserving ones health and sense of well-being. It has to be included. An inactive (hibernating) animal has no need for food. Many of us are close to hibernating these days. We are either sitting or lying nearly twenty-four hours per day. No wonder the pipes get clogged, the joints creak, we can't handle our food (diabetes), and turn into blobs. Humans were not meant to live like that. Healthy bodies and bones need movement and weight-bearing exercise. Performed regularly, such activities are an important aid to weight management.

A recent study[1] has confirmed substantial decline in physical activity during adolescence of both black and white girls. This drop was estimated to be as much as 50 percent in earlier studies. At that crucial time a girl is building the body and forming the habits that will more or less define her for life. Exercise is an excellent inclusion in almost anyone's life style.

Speaking of hibernating, there are subtle forces at work. When one watches television, a form of mental hibernation not necessarily involving sleep may be going on. The brain normally utilizes about 20 percent of ones blood glucose—a rather remarkable figure. Considering that an average person weighs over 100 pounds, that means a mere three-pound mass is using an important fraction of ones total calories. Assuming that most television watching is not heavy brainwork, we may have yet another way to put on weight.

Health Advisories

If we pay regular attention to the news media, we receive health advisories just about every day. These fall into several categories. There are reports on epidemiological studies and smaller human trials regarding health factors. There is the more or less extensive review of a health consideration, such as, what is known about obesity and its prevention. There also are the regular recommendations and reminders from or by health professionals that we will be better off if we do thus and so. Reports on human studies concerning aging, longevity, beneficial, or detrimental effects of foods, new drugs, life style, etc. are usually of great interest because they involve fresh information. The news people are adept at attracting our attention to them and the results can be very compelling. We may be implicated in them and derive a take-home lesson. But how reliable are the results of such studies?

Epidemiological Studies

One of the fields of study which helps us to have a better understanding of our health is called epidemiology. Those who work in epidemiology collect data on incidence of diseases, numbers and causes of death, and investigate relationships between many factors and human well-being. Any group of people, at any stage of life, of either sex, anywhere in the world can be studied with respect to any factors in their lives. This is how we came to understand that high blood cholesterol levels are associated with heart disease *in some people*. So in that instance, thousands of people have had their blood cholesterol concentrations determined and it has been observed that those who contracted heart disease tended to have higher values than those who did not. The correlation was not perfect in that some people with high cholesterol levels did not get heart disease and some with low cholesterol did. But taken together with the fact that cholesterol was found to be a component of plaques constricting blood vessels in heart patients, the evidence was considered by medical authorities sufficient to render blood cholesterol level a risk factor in heart disease.

It can be appreciated that epidemiological studies can evaluate an almost infinite number of health factors using this kind of association analysis. Beyond the confounding complexity of the science involved in such studies, there can be subtle and not so subtle factors influencing how data are collected and the way the results are presented. Just dealing objectively with all the natural variables that a group of people presents is challenging. For example, there have been a number of studies indicating that wine drinking is beneficial to heart health—lower cholesterol, fewer attacks, and so on. Now this result is being questioned because a recent study finds that wine drinking also is associated with greater intelligence, wealth, and education, and people with those attributes tend to be healthier than the average whether they drink wine or not. Cardiologists still feel that drinking wine is good for the heart but it may take additional studies, in which such variables as the foregoing are controlled, to resolve the matter.

So the science itself can be a problem; but then, financial, political, and philosophical/religious considerations can further complicate the situation. Let us say we are going to test for some specific health effect of a food or drug on a group of people. It is not advisable to have anyone with a financial interest in the food or drug directly involved in design, execution or data interpretation of the study. Such individuals might have every intention of remaining neutral regarding possible outcomes, but they should be excluded because revelation of their possible vested interest could render the study results suspect. For example, could one have confidence in the results of an epidemiologic study of health in relation to meat eating under the direction of strict vegetarians? Even scientists who conduct epidemiological studies are not always completely above the battle. They need money to live on, to support their work and further their careers. Usually the easiest place to get money to carry on a study is from those who may benefit financially from it, depending on the outcome. So we must analyze and sift these matters as best we can, including seeking the advice of experts we trust.

Although for the most part epidemiologic studies yield very useful information, they can be a mixed blessing. They mainly generate data about associations (correlations), which are not necessarily causal, and they seldom establish cause-and-effect relationships. Thus, epidemiological studies can make factors—conditions, states, and actions—that tend to coexist with particular ailments easy targets of unjustified accusations. Such factors, are not necessarily the absolute causes of ailments with which they have been associated. Associations may be purely a result of sample selection or of an association with other coexistent factors. Or the factor in question may be a joint or secondary cause, or just an aggravator of the disorder. The aggravation of some cases of prostate cancer by dietary calcium (p. 138) is an example of the latter.

Often, shortly after a scientific study has generated findings of an association between a disease and anything else under investigation, researchers attempt to duplicate the study and/or to verify its findings. Quite often, such follow-up studies yield findings that are considerably different from, or even contrary to, the findings of the earlier study. Such a turn of events might not deter disreputable and/or intellectually lazy persons and organizations from citing the earlier findings deceptively. Following are some findings from recent epidemiological studies: (a) following a low-fat/high-fiber diet is unlikely to reduce one's risk of developing colon cancer, (b) estrogen hormone replacement therapy does not reduce the risk of having a heart attack, (c) dietary fat is not a factor in the incidence of breast cancer, and (d) ample consumption of fruits and vegetables does not contribute to preventing breast cancer. All those results, a-d, counter-findings from earlier studies. The fact that the a-d areas have produced opposing and controversial research findings is common knowledge in the health care field. The purpose here is not to involve the reader in the to-and-fro details of a-d research, but to caution against blind embrace of findings from any study, new or old.

Recently, ample intakes of bioflavonoids, pigments that are widespread in plants, have become popular. From epidemiological studies, it appears that ingestion of bioflavonoids contributes to preventing cancer and heart disease. But other epidemiologic findings suggest that there may be a correlation between generous ingestion of bioflavonoids and some forms of leukemia. Evidence from other studies suggests that isoflavones (e.g., from soy) may be a risk factor for breast cancer. These findings alone, however, do not warrant recommending that all humans forgo consumption of plant-type foods of any kind. Yet opponents of milk have been doing just that with wild cries such as "Milk causes cancer!" Components of plant foods include varied allergens, toxins, and carcinogens which are at concentrations that appear harmless to most people. So, as a matter of principle, moderation and variety in what one eats, are helpful in case particular foods carry unknown detrimental components for the individual. We are now asking that the food we eat carry us in good health to our eighties and nineties or better. Actually, we know very little about the lifelong effects of regularly ingesting particular fruits, vegetables and grains, or animal foods for that matter.

What are the Numbers?

As a teacher, the writer has a tendency to deal in ideas. Generally, students are accommodating of this approach, but sooner or later one of them may insist that the focus be on the numbers and critical details. For example, I might say, "Do you know that milk is an excellent source of vitamin B_2 (riboflavin)?" A probable come back might be, "Yes, and precisely how much, and as compared to what?" I should respond, "1.6 mg/qt which is the daily requirement for an average individual." My guess is that I would get hit at least once more, such as—"What is an average individual?" or "Why is there so much vitamin B_2 in milk?" The approach of these questioning students is precisely the way we should analyze health reports directed at us by the news media. Otherwise we are liable to be overcome by some emotion-laden headline when the real story is in the details or lack of them. For example, if eating a certain food doubles the risk of incurring a particular disease, it sounds pretty bad and we begin to think in terms of avoiding that food. But if the normal incidence of that disease is one person in 25,000, the food only increases the risk to two people in 25,000 - not very devastating. Another example showing how the numbers count, is the childhood vaccination program for a host of serious diseases. A few children are sickened by the vaccines, but millions are protected by them. Thus, the risk is readily accommodated.

A further aspect of the numbers problem and health is in relation to genetics. There is obviously something different about the 15 to 20 percent of people who experience a rise in their blood cholesterol when they ingest foods containing cholesterol. In all likelihood, the difference is due to genetic factors. In all of the serious diseases of humanity, such as cancer, heart disease, and diabetes, there are genes involved. We need to know how many people and what genes carrying how many and what mutations? It has been obvious for sometime that heart disease is very complex and involves protective as well as promotive genes. Cholesterol and saturated fat were declared risk factors in heart disease without anyone knowing to whom specifically the risk applied. Perhaps genetic diagnostics will eventually allow us to define how many different ways people are at risk of heart disease and precisely who is involved. Yes, we need to insist on the numbers and the details.

Health Topic Reviews

One of the more reliable and helpful ways the media have of communicating health information is by way of reviews. Such presentations attempt to focus and bring up-to-date the knowledge of diseases and health considerations of all kinds. They may be done simply as educational contributions or in connection with news releases from new studies on the subjects involved. In the latter case, it is very helpful to have the review so that one knows where and how the new information fits, or does not fit, with what is known. With such background, there is less chance we are going to be alarmed or misinformed by some new information out of context, which often is a favorite media maneuver to get ones attention. My own preference is for the written account because it allows one to study the material. As they say, the spoken word can be "in one ear and out the other." A further advantage of the written piece is that the original report of a study is usually cited. This does two things: it enables one to look up the original work and come to ones own conclusions about it; and it allows one to estimate the quality of the work based on the reputation of the publishing journal. For example, the *Proceedings of the National Academy of Sciences of the USA* (*PNAS*) is a highly prestigious journal. Manuscripts submitted for publication to its editors must first be reviewed to determine their acceptability. This so-called peer review is all done by leading scientists in the subject matter of the article. Without going into all the shades of acceptance or rejection, if authors are fortunate enough to receive acceptance of their manuscripts, it will almost always require some revising. So the mere fact that a paper is published by *PNAS* suggests science of good quality. This is not to say that there aren't many other excellent peer-reviewed science journals or that *PNAS* never errs in what it publishes; but journal reputation is a quality indicator of published science.

Newspapers that take the trouble to enlighten readers by means of such reviews perform a very valuable service. Just this morning I read an excellent article on what is known about cancer genes and how to go about being tested for them. Health is becoming more of a concern to many people, and such articles, while providing news, are also educating us. It is true that the science in them is a little demanding of us at times, but we must keep trying to grow in these realms. Learning is a life's work, especially in our current culture, the information age. Our doctors often don't have the time to explain these things to us, but if we understood health matters better, it might save their and our time as well as medical costs. It may also enable us to ask them truly intelligent questions.

The Health Reminder

Another important level of health information is the health reminder, which is telling one what to eat or do to stay well and live a long life. Obviously this kind of advice can't be any better than the people giving it and any relevant data from which they are working. But the main problem is that the suggestions have a tendency to be trendy. By that I mean they are based on the latest findings and are based on what other health professionals are saying and writing at the time. This is all fine as long as the supporting information is solidly established, but as we have explained above, the latest information may be erroneous, inadequate or debatable and the popularity of giving the particular advice truly unfortunate. For example, the market for eggs, an excellent food relatively rich in cholesterol was incredibly devastated by the dietary cholesterol scare. This fearful concept was not something borne forward by medical experts alone. It was spread in the news media for years and continuing discussions throughout the general public helped mightily in reinforcing the situation. Who has never spoken about cholesterol levels? There is convincing evidence[2] that in most people (80-85 percent) dietary cholesterol has little if any effect on blood cholesterol levels. It is not possible to put and accurate figure on the loss of business in the egg, dairy, and meat industries as a result of the cholesterol scare but it must be huge. This has also involved the loss of the high quality protein of eggs, milk, and meat in the diets of those driven to avoid cholesterol.

Another health dictum that has recently come under question is breast self-examination. For years, women have been urged to do it regularly. A large trial[3] was conducted in China to determine whether many thousands of women who were intensively instructed in breast self-examination would be better off with regard to breast cancer mortality than a control group who did not practice self-examination. The results revealed no significant difference between the two groups. It would seem like the earlier one detected an abnormality in breast structure the better. However, a rather disturbing implication from the study is that by the time one can feel a lump, it may have been growing and spreading throughout the body for eight or ten years—too late. This issue and whether to get a mammogram are under review at the moment. That status reminds us that health advisories may be subject to revision.

* * *

In conclusion, it is worth knowing something about nutrition because it will be information one can use to foster his/her lifelong health. Caution should be used in the application of new health information as it may apply to ones diet. There are indeed irrefutable facts born forward from centuries and even millennia of human experience, and from repeatedly confirmed findings of scientific investigations. The rest may be subject to revisions of varying degrees at any time. In considering the following section on antagonism to milk and the following chapter on healthfulness of milk, think about the quality and reliability of the relevant information.

2. Critics and Criticisms of Milk and Dairy

Critics

Despite the fact that Western civilization has benefited from the use of cow's milk as human food for thousands of years, provocative outcries about milk being bad and even poisonous are carried increasingly in the news media. Basically this strange phenomenon has complex roots in the current culture of America. Hungry or starving people do not complain about food that is palatable and nutritious. Actually much of the negativism is not because of concern about milk's healthfulness; it has a lot to do with advancement of activist causes, particularly getting attention, creating converts, and obtaining financial support for those causes. The reason why milk makes such a fine scapegoat is because it has had such a wonderful image and everyone knows about it. Before discussing the specifics of attacks on milk, we need to consider the circumstances under which they are arising and the role of epidemiological studies in evaluating the nutritional benefits and limitations of milk.

Our Current Culture

A nineteen-year-old granddaughter was expressing to me her satisfaction about my writing this book. She had been reading some segments of it in the rough-draft stage. She said, "I tell my girlfriends they should drink milk, and they say they have heard that milk isn't so good for you." In a nutshell, there is one major aspect of the problem. Milk, which has more essential nutrients than any other food and is arguably the best single food we have, has an image in the minds of teenage girls as "not so good for you." These girls are at a time in life when their bone formation is at a critical stage that will be determining bone strength for the rest of their lives, and they are under the impression that milk, the best dietary source of calcium for bone building and many other benefits "is not so good for you." How does such misinformation get so widely spread? Consider the following forces at work in our culture.

Freedom of speech. In the ideal, such freedom is wonderful. Unfortunately, it can also help people to evade responsibility for the truth, and in unethical hands, it's a problem. Which leads us to...

The news media. They desire to attract attention in order to develop and maintain demand for their programs and publications. How do they do this? One way is by fostering worry and controversy. Why dispassionately present rather colorless facts when you can stimulate great concern with conflict, scary hints, rumors, and half-truths?

The information explosion. This in turn aids the news media. Among other news, there is a continuous outpouring of new scientific findings, which can be quickly sent all over the world in seconds. Often results and opinions are conflicting; people are baffled, confused, and don't know what to think. This can also be called the misinformation explosion. One wonders who is checking for the truth.

Widespread prosperity. America has well over half of the world's wealth. Many Americans are no longer thankful to have the basics and essentials. They want new, more, and better everything. They are also quite concerned about their health, how they look and how long they will live. They provide a marvelous audience for the media who keep them worried and wanting.

Activism. Continuing prosperity, peace and freedoms in the U. S. have given its people a strong sense of security and independence. They feel free to speak their minds and to aggressively support or oppose causes and to become activists. With the news media stirring things up, Americans have developed powerful antagonisms and partisanships. Unfortunately, sometimes activists' singleness of purpose, doesn't let facts or reason stand in the way of the cause; and what they believe in can take on the character of a religious fanaticism.

One would not think that anything as bland and beneficial as milk would get swept up in the foregoing vigorous forces promoting controversy, but it has. Over the past couple of decades, there have been a growing number of articles that clearly infer, if they don't boldly state, milk causes cancer, milk causes heart disease, milk is poison. No wonder my granddaughter's friends have heard "milk is not so good for you." First let's consider the origins of this misinformation and then look at some relevant facts in the matter.

To understand the current antagonisms toward milk, it is helpful to identify major sources of them. There are at least four groups involved in the anti-dairy activities: the animal rights activists, some vegetarians, some environmentalists, and some adversaries of corporate/industrial America. None of these people are all that concerned directly with the healthfulness of milk. They simply see any negative evidence about milk as a means of furthering their more immediate goals, particularly those of getting attention and support for their causes and eliminating the dairy industry. It is clear that sympathizers and activist members of these groups are wide spread and can also be found among news media personnel and health science professionals. Thus, it is little wonder that objective evidence about the healthfulness of milk is hard to find and some people are worried about drinking it. However, most are not fooled; they know it is an excellent food even though a few have problems with it.

The Animal Rights (AR) Movement

Among the various coordinated efforts to discredit milk, that of the animal rights activists is the largest and most aggressive. This group is well organized and heavily funded. Its concerns about the way animals are treated have focused on destroying the good image of milk. It is not really that milk, as such, is bad, it is just a means to an end for them. Their strategy is to attack the dairy industry, which they claim mistreat animals, by doing everything they can to discourage the use of milk and the cow to meet human food needs. If milk can be sufficiently damaged in the eyes of the public, sales of milk and milk products will fall and the dairy industry will collapse, or so they hope. Such failure would reduce, if not eliminate the imputed mistreatment of cows. For the same reason, these people are dedicated to bringing about the failure of the meat industry. These activists are strict vegetarians, also known as vegans.

In order to better understand motivation of the animal rights movement, really it is a religion, one must grasp key elements of that faith. One assumption is that animals are just as important and deserving of respect as humans. In fact, careful analysis reveals that animals are more important to them than are humans. In essence, it is a form of animal worship. Another tenet is that animals were not created for mankind's use. This exalted view of animals and debased conception of humanity implies that Western culture was in grave error from its beginning. Animals should never have been domesticated and all self-considered uses of animals in contemporary culture are tantamount to sin. This includes use for food (meat, milk, fish, eggs, and all products containing them or made from them), clothing (wool, fur, leather, etc.), transportation (plowing, pulling, and hauling humans and other burdens), entertainment (zoos, marine worlds, race tracks, hunting of all kinds, horseback riding, cock fighting), security (use of animals to guard, protect, track, hunt, and see, as in seeing-eye, experimentation) and research (all use of animals in science to further mankind's health, knowledge and well-being). Even the use of animals as pets falls under "degrading treatment of animals," but the leadership treads lightly there because pet owners are a primary source of financial contributions to the cause. The little old lady who loves her pussycat or doggie is an easy mark for the animal rights fundraisers. However, if one is going to be consistent about the concept that man should exercise no mastery over the animals, the pets have to go, too. There are also lots of other little consequences. For example, all tennis should be forbidden until something is found to replace (animal) gut for stringing rackets. Raising bees and appropriating their honey is not nice. It may be an extreme, but it is logical,—silk also is out! Those worms should be left alone to go their natural way! Maybe logic isn't a requirement of the animal rights religion but passion seems to be. As most people know, extremists (terrorists?) of the faith have burned up medical research laboratories, destroyed records, and threatened research professionals. The movement tries to disown such terrorism but not very strenuously.

AR—Physicians and Animals

A misleading feature of the animal rights religion is its concerted emphasis on the presence of some medical doctors within the membership. The main purpose of this is to confer respectability and authority on proclamations and news releases issuing from the organization. One might think from this that there is great concern for health and well-being of the public. Virtually all human medical and health advancements have relied on use of experimental animals whether it was the discovery of the vitamins, development of vaccines, or the devising of new surgical procedures. The animal rights movement is dead set against use of animals for such purposes. By involving some MDs, the real objective is to create a respectable, authoritative image for the animal rights movement; but it was not to benefit public health, nor does their efforts to discredit milk have anything to do with human welfare. Simply stated, the objective is to control and restrict people's use of animals.

AR—Drawing the Line. Where?

In all this concern for animal rights, is the whole membership of the animal kingdom of equal concern? That kingdom extends from one-celled organisms, known as protozoa, all the way up to mammals, which include not only humans but whales and elephants. The worms bugs, lizards, and snakes are in the kingdom, too. Do rights concerns embrace them all? Can one swat flies, kill lice, and spray for mosquitoes? Can one get rid of termites and intestinal parasites? What about infestations with rats and mice? Can one hire a couple of killer cats to get things under control?

AR—The billboard campaigns. In response to the highly successful GOT MILK? advertising campaign of the dairy industry, the animal rights people have been using billboards in an effort to advance their cause. One display urged us to drink beer instead of milk. This annoyed parents in general and Mothers Against Drunk Driving (MADD) in particular. The implication that beer is a substitute for milk, nutritionally or otherwise, is, of course, not true. Another of this group's billboard displays carried a picture of Jesus Christ with the declaration, He was a vegetarian - also preposterous. Christ was an orthodox Jew who annually ate the Passover meal, of which lamb was an indispensable component. He also facilitated enormous catches of fish (Luke 5:1-11) and miraculously multiplied the loaves and the fishes (Luke 9:11-17). These activities hardly fit the definition of a vegetarian. Further, regarding the Bible, God informed Moses that a place he described as "flowing with milk and honey" had been set aside for His people and that he, Moses, was to lead them there from their enslavement in Egypt (Exodus 3:7). Obviously, the implication is that a place that has plenty of milk and honey, two animal food products, is a choice place to be. In addition, God gave humankind power over the animal kingdom (Genesis 1:26). The Bible does not seem to be a very good place to find defenses of absolute vegetarianism (veganism). The people in those times had to work too hard obtaining something to eat to be squeamish about what it was. A major fraction of ancient people in the Middle East spent their lives tending animals.

In fact, strict vegetarianism has emerged in relatively recent times and there are few, if any, controlled studies of its health value either short term or on a lifelong basis. One study[4] in the United Kingdom involving 4,898 meat eaters and 5,904 vegetarians evaluated effects of dietary components on mortality. Vegans, that is, those consuming no animal product of any kind including milk, comprised 77 percent of the vegetarians. The results revealed that those drinking the most milk, as compared to those drinking little or no milk, had a reduced death rate ratio for deaths due to all causes. The implication of this finding is that vegetarians can benefit from drinking milk. However, additional studies of vegetarianism, especially the vegan version, as a factor in human health and longevity are needed.

In addition to misusing Christ as an example, animal rights advocates produced two other questionable displays aimed at policing people's diets. A semi-nude model was employed in one and a touched-up picture of a celebrity without his permission in the other. In response, see the billboard, figure 4.1.

Activists for animal rights like to point out that certain populations have been vegetarian since ancient times, such as the soybean-eating peoples of rural China. This is somewhat true because there wasn't a lot else for them to eat. However, the Chinese have not been above eating dogs and farming fish

Figure 4.1

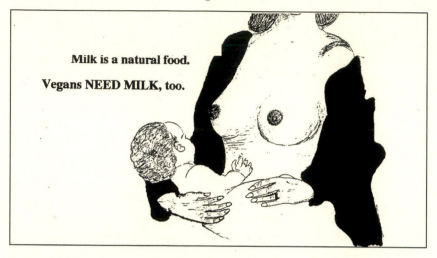

Milk is a natural food.

Vegans NEED MILK, too.

Proposed billboard to promote milk to vegans (strict vegetarians). Milk is the food designed by nature to develop and sustain life. Billboards which attempt to discredit milk don't make sense and are a waste of time and money.

when they could manage it. The whole ancient China-soybean nutrition argument seems scientifically weak. These people did survive, but there is evidence that they were small, undernourished, and short lived by today's standards. They hardly represent a solid data-supported example of what people should be eating to develop and maintain strong bodies and long healthy lives. The irony of it is that milk drinking is becoming popular with the Chinese. They feel milk will make them healthier. Milk production in China has increased over tenfold since 1980 and the market for milk and milk products is growing rapidly.[5]

Eating some fruits, vegetables and grain-based foods *as part of* ones diet is a widely accepted, nutritionally sound practice. But the billboard campaign of animal rights advocates to discredit animal food products seems to be a misguided attention-getting effort. Activist agendas such as that do not provide any basis for establishing what foods (diets) are good for one, nor are they in the best interests of the public's health.

AR—Mediation?

Regarding the ethical treatment of cows, the writer has had considerable contact with dairy operations over a long period of years without ever seeing any intentionally cruel treatment of the animals. At times cows are dealt with firmly to control their movements. That is because half-ton animals out of control are very dangerous. Yes, at some, but not all, dairy farms, cows are contained in relatively small outdoor areas, but it should be remembered that they don't normally mind being close to each other. They tend to herd together naturally even in a spacious pasture. The relatively smaller outdoor enclosures now being used *in some but not all areas* are adequate to provide the cows with fresh air and exercise. In any event, there is no sense in mistreating cows since in all likelihood it would marginalize their milk production as well as create veterinary expenses.

One wonders if there is any acceptable grounds for mediation with the animal rights activists? Let's say I have a nice old pet bossy cow that I milk for the benefit of my family and me. And we treat old Bossy very lovingly. When old Bossy dies, we give her a decent burial and say prayers that her "soul" rests in peace, joy, and mercy in bovine heaven. Would that be tolerable and would the milk from good old Bossy be ok to drink? Working back from that situation, would it be possible to apply those principles to herds of cows and have their milk be acceptable? Probably not. Mediation with animal rights activists does not look promising. If the differences could be settled, it might be a fatal blow to their movement. At least some animal rights activists view human manipulation of cows to give milk as demeaning of the cow and that is unacceptable because the cow has no choice. These people have no trouble seeing equivalency between animals and humans—except that you don't hear much from them about the massive mistreatment of humans by each other throughout the world. Yes, there is complaint about feeding grain to animals because of human starvation in various areas of the world, but that is really not out of concern for humanity, it is primarily a putdown of the meat and dairy industries. For more on that subject, see chapter 6. Speaking of humans, one wonders if human milk is an objectionable animal product (figure 4.1)?

In addition to capitalizing on any negative research findings about the healthfulness of milk, animal rights activists, a few of whom are researchers, conduct investigations on milk themselves. Surprise! The results of those studies are never favorable to milk. It is interesting that just within the past year, leading scientific journals are requiring authors of manuscripts submitted for publication to bare their souls as to where their financial support originates and what companies and organizations they are affiliated with that might have a vested interest in the results being presented. This certainly is a step in the right direction. University scientists wear many hats these days. In addition to their main lines of teaching and research for the university, they are also industrial and government consultants as well as captains of start-up and larger companies. Even university administrations are increasingly involved in financial ventures through collaborations with corporations and licensing of university owned patents. Scientific investigations become a farce when the results are slanted, hand picked or falsified to suit special interests. The *full* truth is what counts and investigators need to be as free of bias as possible.

One problem with respect to research on the healthfulness of milk and other animal products is that people sympathetic to the animal rights cause are growing in numbers and are permeating U.S. society. As discussed following, there is actually a coalition of causes involved. Consequently, the quality of research in this area needs to be scrutinized closely, which is one of the objectives of this book.

Vegetarianism

Motivation for vegetarianism, that is, the partial or complete exclusion of animals or animal products from the diet, derives from various origins. Many religions specify avoidance of selected items or groups of foods. Hindus of Asia reject meat in the diet. Orthodox Jews, while not vegetarians, have dietary laws excluding pork in any form from their diet. Some more modern vegetarians are repelled by the idea of killing animals for food. There is a bumper sticker that states: "Vegetarian: Indian word for 'lousy hunter.'" This reminds us that as food has become so tremendously abundant in the U.S., and very few of us have to hunt for it or produce it, we can be choosy about which foods we will accept and eat. Some vegetarians claim they do not like the taste of meat. Others are influenced by continuing reports that meat and other animal products may not be good for one. Actually, the vegetarians are not alone in being picky about their food. *All* foods are subject to criticisms.

There are variations as to which animal products vegetarians reject. While meat, including poultry, is the main defining item, many will accept eggs, fish, and dairy products. Some consume only one or two of the latter; and another large group, the truly devout, known as strict vegetarians, or vegans, exclude all animal material. I presume even honey would be forbidden by their standards. While anyone should be free to select and eat whatever he/she wants, coercing people with misinformation and propaganda to shun selected foods is unethical in the writer's opinion. Using this approach, animal rights activists have converted some otherwise tolerant vegetarians to their aggressive tactics. The fact that vegetarianism is growing in the U.S. is illustrated by the following common experience. In my parents' home and later in my own, we often had company for dinner. Both my mother and my wife have loved to entertain. The people would come, eat, and enjoy what we had to offer, and express thanks when they left. They were joyful situations. Now it is not possible to have a dinner party without first holding a planning seminar. So-and-so doesn't eat this and what's-his-name is a vegetarian, well, what kind of vegetarian?—and Whoozie has allergies. On some recent occasions, we have had guests from out of town tell us at the last minute that they are vegetarians—great news, after one has spent all day shopping and getting their dinner together. Ultimately, people may have to have dinner parties at cafeterias where each person can sight-inspect, pick, and choose every dinner item. Regarding allergies, medical authorities claim they are mostly imaginary and that true food allergies are quite rare. What's happening to us?

Getting back to the billboard proclaiming that Christ was a vegetarian, there now is a movement attempting to convince Jews that they should be and were meant to be vegetarians. This misguided idea is totally out of keeping with the Old Testament. Starting with the book of Genesis and throughout, it mentions the people's ownership of flocks and herds of animals. These obviously were used for food and clothing. The law for the Passover, that great annual Jewish commemoration, specifies the eating of meat and exactly how it should be prepared eaten and disposed of:

> The Lord said to Moses and Aaron in the land of Egypt regarding the whole
> Israelite congregation.....They shall eat the lamb that same night; they shall eat it
> roasted over the fire with unleavened bread and bitter herbs.... (Exodus 12:9)

Clearly, vegetarianism is a contemporary choice, but why base it on distorted versions of religious history and tradition.

Environmentalism

Another group that is providing reinforcement to the animal rights activists are the environmentalists who see domestic livestock as a blight on the land, not as contented animals enjoying a pasture and eating grass which is hardly human food. They claim many things: cattle make poor use of the land which should be used to grow food for the poor (grain or soybeans, I presume, since they are probably vegetarians), feeding grain to animals is wasteful, livestock cause erosion of the land which ruins it, livestock stinks, and milk and meat aren't good for people anyway. So there they are, right in bed with the animal worshipers and the vegetarians. We attempt to analyze these contentions of the environmentalists in chapter 6. Our purpose here is to show there is quite a coalition of activists that are using every means at their disposal to discredit milk as a food. The following sections contain examples further illustrating how these forces are influencing our food consumption.

"Dairy Free"?

The dairy and chocolate industries have common interests and are very important to each other. They use huge quantities of each other's products. There are vast amounts of milk chocolate, chocolate milk, and chocolate ice cream sold and greatly enjoyed, but in these times, unusual forces are operating. Is there "dairy free" chocolate? This story is worth telling because it interweaves cross-currents that are influencing people about their food. There was a time when it was enough if a food was nutritious, tasty and reasonably priced. No longer.

Members of the writer's family came back from a local tourist attraction bearing chocolate bars the wrappers of which carried in prominent bold letters, "DAIRY FREE." Why be stressing "dairy free"? The same company manufacturing the dairy free bar also was offering one containing milk ingredients. It is well known that there are two kinds of chocolate, milk and dark, and that dark does not contain milk. With some foods, distinctions are made, such as, "fat free" or "caffeine free" in order to help people who have specific nutritional needs. However, "dairy free" is not in reference to a single component; it means a whole class of foods based on milk. It is something like saying "meat-" or "vegetable free." It certainly can be interpreted as a thinly veiled hint that milk and milk products are not viewed as good to eat, at least by some people, and that "dairy free" will help sell to a certain segment of the market.

"Cage Free Browns"

While the following short excursion into the world of eggs is not dairy, it is related to the preceding "dairy free" story. It provides another example of how activist agendas are shaping the contemporary markets for foods. Before we consider the production of eggs by cage-free hens, we need to think about what motivates one who is in business. Company leaders of necessity have a strong focus on making money. Not only is that essential to staying in business, it is unavoidable if one is to benefit the hundreds if not thousands of people either directly or indirectly involved with a company. So the motivation is not just greed, as some would have us believe, it also involves a sense of responsibility and a desire to survive in the competitive environment in which virtually all U.S. businesses must operate. Within that framework, business leaders can change things to suit the agendas of others but not without keeping an eye on costs and profitability.

Cage-free brown eggs are an example of this willingness to be flexible and of the enterprising abilities of the businessperson. As a matter of production efficiency, laying hens are normally kept in small cage facilities that supply feed, gather eggs, and collect droppings all by automation. Animal protectionists have complained about this highly confined, unnatural lifestyle for the chicken. To meet this criticism, the cage-free environment with nest was devised. On the carton it states that birds producing these eggs do so in nests and that they are grain-fed and never caged. However, it is notable that supporting a nicer life style for the hen makes these eggs $0.30 to $0.50 more a dozen. Presumably, such terms and production systems as "cage free" and "free range," employed by the poultry industry, make for a better public image and justify the higher costs.

Antagonism to Corporations

There seems to be rising dissatisfaction among the public with corporations despite the fact that they are the most effective means the world has devised for producing goods and services. It is the main reason that standards of living have risen both in the U.S. and many other countries. If, as most of us pray, the poor of the world are to be better fed, clothed, and housed, private corporations seem to be the best hope. Unfortunately, corporate enterprise has carried abundance via the American life style to the point where people are not simply happy with their nice comfortable existences. Some now have the time, the freedom, and the desire to bite the hand that feeds them; and abroad, we are viewed with envy because of all that we have. This is not necessarily bad. One can hope that criticism might make a good thing even better. However, reckless persistence in a misinformed cause can ruin a good thing. Actually, there are many thousands of corporations in America and they vary in size, effectiveness and goals. Usually, it is large corporations that are the basis of complaints which include dissatisfaction with their imputed greed, power, and degradations of the environment. There is no question that the wealth and power of some large corporations is absolutely awesome. Financing of politicians, lobbyists, and scientists to smooth the way for their products and activities is standard operation. For certain, we need to keep a watchful eye on them; but efforts to trash whole industries does not seem like a very constructive activity.

The economics of corporate profitability makes for both greed and efficiency. Although business motivation usually gets down to money, it is not always easy to read. One might think the dairy industry suffered from all the negative publicity about dietary fat. Indeed they did; medical speculations and misinformation in that area have strongly influenced the public against milk fat. But the industry recognized possibilities in their manufacturing and marketing flexibility. They have brought out graded fat levels of milk and milk products that permit customers to choose what they want. So, for example, one can buy "fat-free," "low fat (usually 1 percent)," 2 percent, and whole milk, which is at least 3.25 percent fat. Before World War II, skim milk was in such limited demand most of it was fed to animals or run down the drain. So the industry has gone from selling whole milk to three additional versions of varied fat content. My guess is that this has not hurt sales. Somehow, I doubt that there is too much worry among dairymen about the fat issue, especially as research continues to reveal unique health values of milk fat.

Another example of business motivation not being quite what it seems arose recently regarding development of a diabetic ice cream. The main problem in diabetes is elevated blood glucose which can lead to all kinds of health complications. Since regular ice cream contains about 15 percent sucrose and 6 or 7 percent lactose, both of which generate blood glucose on digestion, it is not an ideal food for diabetics. An ice cream with less blood glucose potential but the same excellent palatability should have a market among the growing millions of diabetics. It was pointed out by some dairy specialists that the introduction of a new form of ice cream conveys the implication that there is something the matter or limiting about the old (regular) ice cream and thus would conceivably hurt its sales. True, but that's progress. The likelihood is that the new ice cream will bring new customers into the market, and that in the end, more ice cream than ever will be sold. Right now what the United States public needs are foods, which when consumed in reasonable amounts, will not cause weight gain or type 2 diabetes. A good, widely available diabetic ice cream could help.

We should focus at least briefly on the dairy industry as a public benefactor. The purpose is not to overwhelm the reader with statistics about economics and far reaching benefits to the public from the corporate dairy world; but as an example, here are some facts about the industry in Pennsylvania, the fourth largest state in the production of milk. It has 9,700 dairy farms of ten or more cows producing close to 11 billion pounds of milk a year with a value at the farm of $1,716,167,000. There are 616,000 cows and they average sixty-four per herd. Over 17,000 people are employed on Pennsylvania dairy farms.[6] While farm production of milk is only one part of the industry, clearly it is no single corporate monster. Over the country as a whole, it involves thousands of individual farms and millions of cows and people.

Please bear in mind that the dairy industry, as well as the meat and poultry industries, is one of the most heavily monitored segments of the U.S. economy. It is controlled by thousands of laws and regulations at many levels of government, local, state and federal. These restrictions are applied all the way from milk production on the farm, to what the farmer will be paid for the milk, to its processing in the plant and its sale in the supermarket. This is not some operation run by a bunch of robber barons. Your interests are under consideration every step of the way. The surveillance may not be perfect but mostly, it is very good.

We have a tremendous amount at stake in the success of corporate enterprises that make up the dairy industry. It is not just a matter of some critical decision-making executives who are being highly paid to run the companies. There are also millions of other people for whom the dairy industry provides jobs; other millions who own stock in the companies, dairy plants, and farms; and other businesses who sell equipment, supplies, and trucks to the dairy industry, yet other business who sell milk and milk products. Finally, there are millions of consumers in the U.S. and abroad who benefit from the diverse high quality foods made available by that industry. When politicians rail against corporations, I wonder if any man-in-the-street-type voters realize how closely the interests of all of us are identified with corporate success. If the corporate culture fails, our consumer products, our jobs, our investments and our life of abundance will suffer as will our hopes for the underprivileged of the world. Anyone can understand negotiating for improvements in the way the dairy industry operates, but efforts to sabotage it and all those who depend on it and benefit from it are hardly constructive activities.

Criticisms of Milk

Individuals who object to milk have a variety of explanations for their objections. An unquestionably valid one is, "I just don't like the taste of it."

Actually good fresh milk should not have any strong flavor. Nonetheless, some detect flavor compounds they don't like. Another version is, "I don't like the way it feels in my mouth." Still another is, "It leaves a bad aftertaste." These are things that some proportion of the population may say about any food. Such responses simply demonstrate the existence of individual differences. The flavor of milk and how to improve or modify it are discussed in chapter 8. Another commonly heard complaint about milk is that, "it doesn't agree with me." When this is a consistent well-established pattern with the individual, it is likely due to either lactose intolerance or allergy.

There is a class of objections to milk that are efforts to exclude it, such as, "milk is for kids," "drinking milk is unnatural," and "milk is for calves." There is also the subtle criticism of milk by simply not serving it or making it available—a sin of omission. It is as though milk has become socially or culturally unsuitable under the conditions. In the food service industry, this may lead to inadequate sales, so managers ask, "Why carry it?" Finally, there are the mostly devious allusions that milk will make you sick in any one of a variety of ways. Consideration of these various criticisms follows.

Milk is for Kids; Milk is for Calves; Drinking Milk is Unnatural...

Some of the complaints about milk are so contrived, one wonders if the expressed objection is what the person really had in mind. For example, even a superficial knowledge of nutrition would suggest that if milk is good nourishment for a child, it certainly wouldn't hurt adults. One wonders if such people were not hounded a little too much to, "Drink your milk!" when they were young. The substantial value of milk for adults is discussed at length in the next chapter.

The idea that drinking milk is unnatural hasn't much substance either. Considering the extreme spectrum of foods consumed by humans throughout the world, the meaning of natural may be somewhat uncertain, but milk, more than any other plant or animal matter, is food by natural design. That is the purpose for which the mammal mother makes it. In our own self-interest, we do all kinds of unnatural things—drive cars, fly planes, operate computers, etc. We've learned to do a lot of things that are not natural to us but have become so because they are beneficial. Could cow's milk benefit humans as well as calves? Obviously, it does. The essential nutrients that make a calf thrive are the same ones that we need. In fact, many of our nutritional requirements were defined by research on farm animals. Are we in danger that by drinking cow's milk we will develop horns and weigh half a ton inside two years? Pretty unlikely. Viewing the human as just another animal doesn't work. We have achieved a level of intelligence that empowers us for better or worse to manage nature. A rather perverse example is the breastfeeding of baby pigs by women in New Guinea. That is not exactly natural, although cross species nursing is well known. But under the circumstances in which these women live, the nursing is well worth doing. A piglet is a prized possession because when mature, it will provide a lot of food or more pigs, and human milk provides good insurance that it will get there.

The Sin of Omission

A subtle criticism of milk is to just simply omit it from dietary recommendations and serving occasions. Some nutritionist/dieticians are and have been in a frenzy recommending fruits, vegetables, and grains to the virtual exclusion of any other foods. This simply could be driven by fear that any other foods will lead to obesity and poor health, or by vegetarianism, maybe both. In any event, there is *no* sound basis for the general exclusion of milk and milk products from the human diet. On the contrary, it could be quite detrimental to omit them. And milk does *not* normally cause obesity, see p. 123. Another sin of omission, one often cannot get milk in any form on the airlines or in restaurants. There seem to be two excuses: one is simply that "we don't have it," and the other is that "we must save what we have for children." Both of these explanations are versions of the milk-is-for-kids thinking. It is quite clear that at many adult functions such thinking has won out. Milk just isn't served.

No doubt there are also psychic factors that dictate the exclusion of milk. In most occasions where alcohol or soft drinks are served, milk is ordinarily not found. Soda is 'in' under many circumstances with teenagers; and because of peer pressure, one can readily understand that to ask for milk when everyone else is having soda could be awkward. Soda comes in two forms, diet or sweetened with sugar. The diet form, which is artificially sweetened, contributes no nutrition and is simply a nice tasting drink of carbonated water. The sugar-sweetened version does provide calories in the form of the sugar and has become something of a concern regarding the nation's growing overweight problem. According to the USDA, most kids, 74 percent of boys and 65 percent of girls, drink at least one soda a day. In some of these situations, parents are co-conspirators because they bring the soda home from the grocery store. Another source of soda for kids is their schools. Obviously, there is nothing the matter with anyone drinking an occasional soda. If it is consumed to a degree that it interferes with a person's receiving a balanced diet, then it is unfortunate.

We like to think that the public school lunch programs in the U. S. are a wonderful institution. You know, the idea that the kid is getting at least one good meal a day, and that such good things as surplus milk, cheese, and butter are donated to these programs. Come to find out, nutritionists in California have felt that the school lunch programs are so bad that they have sought corrective legislation. The main problem is that the schools are in very profitable arrangements with the soda and snack food suppliers and they feared that changes would take away millions of dollars and possibly bankrupt school cafeterias. Associations of school administrators and cafeteria employees lobbied heavily against the legislation which was finally passed in watered down form and signed by the governor. In essence, it imposes some standards in elementary schools, bans the sale of soda until after lunch in middle schools and changes nothing in high schools. So the soda and snack foods culture in California schools appears to be here to stay because kids like it and the schools and cafeterias need the money. That's another way to make it easy to omit healthy foods, such as milk, during the formative years of life.

Some of the guilt for sins of omission about milk may rest with the dairy industry. Despite the tremendous public service it renders and the effectiveness of such advertising as the "Got Milk?" campaign, there is not much response from the dairy industry to the growing inroads of its antagonists and competitors. Yes, responding to criticism can be a way of legitimizing it. But in the meantime some medical authorities dispense speculative and misguided information about milk, fanatics claim that milk causes all kinds of disease, and the public schools push the sale of soda. Those hardly seem like conditions under which the dairy industry can rest on its laurels. While the industry does support research and educational programs, and it does have lobbies to defend it, those efforts seem to be more than matched by the aggressive barrage being leveled against milk in the communications media.

Milk Substitutes

In the sense that milk is a beverage consumed to refresh, quench thirst, and provide a break; there are many substitutes for it. In fact this is a very active area of research and development with steady release of new "health" drinks and addition of milk and new flavors to older beverage concepts. However, under the generic name, soy milk, we have a long standing attempt to closely imitate milk in appearance, flavor and nutritive value. There are now quite a number of soy milks under various trade names on the market. The dairy industry seems pretty relaxed about this category of product and that it probably isn't going anywhere. In a way, soy milk is sort of a compliment to the dairy industry—your product has to be pretty good to have imitators. There is a bit of irony in it, too. Why are the strict vegetarians and milk critics pushing a product that attempts to closely match milk while they say milk is bad for one? What a non sequitur!

Soy milks will never be completely comparable to milk because they were not produced and perfected specifically by mammalian tissue as a food for development and survival of mammals. Even with our existing knowledge of the hundreds of nutrients and bioactive substances in milk, the understanding of what nature has wrought in creating it is far from complete. Man is not simply going to mix up some ingredients and reproduce what it took nature millions of years to perfect.

As with all other processed food products, soy milks have problems—not least of which are flavor, uniformity, and price. In its rigorous control of these factors as they relate to real milk, there is no question that the dairy industry has a distinct advantage. Nonetheless, soy milks are definitely offering milk increasing competition. Now they are being offered in the dairy case. Their sales, while not large compared to milk, are growing rapidly. Sales of a leading soy milk increased eightfold in just the past three years. Soy milks are prospering as a result of real or imagined lactose intolerance or allergies to milk by some consumers, as well as from the growing cult of vegetarianism in its many forms. Certainly the consumption of soy milks will increase as long as scary misinformation about milk continues to spread uncontested.

As is characteristic of the American way, milk and all of its new and old competitors will go on confronting each other in the market place. Based on its merits, milk should always do well. The real challenge is to keep consumers correctly informed about milk and its competitors. It is interesting how complicated things become in the modern world. As a vegetarian, one might see the soybean versus milk as a very clear-cut issue. It is not so at the level of U. S, agriculture. The same soybean that is used to make soy milk is fed in huge amounts to dairy cows. So, if you like, real milk can be thought of as soy milk, too.

Some Positive Factors about Milk

I often hear various forms of the question, "What's so great about milk?" Sometimes it's the questioner's lead-in to the latest bad news he or she has heard or read about milk. Frequently it is simply a desire to know whether and how milk is of special value as a food. To meet this latter need, the following list is presented. There are many other items that could be added but those given are ones of major significance.

1. *Milk contains more of the known essential nutrients required for human health in greater amounts than any other single food.*

2. *Because of its very nature and purpose, milk contains what is needed to sustain life.* It is unlikely that science will ever be able to give a complete accounting of all that milk offers in that regard.

3. *In terms of good quality, milk is America's most consistent and reliable food—essentially the same any day, anywhere throughout the country.*

4. *Because of its high protein and calcium contents, milk is of exceptional value as a food for the growing human.* This is understood to include ages twenty to thirty during which period bones are still maturing and some actual growth may be taking place.

5. *Milk contains more utilizable calcium, the essential bone building and maintaining element, than any other single food.*

6. *The known capacity of milk to suppress obesity can be of benefit to people of all ages.* This is particularly true in the increasingly sedentary culture of America, and when excess weight is a known pathway to many deteriorative diseases. People's preoccupation with their body images is also of no small importance in this connection.

7. *Casein, the major protein of milk, has the very unique property of beneficially influencing its own digestion as well as that of other proteins fed with it.* Digestion of casein makes absorption of resulting amino acids more efficient and makes possible absorption of some biologically active peptides before they are broken down.

8. *The conjugated linoleic acids (CLA's) of milk fat show strong evidence of suppressing cancer, atherosclerosis (heart disease), and fat deposition in experimental animals.* Preliminary evidence indicates their effectiveness against breast cancer in humans.

9. *Milk is an ideal food for the elderly in that it is highly nutritious and requires no preparation, no precision use of tableware and no chewing.*

10. *The fat and non-fat phases of milk are easily and efficiently separated commercially so that milk and milk products can be adjusted in fat content to whatever is desired including "fat-free."*

11. *Milk fat (cream, whipped cream, butter, butter oil, ghee, samna) is one of the most palatable food components known to man.*

12. *Milk is both a great food and a refreshing beverage.*

13. *Milk can be easily modified to suit individual taste by adding such readily available flavors as vanilla, chocolate, or almond.*

14. *Milk is both a "fast" food and a "convenience" food - no preparation, immediately ready for consumption.*

Perhaps No. 1 on the list is the simplest single answer to what is great about milk. In other sections of the book, we have more to say about the various listed statements and where appropriate, the supporting science is cited. For example, with respect to those dealing with healthfulness of milk, see chapter 5 immediately following.

* * *

Most people view milk as a highly nutritious food and a refreshing beverage. However, for a variety of reasons, some individuals reject milk. Avoidance because of flavor objections or untoward physiological responses is quite understandable. In some social situation, milk may not be the beverage of choice.

Unfortunately the unjustified view that "milk is for kids" misleads many people and blocks or reduces its availability in some circumstances of the adult world. It has many merits in diets for adults of all ages. Sad to say, there are many people with causes and missions who are happy trying to make milk look bad. However, if the facts are allowed to come out, milk can easily hold its own.

Suggested References

Miller, H. I. and Conko, G. Precaution (of a Sort) Without Principle. *Priorities for Health* 13(3):5-14, 36-39. 2001. American Council on Science and Health, New York.

Mason, S. Biting Movement: Animal-Rights Trespassing and What Some Critics Are Saying About It. *Ibid* pp. 15-19, 36.

Notes

1. Kimm, S. Y. S. et al. *New England Journal of Medicine* 347(10):709-15, 2002.
2. Mc Namara, D. J., Cholesterol intake and plasma cholesterol: an update. *Journal of the American College of Nutrition* 16(6):530-4. 1997.
3. Thomas, D.B. et al. *Journal of the National Cancer Institute* 94(19):1445-57. 2002.
4. Mann, J, I., et al. *Heart* 78:450-5. 1997.
5. Chen, K. New Craze Seizes China's Consumers: A Glass of Milk. *Wall Street Journal* 2/28/03.
6. Data courtesy of Tammy Perkins. College of Agricultural Sciences, the Pennsylvania State Univeristy.

5

Nutrition and the Healthfulness of Cow's Milk

General Qualities

In the United States, the dairy industry has grown with the country. The several-hundred-year period since arrival of the early settlers has seen the cow population rise into the millions along with that of the human. At the same time, there have been notable increases in the stature, health and longevity of Americans. Despite their nutritional excellence, there is no absolute proof that milk and milk products were indispensable to those improvements. However, it seems certain that the calcium of milk was important in the increased stature because milk was, and continues to be, the major dietary source of calcium for bone growth. More importantly, and mentioned again for emphasis, it is common knowledge that millions of people during this several-hundred-year period consumed milk and its products as regular and significant components of their diets, *and this was not associated regularly and consistently with any serious disease.* While it is true that there have been sporadic outbreaks of diseases traced to milk, mainly prior to widespread use of pasteurization, none of these were due to milk itself, but to bacterial contamination of it.

Early in the last century, cow's milk reached a zenith in its acceptance. It became known as "nature's most nearly perfect food." The cow was christened "the foster mother of the human race." In that era, nutrition research established cow's milk as having more of the vitamins, minerals, trace elements, essential amino acids and essential fatty acids required by the human than any other single food. To the writer's knowledge, no nutrition scientist has even attempted to refute that fact. There are all kinds of antagonists towards milk these days but they cannot deny that fact. For a summary of milk's main nutritional strengths and insufficiencies, see table 5.1.

Milk is not only a source of the classical dietary nutrients, it also contains bioactive substances that have filtered out of lactating and other cells as well as from the blood into the mammary gland.[1] As explained in chapter 2, blood not

111

Table 5.1
Cow's Milk as a Source of Nutrients

Excellent	Good	Poor
calcium	protein	iron
phosphorus	fat	vitamin C
vitamin B$_2$	carbohydrate	fiber[2]
vitamin D	vitamin A[1]	folate
	niacin	
	vitamin B$_{12}$	

[1]When its precursor, ß-carotene, is included.
[2]Milks of all species are completely devoid of fiber.

only supplies precursors for milk synthesis, a number of its components are transferred as such to milk. Some of these, such as serum albumin and immune globulins, are well known. It is estimated that there are about 2,000 proteins in human blood. Most of these are at very low concentration. How many of them become milk components in biologically important amounts is not known. However, it is well to bear in mind that blood contains the nutrients that nourish all the tissues of the body and that milk is derived from blood. The list of known hormones, enzymes, growth factors, and cytokines in milk that help to sustain life is ever growing through continuing research. Whether all the exquisite mechanisms inherent in milk to develop and maintain the body will ever be completely understood is a moot question. Fruits, vegetables, and grains also are fine foods for the human, but unlike milk, none of them is specially designed for growth and maintenance of mammalian tissues.

Particular Milk Components

In order to more fully appreciate the beneficial impact that milk has on us, the ongoing progress in further understanding the nutritional merits of milk should be taken into account. In this and following sections, some of these research highlights are described.

Casein—remarkable units of nutrition. The major protein of cow's milk, known as casein, is not one but a group of related proteins. These are bound together with calcium phosphate into particles known as micelles.[2] These particles are visible in that they reflect light and give skim milk its bluish-white appearance. This micelle is a most unusual package of nutrition. All in one unit, it contains the essential and non-essential amino acids, as well as calcium and phosphorus needed to build bone, muscle, and tissue in the newborn. Milk of all mammals examined to date, including that of the human, contains these casein micelles. However, bovine milk contains about ten times as much casein as does human milk. The reason for this difference appears to lie in sizes and maturation rates of the two species. The calf is about ten times the weight of the human at birth. It is almost immediately on its feet and physically active upon delivery, whereas the human infant is quite helpless. Further, the calf becomes a massive animal weighing a half a ton within a year or two, whereas the human is notably slow growing.

Human milk cannot be effective as the exclusive nourishment of a baby for much more than six months to a year. But the young human is undergoing growth and development for many years. As discussed following, deposition of calcium into bones of the human continues into the third decade of life. So a profound solution to this (probably unrecognized) need for dietary calcium by some primitive human cultures was consumption of milk, a very rich food source of calcium, from their cattle.

Casein—modifier of digestion. A further feature of the casein micelle is that it is digested, that is, broken down into small peptides and amino acids, by a slow and rather unusual process. The initial step in digestion involves its conversion into curd particles in the stomach. This step is brought about by rennin or pepsin enzymes of gastric juice that cleave a specific peptide from the surface of the micelles which renders them unstable and inclined to self-aggregation. This formation of curd particles, which is the very same process as takes place in the initial step of cheese making, delays breakdown of proteins in the gut with the result that amino acids are absorbed more slowly and existence of intermediate peptides is prolonged.[3] This slower digestion of protein not only improves the efficiency of amino acid utilization by the body, but it also influences the survival time in the gut of other dietary proteins (and their fragments) fed with casein. For example, the absorption of insulin-like growth factor-I into the circulation of the rat was greatly increased by feeding casein with it. The understanding has been that proteins must be broken down by digestion into their individual amino acids before absorption of the amino acids would occur. It now seems likely that small peptide fragments of the protein comprised of connected amino acids can be absorbed, and in some cases, even the intact protein, that is its entire chain of amino acids may pass from the gut into the circulation.

This capacity of casein to slow digestive breakdown of proteins is of interest with respect to the other proteins in milk. Milk of both the human and cow contain many proteinaceous hormones, growth factors, and bioactive substances that might have physiological effects in the consumer provided they escape complete digestive destruction. The fact that such substances are often effective in extremely small amounts and that milk is usually a regular (daily) item of the diet are important factors. A further consideration is that with some of these, the whole molecule is not needed. A peptide fragment may be just as effective. This is the case with the neurotrophic factor, prosaposin, of which milk is a good source. Peptides containing a requisite twelve-amino-acid fragment from the saposin C region of this protein exhibit some of its neurologically related activities including stimulation of nerve cell development and relief of pain. For further discussion of prosaposin, see a following section in this chapter on milk components and the nervous system.

The ability of casein to improve efficiency of amino acid utilization and to facilitate absorption of bioactive peptides qualifies milk as a "functional" food, a term currently applied to foods that benefit the consumer in ways beyond what would be expected from their classical nutrient contents.[4] Regarding other functional properties of milk, see the following section on milk fat and conjugated linoleic acids (CLA).

Calcium. It is hardly necessary in this age to document the importance of calcium in the human diet.[5] Authorities are recommending as much as 1.2 g. of it per day for an adult and frequently more for women because of such considerations as menstruation, lactation and osteoporosis (see following). Milk, which contains about 1.0-1.2 g. of calcium per quart, is considered to be the best dietary source of this nutrient. On average, 76 percent of the calcium in the American diet comes from milk and milk products. Calcium can be obtained from a wide variety of foods but in many of these, it is not as readily available as it is in milk (and its products); and with most of them, consumption of massive quantities would be necessary to meet the daily calcium requirement. In addition, the fact that a food contains calcium does not assure its bioavailability when consumed. Vitamin D is an absolute requirement for digestive absorption of calcium. The lactose of milk also enhances that process. Calcium not only builds bones and teeth, it is utilized in essential functions all over the body, that is, for muscle contraction, secretory mechanisms, intracellular signaling, enzymatic reactions, and so on.

A special consideration about calcium concerns the window of opportunity regarding its deposition in bone. Maximum bone mass is achieved by age twenty-five to thirty. Thus bones will not normally increase in size or strength beyond that age range. One of the major roles of dietary calcium beyond those years is to help suppress calcium loss from bones, a principal cause of their weakening and increased tendency to break. This deterioration, known as osteoporosis, is primarily a disease of women. Men experience only 20 percent of all the osteoporotic fractures. The difference arises from the fact that men by nature tend to consume more calcium, have greater bone calcification, and less (damaging) hormonal fluctuations. For example, menopause seems to stimulate bone loss in women. By age sixty, nearly 40 percent of women show evidence of osteoporosis in bone density measurements. Unfortunately, there are no early overt signs of the disease. While there is some question about how reliable and predictive bone density measurements are, it probably pays women to get one along with their mammograms and Pap smears. In the past few years, hormone treatment programs have become available that will not only stop osteoporosis but will promote new bone formation in older women. Of course, for this to happen, adequate calcium must be included in the diet.

In view of the comparatively small stature of primitive humans, it appears that calcium was chronically limiting in their diet. The writer was privileged to visit an historic settlement in northern Germany some years ago. It dated from about 1200 A.D. and contained a home that was open to the public. Sleeping compartments were built into the walls like berths on a railroad car. They were about five feet in length and could not have comfortably accommodated any but the very smallest modern adults. At the time that Europeans settled America in the seventeenth and eighteenth centuries, they averaged about five feet in height. Since that time, they have added another six or eight inches. While many factors may have contributed to this increase, it is obvious that calcium in the diet would be essential, and that products of the expanding American dairy industry would be the logical source of the calcium enabling this growth. More or less the same thing has occurred in Japan during the past century, namely a significant increase in height, during a notable development of their dairy industry. Of course calcium, while essential to increased bone growth and stature, is not the only contribution that milk would be making in this situation. High quality protein and growth-promoting B vitamins and vitamin D from milk would be other contributing factors. Even with the ready availability of milk and milk products, the most widely consumed food sources of calcium, the element is still limiting in the diet of many today.

In a report[6] published in 1994, it is stated that calcium is undersupplied by up to 50 percent in the diet of German children and adolescents, this in the modern world in a country with relatively abundant food and a good standard of living. The United States is in a similar situation. According to the National Institute for Child Health and Human Development, the majority of American school children, including teenagers, do not receive the recommended dietary allowance of calcium. Children who avoid drinking milk, and there are a lot of them, have low calcium intakes and poor bone health.[7] Milk consumption significantly increases bone mineral acquisition in adolescent girls.[8] It is not hard to believe that primitive humans were relatively undernourished with respect to calcium and that those who adopted milk as food may have been enhanced comparatively in size, strength, and health.

Vitamin D. One of the great human nutrition success stories is the fortification of milk with vitamin D. Proper development and mineralization of the human skeleton requires this vitamin. It enables the absorption of calcium and phosphorus from ingested food into the circulation and their incorporation into bone. Those elements are the principal ones that account for the structure and strength of bone. In the absence of vitamin D, a condition known as rickets develops. This disease, which occurs primarily in infants and children, is marked by bending and distortion of the bones and formation of nodules on the ends and sides of bones. Prior to fortification of milk with vitamin D starting in the 1920s, rickets was not uncommon in America. Fortification was proposed because there are no foods that are good natural sources of the vitamin; and since milk is a rich source of calcium and phosphorus, it would make available in a single food the essentials for development and maintenance of the human skeleton. During the 1930s, vitamin D fortification of milk spread rapidly with the result that rickets was virtually eliminated. Currently in the United States, 98 percent of the milk supply is fortified with vitamin D at a level of 400 IU (10 μg) per quart which amount is the current recommended daily allowance (RDA) or daily value (DV) for the vitamin.

One of the confounding aspects of vitamin D nutrition is that exposure of the human body to sunlight generates vitamin D from 7-dehydrocholesterol, a precursor in the skin. It is the ultraviolet (uvB) component of sunlight that accomplishes this reaction. Vitamin D produced by this means is effective in meeting the body's needs for the vitamin. Unfortunately there is a great deal of variation in how much each of us in various geographic locations and times of the year will be exposed to sunlight. For example, in northern latitudes such as in Scandinavia during the overcast short days of winter, there may be little exposure day after day. So light induction of vitamin D is not a very precise or reliable way of acquiring the vitamin.[9] A further problem is that too much exposure to sunlight in the case of certain ethnic groups and skin types causes the skin to age and become cancerous.

The foregoing limitations not withstanding, there is extensive evidence that exposure of the human body to ultraviolet light is beneficial. Such radiation is known to decrease blood pressure in hypertensive individuals. Living in sunnier climates is associated with a reduced risk of major cancers (breast, colon, prostate, ovarian). The primary evidence of this is from epidemiological studies comparing incidence of these cancers among people living at various latitudes. Vitamin D is also associated with suppression of osteoporosis. As a result of these and other observations, some health specialists think that the current RDA of 400 IU (10 μg) for vitamin D is too low.[9,10] If they are proven correct, drinking milk would be one way to increase somewhat ones intake of the vitamin. However, daily dosages as high as 100 μg of vitamin D_3, which is ten times the current recommended daily intake, have been suggested.[10]

Skin color and vitamin D involve nutrition in another important way. Overexposure to sunlight can destroy the essential nutrient, folic acid, in the human circulation. Folic acid deficiency can cause faulty development of the spinal chord and vertebrae in a fetus, and infertility in adults. Human skin pigmentation throughout the world has evolved to be dark enough for protection of folate but light enough to enable vitamin D formation[11]. Of course, this may have been alright in the days of primitive man, but with people of diverse skin colors migrating all over the world and living increasingly indoors, exposure of the skin to sun is a rather confusing health and nutrition consideration today.

Milk fat and conjugated linoleic acids (CLA). The fat in milk contributes to human nutrition and well-being in many ways. In addition to its basic function as a source of energy, it is a carrier of vitamins A, D, E, and K; it also contains essential fatty acids, as well as important flavor and aroma substances. In general terms, we need to bear in mind that humans have been consuming animal fats in their diet from prehistoric times. We evolved with a capacity to benefit from such fat in our diet and from plant fats as well, including those in vegetables, fruits, nuts, and seeds. However, processed polyunsaturated and hydrogenated vegetable oils only started entering our diets in serious proportions sixty or seventy years ago when the consumption of margarine began to increase, polyunsaturated fats were given a big boost by medical authorities and hydrogenated vegetable oils began to be used extensively in processed foods and food preparation. It may be more than coincidence that this period of rising processed vegetable oil consumption has led to an era when heart disease has become increasingly problematic.

Research findings that milk fat contains conjugated linoleic acid (CLA), discussed in several reviews,[12-14] have proven to be a very significant breakthrough with regard to the healthfulness of milk. There is evidence that a number of different forms of this acid are present in milk and that two of them may have inhibiting capacities for some of the most important human diseases (cancer, atherosclerosis, and obesity). Findings are also suggestive that CLA may strengthen our central disease fighter, the immune system. As a consequence, there has been great interest within the nutrition research community regarding CLA.

First, what is linoleic acid? It is a major component of the fatty substances in plants including vegetable oils. Since cows ingest grasses, grains and other plant materials, they normally have a fair amount of linoleic acid in their diet. As discussed in the next chapter, the cow's ingested food goes first to the rumen, or first stomach, where it is exposed to the fermenting action of resident bacteria. As a consequence of this action, the linoleic acid is converted into a number of other acids closely related to it in structure. These acids subsequently enter the cow's circulation and are incorporated into the fat of her milk and of her body. This is why the fat of cow's milk is unique in comparison to any other fat or oil; and as we shall see, this uniqueness may relate in important ways to the healthfulness of milk fat and milk products.

A number of the fatty acids formed from linoleic acid in the cow's rumen are conjugated forms of the acid, CLAs. When these acids are fed, the amounts of each form of CLA is usually not specified. Thus the term, CLA, represents a mixture unless otherwise stated. Two of the principal CLAs of the rumen have been given the common names rumenic and depressic, the former being based on origin and the latter on its action. Rumenic acid represents 80 to 90 percent of the total CLA formed in the rumen. The structural nature and production of these acids are discussed at greater length in the notes for this chapter.

Rumenic acid in the diet has been shown to suppress cancer in experimental animals.[15] Depressic acid is a potent inhibitor of milk fat synthesis in the cow.[16,17] When ingested, that form of CLA also has a capacity to suppress fat deposition and favor muscle mass development in animals.[18,19] If it has a similar effect on fat synthesis in the human, it will be a remarkable discovery with regard to possible control of obesity. In a review of dietary CLA effects in animals and humans, Jahreis et al.[20] report that a few human studies have shown increased muscle mass and reduced body fat as a result of CLA intake. But as they state, the data are suggestive at best and much more extensive and rigorous investigations are needed. When fed to rabbits, CLA suppresses and, even to some degree, reverses atherosclerosis, a principal manifestation of cardiovascular disease.[21] It is not yet known whether only one or both forms of CLA are involved in this latter effect.

Thus far, most research on CLAs biological effects have employed experimental animals. However, an unpublished investigation in France revealed an association of breast cancer with reduced tissue levels of CLA. In addition, elevated dietary and serum CLA have shown a correlation with reduced risk of breast cancer.[22] As noted in a following section, consumption of milk and milk products accompanies a reduced incidence of breast cancer. According to a report[23] of the National Research Council, CLA (rumenic acid) is the only dietary fatty acid shown unequivocally to inhibit carcinogenesis in experimental animals.

The CLAs have been an intensely active area of research during the past fifteen years. It is hard to imagine how any substances in milk could be more potentially meaningful in the realm of human health - a group of related fatty acids that appear to suppress cancer, control weight/body composition and discourage heart disease. No doubt, the many encouraging investigations involving CLA feeding to experimental animals will in time be extended to well-designed human trials.

Milk components and the nervous system. Brain and other aspects of the nervous system are developed and maintained by general nutrients, such as protein, lipids, and carbohydrates, and by substances that are of specific benefit to neural cells. In chapter 3 we touched on the importance of human milk to the developing brain. Beyond the general nutrients of cow's milk, we do not know whether components of it specifically aid the development and maintenance of the human nervous system. This area should be the subject of extensive research. However, it is worth noting that milks from a number of species contain several important support substances for the nervous system; namely, nerve growth factor (human and mouse[24]), prosaposin[25] and insulin-like growth factor-1 (IGF-1)[1]. The observed gastrointestinal stability and absorption of IGF-1 aided by casein in the rat,[26] and its ability to increase myelination and size of the brain in the mouse[27] appear particularly relevant. Prosaposin, a multifunctional protein also stimulates myelination, the process that puts insulation on nerve cells (neurons) thus rendering them capable of transmitting nerve impulses. Prosaposin also contains a peptide sequence that stimulates sprouting (maturation) of neurons and that relieves pain.[24]

Another component of human milk, now known to have neurotrophic effects, is erythropoeitin. This protein is required for production of red blood cells (erythropoeisis) by bone marrow; and more recently, its capacity to promote growth, differentiation and survival of various neural cells has been shown. Evidence has also been obtained recently that eythropoeitin of human milk survives digestion in the infant gut.[28] Like prosaposin, erythropoeitin retains some of its neurotrophic effects in a small peptide fragment of its total structure.[29] This property may be important in allowing the active portion of the protein to survive digestion (of milk) and be absorbed into the circulation. Such neurotrophic peptides may aid in development of the nervous system in the newborn. In the adult, they may help maintain the nervous system and ward off senile dementias such as Alzheimer's and Parkinson's disease. While erythropoeitin has not been reported as a constituent of cow's milk, I am unaware that anyone has attempted its detection there.

In a rather ironic twist of events, some of the strongest evidence that protein components in foods can reach and influence the brain is the findings regarding mad-cow disease. In that case, an ingested protein with relative molecular mass of about 27,000 escapes digestion in the gut and somehow reaches the brain where it destroys cells[30]. We consume many different proteins of roughly that size in foods every day of our lives. The crucial fact is that not very much of such proteins escapes digestion, gets into the circulation, and reaches other parts of the body. While the foregoing is evidence of the negative effect of a protein consumed in food on the brain, it does provide evidence of a food protein-to-brain pathway.

Scientist had long thought the adult brain has no capacity for renewal. However, there is now increasing evidence that old cells are dying and new cells are being produced there on a daily continuing basis.[31] The latest observations concern the hippocampus (in rat), a part of the brain involved with learning and memory. Learning efforts prolongs the life of newly generated cells in the adult hippocampus. Thus, with respect to keeping in shape, learning appears to be to the mind what exercise is to the body; or as they say, "Use it, or lose it."

Natural antibiotic activity of milk. The term, antibiotic, means literally antagonistic to or against life. Common use of the word is in application to widely used drugs that suppress disease-causing bacteria. Penicillin is a classic example. Such drugs have come to be of great importance in the nation's health. Since one of milk's major purposes is to protect the newborn from diseases, it is not surprising that milk has antibiotic activity. Mucins and antibodies of human milk are known to help regulate bacteria in the infant intestinal tract and to protect against diseases as discussed in chapter 3. Fresh cow's milk is bactericidal, that is, antibiotic. Its low initial bacterial count often diminishes during the first several hours after milking. There is a complex of factors contributing to this state in milk, and one of the factors is the glycoprotein, lactoferrin.[32] It suppresses bacterial growth by tying up iron needed by the microorganisms to grow and multiply. It also inactivates them by a second mechanism involving the permeability of their outer membrane. By binding to this membrane, lactoferrin is able to interfere with uptake of nutrients and discharge of waste products by these organisms. It also renders them susceptible to other antibiotics.

Of great interest is that digestion of lactoferrin by the enzyme, pepsin, increases this antibiotic activity. Resulting peptide fragments from lactoferrin are tenfold or greater more effective than intact lactoferrin regarding this antibiotic action.[33] Pepsin is secreted for the purpose of protein digestion in the stomachs of all mammals including the human. Thus, as a result of peptic digestion, milk may impart greater antibiotic activity than it has when secreted. A wide variety of bacteria are inhibited by the peptides derived from lactoferrin including numerous food born pathogens and food spoilage organisms.[33, 34, 35]

Another report that alerts us to the potential importance of antibiotic peptides from lactoferrin is one showing that they induce apoptosis (programmed death) of human leukemia cells and other forms of cancer.[36] So lactoferrin seems to be a cancer antagonist as well.

Before we can take joy in this additional protection against disease that milk may be providing us, a lot more research is required. While pepsin in the stomach may generate potent antibiotic peptides, other digestive enzymes may destroy them. So the question is how stable in the gut contents are the peptides from lactoferrin? In addition, to what extent are those peptides entering the circulation and reaching other parts of the body? The same questions were raised regarding neurotrophic peptides in the preceding section. Research regarding human digestion-absorption processes is somewhat neglected because that region of the body is relatively inaccessible and probing it is unpleasant for the subject. To get the idea, think stomach tubes, blood sampling and filling out human subject forms for the government. Then there is the problem of trying to find traces of key substances using highly sophisticated analytical techniques. Nonetheless, it is important to know whether bioactive peptides derived during digestion of our food are active in the gut, the circulation and/ or the far reaches of our bodies.

The larger significance of antibiotic activity derived from lactoferrin is in the principle involved. It appears that the health value of milk is not just based on its content of many nutrients and bioactive components. It also depends on functional substances produced from milk components during digestion. As compared to other foods, this seems particularly plausible in the case of milk, which is specially designed by nature in many ways to promote and protect life. Thus, when the bioactivities of peptides derived from milk proteins during digestion are considered together with the stability provided them by unique digestive conditions induced by casein, it is evident that an entirely different additional health benefit is operative from milk. Even though the peptides in question are intermediates in a further degradation process, they only need to be protected by the casein phenomenon long enough to do their work in the digesta or to be absorbed into the blood to do work elsewhere in the body.

Milk is also for Adults

Despite the fact that it is an excellent food at any age, the thinking, "milk is for kids" prevails in the minds of many adults. This implies that milk is ok while one is growing but that adults don't need it. Maintenance of the body is not unique to adulthood. Existing tissues and bone must be nourished also throughout infancy, childhood and adolescence. Milk can and does contribute strongly to this requirement. Further, there is good reason to believe that milk benefits growth, replacement and repair processes in the adult. The best current evidence indicates that calcium deposition into bone proceeds at least until the late twenties. Moreover, there is constant turnover in most cell types of the adult body. Finally, as everyone can see, body maintenance in the senior years is a serious business. Things are breaking down, organ functions are dwindling, bones are thinning and muscles wasting. One needs foods with proven capacities for tissue maintenance such as milk. Of course, this is not to say that milk can solve all the problems of aging, but *there is no reason to believe that most older people can not benefit from its inclusion in their diets.*[37]

One often cannot find milk in restaurants, on airplanes and at adult gatherings. Sometimes it is carried but must be specifically requested. When requesting it on airplanes, the writer has been told, "Sorry, we are saving it for children." The assumption seems to be that adults only drink coffee, tea, soda, or alcoholic beverages. This results from the fact that many adults give up milk drinking by early adulthood. There are a number of reasons why adults can benefit especially from drinking milk.

The number of elderly in the U. S. is increasing. According to the latest census (2000), there are close to 17 million people over seventy-five, an increase of 3.5 million over the 1990 census. This is a notable increase but it will be much greater when the "baby boomers," who are now an 82.8 million swelling of the population between the ages of thirty-five and fifty-four, get up into the seventy-five-and-older group. According to the 2000 census the thirty-five-to-fifty-nine-year-old group grew by a whopping 20 million. That accounts for close to half of the population growth between 1990 and 2000. And a lot of those boomers are going to get to be seventy-five. As of 1998, the average life expectancies of men and women were 73.8 and 79.5 years, this in comparison to 71.8 and 78.8 years, respectively, in 1990.

In keeping with those figures, there is a strong desire in many adult Americans to want to live "forever." However, it is necessary to keep in mind that the human lifespan has limitations. The following is something of a worst-case scenario for eating and the older person, but some of it, sooner or later, touches everyone who gets there. Failing senses and bad dietary habits of older people often create grave risks to their health. It is a time of life when food digestive/absorptive capabilities tend to dwindle. In addition, the senses of sight, smell, and taste, which are highly essential in judging food freshness and quality, may progressively lose their edge at that time. The abilities to detect signs of spoilage, such as off-flavors, off-odors and mold growth, become dulled. A recent study[38] found that 62.5 percent of people between the ages of eighty and ninety-seven have olfactory impairment, that is, significantly diminished ability to perceive odors and flavors. Forgetfulness of the elderly can overlook how long a food has been in the refrigerator, or just as importantly, how long it has not, but should have been there. "Doggy bags" brought home from the restaurant have been several hours at nice growing temperatures for bacteria and are already on their way to spoilage. They should be used promptly. For any food that appears marginal, disposal is the safest thing. It isn't worth risking food poisoning.

Chewing and swallowing can be problems for the elderly. The good teeth and muscles that actuate the jaws and throat may have become a thing of the past. Eating can become a chore. It takes longer to get the food chewed finely enough for swallowing. When eating with others, this can become an embarrassment because everyone else has finished with their main course and there you are still chewing away—and don't stop to enter the conversation since it will only put you that much further behind. Another embarrassing condition is the shaky hand. This makes it possible to get as much food on you as in you. Stains on clothing are a further giveaway of this trying condition.

Perhaps most serious of all, these difficulties reduce ones pleasure in eating at a time when appetite is in decline. As a result, food intake diminishes and undernourishment, which should be avoided at all cost, may begin to set in. One of the most certain ways to expedite ones demise is not to eat properly. This leads to a lack of energy, weakness, and less inclination to move. These conditions become a downward spiral and difficult to reverse. As we know these days, exercise is almost as important for well-being as food, and without food there will not be enough energy to sustain exercise. The less one exercises the less one can exercise—and so it goes.

Milk, as produced by the U. S. dairy industry can be a great help in dealing with most of these food-associated trials of the elderly. As obtainable from supermarkets and other retail outlets, it is a first class convenience food—cold, clean, refreshing and ready to be consumed. Other than pouring, it requires no preparation. As a liquid, all one needs to do is swallow it. As we have noted (p. 118), it contains more of the required nutrients for the human than any other single food. Along with a one-a-day mineral/vitamin supplement, a couple of glasses of milk a day are particularly good backup nutrition for the elderly because they are often disinclined or unable to prepare food.

Another good reason why adults both young and old should drink milk is in order to keep their bones in good shape. It is a well-established fact that milk is an excellent source of calcium for building and maintaining bone structure. As an elderly person, the condition of one's bones is influenced by what one has eaten and done all of ones life. Broken hips are the beginning of the end for 340,000 elderly Americans every year. One in four of those die within a year of their accidents and half never walk unaided again. The vast majority of hip fractures are among women who have osteoporosis, a weakened condition of the bones (for further discussion, see following).

It is true that some older people to varying degrees lose their ability to digest the lactose of milk (lactose digestion capability [LDC]). This may come about as a result of aging in the same manner that many other human abilities eventually decline. It is also possible that LDC may be subject to the "use it or lose it" syndrome. If one quits drinking milk at age twenty-five, it may not find a happy home in the stomach forty or fifty years later. Keeping ones LDC functional by drinking a glass of milk a day might not be a bad idea. Of course, some adults have never had LDC, but as noted in the following section on issues and in chapter 1, there are a number of easy ways of handling this problem. Perhaps the simplest is to drink small increments of milk periodically throughout the day as opposed to quickly consuming a full glass. Regarding the healthfulness of milk, continued strong endorsement of it for children and adults by leading health organizations including the National Institute of Child Health and Human Development, American Academy of Pediatrics, American College of Nutrition and the American Academy of Orthopedic Surgeons is unbiased support from thousands of health professionals. Such organizations are counseling us to drink more not less milk.

Milk and Weight Control Diets

Diet may well be the most popular book subject of all times. There are diets based on reduced calories, low fat, high protein, low carbohydrate, and all kinds of supplements. Real fame is to have a diet named for one. Despite all this outpouring of recommendations, Americans continue to get heavier. The latest figures indicate that more than half the population is overweight. Further, gaining weight may only be the beginning of ones problems. Obesity, diabetes and heart disease go hand-in-hand. There is a very strong consensus among health authorities that Americans eat too much and exercise too little. According to a recent statement of the American Heart Association, one-third of those afflicted with heart disease could be successfully treated by proper diet and exercise.

While exercise is unquestionably part of the answer to weight control, simple dietary measures for dealing with the problem do not yet seem to be at hand. However, several characteristics of milk suggest that it can help with weight control. To summarize from the foregoing in this chapter, the relatively slow

Figure 5.1

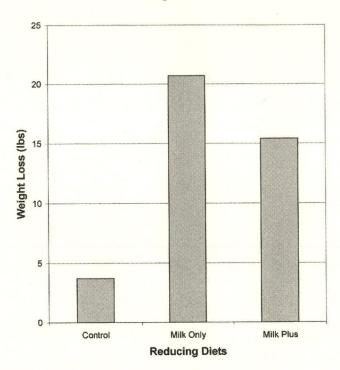

Average weight loss by 31 obese outpatients during a 16-week period comparing three reducing diets: a standard (control) reducing diet (n=9), a milk only diet (n=11) and a diet of milk plus one other optional food (n=11). For details, see the report of the study (Summerbell, C. D. et al. Br. Med. J. 317:1487-9. 1998.) from which these data are adapted. Graph courtesy of William Fisher.

digestion of milk casein tends to sustain a sense of fullness. This is also aided by the high volume (87 percent water) to low calorie content of milk. There is also the evidence that dietary CLA in milk fat may suppress fat deposition. In addition, it seems well established that the calcium of milk and milk products inhibits weight gain.[39] Just how calcium brings about this regulation of fat metabolism is the subject of continuing research. An additional consideration may be calcium's formation of insoluble, and thus unabsorbable, complexes with fatty acids during digestion. Instead of entering the circulation for use or storage (fat) in the body, these fatty acids are passed on through us.

Thus, it is not surprising that milk is a useful component in dietary treatments. An English investigation[40] of three weight-reducing diets for obese outpatients is a case in point. The three diets were a conventional reducing diet of 810 calories, a milk only diet of the same calorie content and a milk plus diet that allowed the patient to include one other food selected on a day-to-day basis. This latter diet averaged 1,339 calories per day. The milk only diet, equivalent to five glasses (1/2 pints) of milk a day, was clearly superior. The results regarding weight loss by the end of the sixteen-week program, figure 5.1, make clear that milk can be very effective in simple treatment programs for weight reduction. Before undertaking any effort to reduce weight by means of radical changes in diet, a person should consult an expert on human nutrition.

Another pertinent report[41] indicates that consumption of milk and milk products suppresses the insulin resistance syndrome, a condition characterized by obesity, abnormal glucose homeostasis, hypertension and dyslipidemia (Low HDL cholesterol and elevated serum triglyceride concentrations). All of these latter are signs pointing toward diabetes and heart disease. So the fact that they are reduced or eliminated as ones intake of milk and dairy products increases is another indication of milk's healthfulness. The study was a ten-year follow-up on 3,157 young (18-30) adults. The subjects included blacks and whites of both sexes.

In addition to passing up a generally nutritious food, girls and young women who exclude milk from their diets enhance two serious risks: weight gain and poor bone structure. Such deficiencies are not the type that quickly and clearly make themselves evident but they can be very detrimental over the years.

Issues

In the foregoing chapter, the need to carefully sift reports, claims, and criticisms in the health arena was emphasized. This is particularly true of publicity from the anti-milk activists who are not at all hesitant in their efforts to spoil the good image of milk as a means to other ends such as eliminating all animal agriculture. It is also worth noting that major public health problems such as heart disease, cancer and osteoporosis are primarily afflictions of older people, and the older one gets the greater ones chances are of contracting one or more of them. By the same token, one may survive into old age in part as a result of having consumed milk regularly, a sound nutrition practice. So logically, milk drinking might well be associated with the incidences of these major diseases of the elderly, but not as a result of any cause and effect relationship.

Another ironic twist is that even essential nutrients aren't always problem-free. Some examples: In two recent studies, higher intake of vitamin A, without which we can not survive, was associated with a greater incidence of hip fracture in older women; at the same time we need calcium in our diet, it has been associated with prostate cancer in some studies; linoleic acid, the principal form of essential fatty acid, promotes growth of cancers in experimental animals, and is also subject to oxidation and may elevate 'bad' cholesterol-carrying LDLs in the blood. Linoleate is also a precursor of substances inducing inflammation in the body, a response that can be both good and bad. As discussed following, homocysteine, a risk factor for heart disease, is derived from the essential amino acid, methionine. There is no way we can give up methionine in our diet! Thus, if these dietary components, which we must have in order to survive, can be problematic in certain individuals, why should we let anyone try to tell us it is a catastrophe when a few people have some problems with milk?

As previously stated, there is no perfect food. Humanity represents such a spectrum of physiologic, immunologic and genetic functionalities that there are always individuals who will not be able to accommodate a given food. We are not questioning that fact in regard to milk. Despite millions of happy customers for it, there are some who can't take it. Moreover, there are some legitimate issues about the healthfulness of milk. The pros and cons of these need to be discussed, especially as fresh, relevant information develops. Some epidemiological studies have implicated milk consumption as a disease-related factor. Unfortunately, such limited information is treacherous in the hands of anti-dairy activists providing them with the means to scare people about consuming milk and milk products. *The fact is that no cause and effect relationship has been established between milk drinking and any major disease.* Those for which associative evidence has been presented are heart disease, cancer and osteoporosis. All three are highly complicated and the subjects of vast continuing research efforts. Following is an attempt to analyze concisely where milk stands with respect to them. Lactose intolerance, allergy and less common ailments sometimes attributed to milk are also discussed.

Heart Disease

July 16, 2002 is a date of historic importance regarding heart disease. On that date, the American Heart Association (AHA) went on record in the journal, *Circulation*, that every person in the United States starting at age twenty, should be regularly evaluated for the risk of having a heart attack or stroke. Why is this proclamation important? The Association explains that because of current life style, diet and genetic considerations, all young Americans need to be regularly assessed for heart health. There is another very good reason for the proclamation. Instead of implicating whole segments of the food industry as producing products that are heart unhealthy for the entire population, the medical community is now recognizing that certain specific individuals may need to be guided not to eat too much of particular foods or too much food in general. Because of the cholesterol scare, many Americans have been anguishing for years whether it is safe to drink whole milk or eat an egg, probably the two most healthful foods known. It has been the era of falling milk consumption (see p. 34 of Miller et al., suggested references) and no-fat, low-fat foods while, at the same time, incidence of obesity and heart disease have been increasing. Clearly there are some inconsistencies here. The vast majority of people are not at risk of heart disease for including a reasonable amount of milk, eggs, or fat in their diets. In fact those things will be good for them. So carrying out the AHA proposal will help define who among us have special problems and need to take special precautions.

Because heart disease is such a central issue in diet and health for all of us, it is treated here at some length. There is no intent in so doing to preempt the medical profession; but to the extent that milk and milk products overlap into health considerations, the issues deserve discussion. Of course, as the AHA recommends, all of us should be checking periodically with medical specialists regarding possible heart problems.

Cardiovascular disease (CVD), the common major heart problem, is the number one cause of death in America. In 1999, it accounted for nearly a million deaths or 40 percent of the total. It is estimated that 62 million Americans suffer from CVD. The blood vessels of our body represent a system of tubing which in CVD becomes narrowed or even blocked preventing flow of blood. We are told that on autopsy, no matter what the cause of death, almost everyone shows evidence of CVD. However, the picture is changing somewhat. While CVD remains the leading cause of death in the U. S., the number of deaths due to it have been falling markedly according to statistics of the National Institutes of Health. From a high of close to 500 deaths per 100,000 people in the late 1960s, the rate is now around 200 deaths. The experts have not pinpointed any one thing in particular as the cause of this change but there is no question that improved treatments and better drugs are contributing. It appears that the impact of the disease in many is being delayed into later life. There is even some question of whether the obesity epidemic will have much of a bearing on the matter.[42] It is one of those changing situations about which we have to "stay tuned."

It has been proposed by the American Heart Association that one-third of all CVD can be successfully treated by proper diet and exercise. The implication is that the other two-thirds does not involve diet and of the one-third that does, we don't know how much could be corrected by exercise alone, by simply eating less or both. So, taking into account the need for exercise, in reality a minor fraction of CVD seems to involve diet. As discussed following, milk may actually protect against CVD.

Cholesterol, and saturated fat. Cholesterol, a waxy fatty substance, is an essential structural and functional element in all the cells of our bodies, especially in the membranes of those cells. It is also an important component of the brain and is a precursor of steroid hormones required in the metabolism and genetics of the body. Cholesterol needed by the cells is supplied either by their own production of it or by uptake from the blood lipoproteins which transport cholesterol of dietary origin as a complex with proteins and other lipids. In the normal, healthy individual, these two sources are balanced to meet the body's demand. In other words, cellular synthesis increases or decreases in response to the amount supplied by the blood, and in this way a more or less constant level of blood cholesterol is maintained—but not for everyone.

Despite many unanswered questions and the expanding complexity of heart disease, cardiologists still strongly urge all adults, especially young adult males, to strive for low blood cholesterol levels. The original simplistic view was that cholesterol in the diet is transferred via digestion and absorption to lipoproteins of the blood and, because of oversupply there, it deposits in walls of blood vessels. Such cholesterol then becomes a main constituent of plaques which narrow arteries and predispose them to blocking by clots and closure, that is, CVD. Since tissues need continuous perfusion with fresh blood to live, choking off vessels leads to death of tissues downstream from the blockage When such a restriction occurs in an (coronary) artery feeding the heart muscle, it can weaken or destroy heart (beating) function and cause death. Under that scenario, all cholesterol was "bad."

One may wonder, what is this "good" and "bad" cholesterol story? Research has slowly but surely produced a more detailed, far more complex, and somewhat different picture. It is now known that there are two major players in the blood cholesterol drama. One is the high-density lipoprotein (HDL) and the other, low-density lipoprotein (LDL). HDLs tend to scavenge excess cholesterol in the circulatory system and carry it into cells of the liver and peripheral tissues for disposal or recycling. Thus HDL cholesterol is known to be nonproblematic or "good." LDLs also carry cholesterol which normally can be handled satisfactorily by pathways in the body but if the lipids are either oxidized as ingested or becomes so while in the circulation, the LDLs carrying them may be diverted into walls of blood vessels where they contribute to plaque buildup. Thus, cholesterol of LDL's has become known as "bad." Removal of the bad LDLs from the circulation may be accomplished in part by macrophages that are part of the resident cell population in the walls of blood vessels. These garbage-disposal type cells recycle virtually everything constituting the LDL except its cholesterol that simply accumulates as a metabolic clinker. This is one of the newer rationals as to why vascular (atherosclerotic) plaques are full of cholesterol. Inflammation, as discussed in a following section, is another.

The other reputed bad actor in the fear of CVD is saturated fat. However, the causative link between saturated fats and CVD, if one exists, is indirect. The saturated fatty acids, derived by digestion of saturated fats, have been designated a risk factor in heart disease. This risk centers mainly on two such fatty acids, that is, myristic (C:14) and palmitic (C:16) acid.[43] They are significant components in a number of fats including milk fat. The current hypothesis is that these acids down regulate LDL-receptors in the liver thus keeping the LDLs in the circulation longer, thus increasing "bad" cholesterol and the chances that the excess LDLs will enter macrophages in the walls of blood vessels, a step in plaque buildup.

A coincidental implication about fats in the diet and CVD risk factors emerged from an extensive analysis of low-carbohydrate diets regarding their effects on weight reduction.[44] This involved 107 research articles reporting ninety-four dietary interventions involving 3,268 participants. The principal finding was that weight loss, when evident, was related to reduced caloric intake. A consequence of lowering the proportion of carbohydrate in a diet, if it is to be isocaloric with a control, is that protein and fat content would increase. In fact, low-carbohydrate diets are also known widely as "high-protein, high-fat diets." Those conducting the analysis reported that these diets had no adverse effects on serum lipids, that is, triglycerides, LDL-, HDL-, and total cholesterol. Apparently saturated fats were not behaving like a CVD risk factor in these diets.

While all of the foregoing remains a part of the evolving heart disease story, there is more. Actually most of us are able to make new blood vessels that can supplement and bypass those that are diseased and no longer working well. It is also possible for some of us to reverse plaque formation by proper diet and exercise. In addition, heart disease appears to involve a primary causative phenomenon; namely, inflammation.

Inflammation. A perennial problem with the longstanding cholesterol-saturated fat theory of CVD has been that some people with high cholesterol values get along fine and a substantial number of those with normal or low values suffer heart attacks. This and a lot of accumulating evidence has lead cardiologists to embrace a new outlook on the cause of CVD; namely, that inflammation is the principal factor, see *Atherosclerosis an Inflammatory Disease* by R. Ross and *Atherosclerosis: The New View* by P. Libby in the suggested references at the end of this chapter. More particularly, injuries to the walls of blood vessels brought about by chemicals such as from smoking, viral and bacterial infections, high blood pressure, disruptions of plaques, etc. produce immune responses and inflammation. This may lead to several types of unfavorable events: blood clots may form at these sites and either constrict blood flow locally, or they may break loose and block flow at other locations; in addition, blood coagulation factors may be released from these injuries which enhances the tendency for clots to form at other sites in the body; and in the course of repairing such injuries, macrophages (white blood cells) become engorged with cholesterol from fragmenting tissue and plaque material. It is theorized that their eventual death (as foam cells) leaves residues of cholesterol that serve as a focus for plaque buildup and structural instability.[45] Of course, thickening and clotting of blood within vessels is an extremely serious concern in both CVD and stroke. Scientists are of the growing belief that arterial inflammation is even more important than classical bad cholesterol in causing heart attacks and strokes. Who would ever believe it after all the furor about cholesterol?

There are a number of blood markers of inflammation and vascular injury that are elevated in those afflicted with CVD. They include C-reactive protein, MPO (an enzyme), interleukin 6, and homocysteine. C-reactive protein has been found to be a better predictor of CVD than LDL cholesterol.[46] Another significant inflammatory marker in a large study of healthy postmenopausal women with no symptoms of heart disease was serum albumin in the urine. Those who had the highest levels had a death rate for CVD 4.4 times those with no albumin in their urine. It is speculated that albumin arises in this circumstance from bleeding in the linings of arteries.

The importance of inflammatory phenomena in CVD is also supported by the efficacy of anti-inflammatory and blood-thinning drugs in the treatment of heart disease. Even the cholesterol-lowering drugs, the family known as statins,[47] have anti-inflammatory and blood thinning activities which raise the question, is it cholesterol lowering, blood thinning (anti-clotting), anti-inflammation or all three that make those drugs effective? No matter what the answer, the drug manufacturers and the medical profession focus on cholesterol lowering because that is the concern we have all been taught to have.

Genetics. One of the most important single factors in heart disease is predisposing genetics. This is especially true of the disease as it occurs in young and midlife individuals. Doctors invariably ask someone with elevated blood cholesterol or chest pains, "Is there any history of heart disease in your family?" Information is growing steadily with regard to specific genes associated with CVD. One of these is the gene for a blood clotting factor carried by 20 percent of middle-aged white males that elevates their risk of dying from sudden cardiac arrest. Another gene, just identified, is involved in erratic heartbeat. Others cause elevated serum cholesterol, elevated serum triglycerides and high blood pressure. Considering the complex structure and functioning of the cardiovascular sytem, there must be many crucial genes involved. Eventually we will have much more detailed information and that will be good. Rather than scare everyone into avoidance of dietary cholesterol and saturated fat, we may learn precisely for whom they are a problem. There is hope that gene therapy and genetic counseling also will be able to help some people. It is reported[48] that there are no less than five genes that can cause elevated serum cholesterol, the latest being one which regulates conversion of cholesterol to bile acid.[49]

There is one gene called APO-E which codes for a protein, apo-e that coordinates uptake of triglyceride (fat) from blood lipoproteins into cells throughout the body. There are three genetic variants of this protein one of which, apo-e_3, does its job well and tends to keep blood triglyceride concentrations low. However, the apo-e_4 version is relatively inefficient and promotes unhealthy prolonged circulation of lipid-laden proteins in the blood with the result that they eventually are taken into vessel walls and contribute to plaque formation. Thus APO-E_4 is a risk factor for early development of CVD. Southern Europeans have a notably lower incidence of APO-E_4 as compared to other populations.[50] Could it be that the "heart healthy" Mediterranean diet is in part the "heart healthy" APO-E_3 gene?

There is a well-known difference between men and women regarding CVD. The onset in men is earlier and it was thought that the factor sparing women is estrogen because they catch up with the incidence in men soon after the hormone is reduced as a result of menopause. As mentioned in chapter 4, not all studies could confirm that hypothesis and it is now believed that there are genetic factors involved. Defining the genetics of this situation, especially to aid diagnosis, is a current research objective.

Homocysteine. The story of this risk factor and marker of heart disease is instructive in a number of ways. In the late 1960s there was a medical researcher, Dr. Kilmer Mc Cully, who proposed that homocysteine, a metabolic product derived from methionine, is a cause of CVD. Methionine is one of the *essential* amino acids. We must have it if we are to make the thousands of proteins for developing and maintaining our bodies' structure and functions. So the idea is that something you absolutely require in your diet may be a factor in the disease. At the time of Mc Cully's proposal, the cholesterol theory of CVD was widely accepted by the health care world and no one had much sympathy for his hypothesis, although it was justified by substantial evidence. For example, people who have a defective gene that makes them incapable of properly using homocysteine manifest CVD early in life. Over the next couple of decades Mc Cully kept working and the evidence that he was right became overwhelming. Homocysteine is now recognized by the American Heart Association as an independent risk factor for CVD. Elevated levels of the compound in the blood, which goes by the fancy name of hyperhomocysteinemia, can produce damaged blood vessels and heart attacks.

In order to keep us from accumulating homocysteine, it is necessary to have an adequate intake of B vitamins, especially $B_6 B_{12}$ and folic acid. In that regard, the government mandate in 1998 to fortify wheat flour and other grains with folic acid should be a help. As with other causitive factors for CVD, specific genetic disorders can also produce elevated blood levels of homocysteine and attendent CVD symptoms. The limited studies to date indicate that milk in the diet lowers blood levels of homocysteine. Analysis of blood for homocysteine concentration is now done routinely along with assays for many other blood constituents.

While the modes of action of homocysteine in producing CVD are the subject of continuing research, possible pathways involve its oxidative effects on LDL lipids, inflammatory effects in blood vessel walls, and its interference with blood vessel dilation. The oxidative effect on LDL lipids would implicate homocysteine in the previously discussed pathway that carries cholesterol into plaques. Some details on formation and structure of homocysteine are provided in the notes (for chapter 5). For further discussion of homocysteine as a CVD risk factor, see the selected reference at the end of the chapter.

There are two human-interest aspects of Mc Cully's research efforts. They once again teach us how valuable it is for a researcher to be relentless. His findings were being put down, overlooked, ignored, and rejected for years but he refused to quit and eventually prevailed. The other notable twist is the lack of open-mindedness in the medical community that required McCully to hammer away for twenty-five or thirty years to gain acceptance of his findings. Now it would be nice to know, what proportion of CVD is, and has been, due to elevated homocysteine?

Omega-3s or vote "yes" on fish. In the early 1950s when the gospel was emerging that saturated fats are "bad," the vegetable oils rich in linoleate (18:2), such as corn, soybean, and cottonseed, were widely recommended as "good" because of their capacity to lower blood cholesterol. Fish oils were also studied as dietary components at that time because of their polyunsaturated fatty acid content. It had come to light that Eskimos living almost exclusively on diets of fish had no heart disease; in fact their arteries were found to be smooth and completely free of plaques. Despite this effectiveness of fish oils, they never got the attention or market demand of the vegetable oils. In the intervening years an important set of health related differences has been revealed between the vegetable and fish oil polyunsaturated fatty acids based on their structures. The common vegetable oils contain primarily what are known as omega-6s, particularly linoleate, while the fish oils have mainly omega-3s.[51] It develops that inclusion of omega-3s in the diet yields unique benefits in protecting against CVD as discussed following. Both -3s and -6s are important in growth, development and maintenance of the body. Both are required in the structure and function of membranes throughout the body. However, there are vital differences in some of their functions. Omega-6s are precursors of eicosanoids, molecules that promote inflammation, blood clotting, and blood vessel constriction, all of which are essential in some circumstances but complications in CVD. From a cardiovascular standpoint, omega-3s reduce the tendency of blood to clot, lower serum triglyceride levels, suppress atherosclerosis, alleviate irregular heart beat and decrease incidence of sudden death. As a result of the dietary emphasis on reducing cholesterol and saturated fat in the American diet, it appears we may have gone a little overboard regarding consumption of polyunsaturated vegetable oils containing omega-6s. This is not a little ironical in that we increased consumption of them to help eliminate heart disease.

One wonders how we developed this need for a balance in our dietary supply of these two structurally and functionally unique classes of fatty acids. It is interesting that the cat family is known to have an absolute requirement for DHA. Cats cannot make DHA from suitable omega-3 precursors by carbon chain elongation and desaturation as we can. They must have it in their diets and two common sources are fish and animal brains. I suspect the following story illustrates their instinct in that regard. My family like many others has been a lover of the domestic cat. Thus for generations I have been coming home to find headless mouse trophies on the doorstep. Nothing but the head will have been eaten; and what is in the head? Brains. And what is in the brains? Lots of DHA!

The need for water must have always been an important human priority. One can imagine primitive human settlements near bodies of water for purposes of washing, bathing, drinking, and *fishing*. In all probability, fish have been human food throughout our evolution. As a consequence, nutrients provided by fish could have become essential to the human during prehistory—not in the sense of a minimum daily requirement, but with respect to periodic inclusion in the diet for purposes of long-term health. This would make sense regarding fish lipid components, such as the omega-3 fatty acids. Following ingestion, they are storable at least in part in adipose tissue, and thus could be retrieved and used as needed by the body. A rather striking speculation is that humans split off from the apes because of fish eating in which we persisted. This eventually made us smarter than the apes because of our greater omega-3s consumption and consequent further brain development.

Probably if man had continued living primitively, details of the healthfulness of omega-3s might have remained hidden. However, because of the division of labor and abundance of food in America today, exceptionally selective diets are possible. So one could limit intake of fish or other suitable sources of omega-3s all ones life. Further, it appears that the deficiency symptoms are slow in manifesting themselves and show up mainly as a variety of deteriorations (aging), including heart disease, in the adult. In addition to suppressing cardiovascular disease, omega-3s also inhibit cancerous tumours. Inadequate intake of omega-3s is associated with numerous other human pathologies. For a review, see A. P. Simopoulos in the list of suggested references. The human infant needs the omega-3, docosahexenoic acid, also known as DHA, for growth and development, in particular for the brain, vision and intelligence. The supply of omega-3s via human milk and infant formula, the latter by fortification, is discussed in chapter 3. As a dietary source, cow's milk is relatively low in both omega-3s and -6s. Recognizing that good sources of -3s are limited, the American Heart Association has recommended inclusion of at least two servings of fish per week in the diet. The AHA Dietary Guidelines:—Revision 2000, are published[52] and can be seen at: <http://circ.ahajournals.org/cgi/content/full/102/18/2284>

Blood pressure/stress. There is this classic picture of the driven, overweight businessman. He has a high-pressure life, his face is florid, and when he has a heart attack, people say, "Of course." While CVD is not quite that simple, there seems to be little question that stress and high blood pressure, that is, greater than 140/90, are risk factors for heart disease. Stress tends to raise "bad" cholesterol and high blood pressure can cause injury and inflammatory damage to the walls of blood vessels. Over 50 million adult Americans are estimated to have high blood pressure and half of the population has blood pressure high enough to be considered at risk for heart disease and stroke. It is said that living in America is relatively stressful. What does that have to do with milk? There are a couple of points.

We are frequently being told that populations in other areas of the world are healthier than Americans because of diet. The fruits, vegetables, especially soybeans, and wine consumed in those other countries are supposed to be much better for one than the milk and meat that Americans include in their diet. Unfortunately, the populations being compared differ rather markedly in genetics, life styles and attendant stress, which all need to be taken into account. In many countries, rigorous exercise is demanded in the pursuit of daily bread, in some others an after-lunch nap is in order. Physically demanding jobs are dwindling in the U. S., and a siesta has never been widely accepted in the American work force. Comparing various populations throughout the world with respect to their health is obviously fraught with difficulties because of the many complex factors involved. For example, see the preceding discussion of the APO-E genetic variations in Europeans.

The general consensus is that milk and the calcium of milk products tend to suppress high blood pressure and weight gain. Both these latter are well-known risk factors for CVD and stroke. Not only is there no evidence that consumption of milk or milk products is a cause of heart disease, the practice may actually have a number of preventive benefits, see the preceding discussions and documentation of milk in relation to CLA, calcium and weight loss. Regarding high blood pressure (hypertension) in particular, recent research[41] shows that consumption of milk and milk products are preventive. This further confirms longstanding evidence to that effect (see Miller et al. pp. 117-154 in the suggested references).

Milk not a problem. It can be seen from the foregoing that a lot has been learned since the days when heart disease was simply and directly equated with blood cholesterol levels and that consuming polyunsaturated, instead of saturated, fats would lower cholesterol and solve the problem. It is now evident that inflammation, injuries, and blood thickening/clotting activities in blood vessels are very important immediate symptoms of CVD as are impaired capacities to clear lipids, especially cholesterol and triglycerides, from the blood. Oxidation of dietary polyunsaturated fats may be as big a problem in cholesterol metabolism as are saturated fats. Milk does contain a small amount of cholesterol, 0.30 to 0.35 percent of the fat or about 35 mg per eight-ounce glass. The recommended daily intake of cholesterol is not to exceed 300 mg. Consumption of the skim milk phase of milk tends to lower blood cholesterol; so the overall contribution of whole milk to the blood cholesterol level is essentially nil.

Not only is there clear evidence of milk's non-involvement in CVD, actually it seems to afford some protection against the disease. A recent investigation presenting such results is the Collaborative Study follow-up of 5,765 Scottish men aged thirty-five to sixty-four years.[53] These subjects were evaluated before the era in which low-fat/non-fat milk drinking became popular. So the results are meaningful in terms of whole milk. Milk consumption by the subjects was sorted into three classifications: less than 1/3 pint per day, from 1/3 to 1 1/3 pints per day, and greater than 1 1/3 pints per day. The results revealed that those drinking the most milk were at reduced risk of death due to heart disease (relative risk, 0.92) or death due to all causes (relative risk, 0.90) as compared to those drinking little or no milk. The publication containing these findings cites similar results from a number of earlier studies of the same question. While heart disease is somewhat less problematic in women, menopause is said to put women at comparable risk to that of men. A study evaluating milk and milk products consumption in relation to heart disease mortality of such women indicated that dairy foods have a protective effect in women, too.[54]

Concerning the Scottish study, note that milk drinkers were at reduced risk of death due to all causes as compared to those drinking little or no milk. So milk drinkers were not just contending better with heart disease, but with causes of death in general. In a study of vegetarianism involving over 10,000 people in the U. K., those drinking the most milk had a reduced death rate ratio due to all causes.[55] So there is some evidence that consumption of milk is associated with the general health and longevity of adults. Hopefully, there will be much further research effort along those lines. How to live a long healthy life is of great general interest. Life expectancy is increasing for Americans but its growth has slowed somewhat during the past fifty years (figure 5.2).

Figure 5.2
Average Life Expectancy

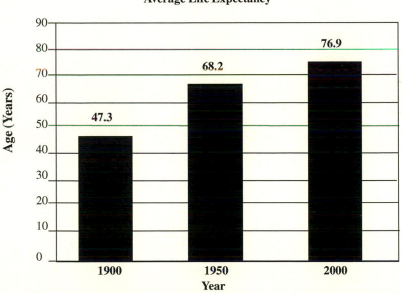

A comparison of life expectations for Americans born in 1900, 1950 and 2000. Data reported by the National Center for Health Statistics. Graph courtesy of Amy Fisher.

Stroke

As with other tissues and organs of the body, the supply of blood to the brain is essential. A stroke occurs when this supply is disturbed to an extent causing damage to some part of the brain. As a result the physical or mental functions controlled by the injured portion of the brain will deteriorate and become partially or completely inoperative. Basically strokes are of two types, one in which a blood vessel has lost its structural integrity and a hemorrhage or leakage of blood into the brain occurs; the other type results from a blockage of blood flow such as by a blood clot. This latter type accounts for 70 to 80 percent of strokes.

The symptoms of stroke often come on suddenly and can be fearful. The most common ones are sudden weakness or numbness, dizziness, dimness of vision, difficulty speaking, powerful headache, and mental confusion. Any one of these symptoms is a well-justified basis for seeking medical assistance, especially if they persist. Stroke can be an extremely serious event. It ranges from temporary loss of a nerve-controlled function, such as speech or movement of some body part, to permanent paralysis and even death. A major problem with stroke is that it is so misleading and distressing, the victim often dies before he or she can get help.

According to the Centers for Disease Control and Prevention about 500,000 Americans suffer their first stroke each year. There were 167,366 deaths due to stroke in the United States during 1999. That places stroke in third place, after heart disease and cancer, as a cause of death in this country. The people who have strokes are mostly, but by no means exclusively, men over sixty-five. There are about 25,000 cases of stroke each year afflicting men in their thirties and forties. Stroke is commonly related to heart disease because the characteristic narrowing of blood vessels as a result of plaque formation, a symptom of heart disease, can facilitate their blockage or rupture. And if either of these occur in the brain, the result is a stroke.

The limited evidence available indicates that milk consumption lowers ones risk of stroke. The one extensive study to date involved 3,150 older (fifty-five to sixty-eight) men of Japanese descent in the Honolulu Heart Program.[56] They were followed for a period of twenty-two years. In this group, drinking a pint or more of milk a day was observed to cut the risk of stroke in half. While these results are encouraging with regard to milk, and confirmed somewhat by the Scottish study,[53] it would be helpful to broaden the understanding beyond Japanese men living in Honolulu, a rather specific focus with respect to gender, nationality, and geographic location.

Cancer

In the anti-milk literature, one reads the flat statement, "milk causes cancer." The purpose of such statements is to get people's attention and to terrify them about consuming milk. Such statements are irresponsible and unjustified. All that seems to be required is for a study to vaguely implicate milk drinking or some component of milk (there are thousands of them) and we suddenly have "cause and effect" from some anti-milk person. Why bother with the fact that the causes of cancers involve complex genetic and environmental factors that are baffling even to the experts? Why bring up the fact that milk contains a variety of anticarcinogens?[13] For the sake of brevity and relevance, the following discussion is confined mainly to what if any role milk may have with respect to breast and prostate cancer. For some background information on breast cancer, see also chapter 3.

Breast cancer. It is the position of the American Council on Science and Health, who carefully investigate such matters, that the cause(s) of breast cancer is not known.[57] By comparing cross-cultural statistics for breast cancer, for example, data for women in China versus those for U.S. women, it is possible to imply that Chinese women have less breast cancer because they drink little or no milk. A far better comparison would involve the milk-drinking variable in the same country in order to eliminate confounding cultural differences. A study of that type, conducted in Finland[58] showed a clear-cut benefit for drinking milk. Incidence of breast cancer in the study was reduced in direct proportion to the amount of milk consumed (figure 5.3). These findings on Finnish women were confirmed by a similar study of 48,844 premenopausal Norwegian women.[59] Cow's milk contains a number of substances known to be anticarcinogenic including conjugated linoleic acid (CLA), butyric acid, sphingomyelin, ether lipids, vitamins A and D, carotene and whey proteins.[13] A

Figure 5.3

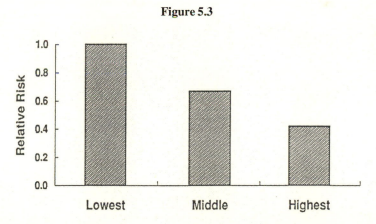

Relative risk of breast cancer as a function of milk intake. Breast cancer risk is reduced (P<.003)in relation to milk intake (Low=486, middle=679 and high=1060 g/d of dairy products). Data adapted by D. E. Bauman from Knekt et al. British Journal of Cancer 73:687. 1996.

study which analyzed breast tissue in women with and without breast cancer revealed that greater incidence and size of tumors was associated with lower tissue concentrations of CLA. CLA has been shown to suppress cell growth in many cell lines from many types of human cancer (breast, prostate, colon, ovarian, lung, melanoma).[13]

In addition to the foregoing impressive indications that milk and dairy products consumption is inversely related to incidence of breast cancer, there are other clues that milk may help. Infants and children, the biggest class of milk consumers, are relatively free of most cancers. It also is notable that dairy cows are essentially free of mammary cancer. There is also the protective effects of human lactation, discussed in chapter 3. In summary, there not only is no credible evidence that milk causes breast cancer, but rather it appears milk is a significant cancer restraining factor.

Prostate cancer. Cancer of the prostate is the second most frequent cause of cancer deaths in men (lung cancer being first). There are about 180,000 to 200,000 new cases reported each year. The precise cause of the disease is not known; and in particular, what makes it change from a relatively benign condition which can go on harmlessly for years to an aggressive malignancy remains a mystery. Virtually every male who is eighty or older has prostate cancer. The chances are that those individuals will die of something else. Detection of prostate cancer is now somewhat more practical and precise due to availability of the prostate specific antigen (PSA) test. However, evaluation of a tissue biopsy is considered essential for diagnosis.

The American Council on Science and Health has prepared a very informative report on prostate cancer.[60] The established risk factors for the disease are increasing age, African-American ethnicity, family history of the disease (genetics) and male hormones. It is the Council's contention that no lifestyle factors, including diet and exercise, have been conclusively established as risk factors. However, there are a number of epidemiologic studies that have shown an association between consumption of milk and milk products and incidence of prostate cancer. More specifically, it appears to be the calcium of the milk that is the associated factor since calcium supplementation of the diet produced a similar association.[61] Thus, it is logical that milk might be involved because it supplies calcium in the American diet. Like most cancer research, that seeking the cause of the prostate affliction becomes more complicated. A number of epidemiological studies show no correlation between milk drinking and prostate cancer, and a large prospective study implies that milk fat contains a factor(s) that reduces the risk for this kind of cancer.[62]

Since dietary calcium is an absolute necessity for life and good health, the fact that it may aggravate prostate cancer poses a dilemma. Obviously every older male does not need to reduce his calcium intake. In fact from the standpoint of discouraging weight gain, osteoporosis and a host of other problems, it would be foolish to do so. However, it would not be unreasonable for physicians to prescribe, on the basis of PSA test results, reduced calcium intake. With further research, it may become clear that raising the vitamin D intake would also be beneficial. Another therapeutic option lies with the flexibility of milk processing. Just as the dairy industry has supplied lactose-free milk for the lactose intolerant, and fat-free milk for the diet/heart/weight conscious, it could also produce low calcium milk. Such processing by ion-exchange has been available for many years. As mentioned in chapter 4, we need to exercise caution in our interpretation of epidemiologic findings. Association of milk consumption with incidence of prostate cancer, a disease of old men, may also imply that milk promotes longevity.

Liver cancer. There is evidence in studies of both humans and laboratory rats that subjects exposed to aflatoxin, a poison produced by molds, may enhance their development of liver cancer when they consume milk. The human association was observed in India among undernourished children who, no doubt because of near starvation and lack of refrigeration, had been eating moldy food. Of course, spoiled food should be avoided. So far as laboratory rats are concerned, it is well known that a standard diet (Sherman) comprised of milk and wheat keeps them tumor-free and in good health. It is relevant here that with respect to milk, the cow is a first line of defense in detoxifying and screening out agents that might get into us from vegetation. For example, this was brought out with respect to radioactive strontium, an atmospheric pollutant some years ago. In being directly exposed to the air during their production, fruits, vegetables and grains have a few drawbacks, too.

Osteoporosis

Osteoporosis, a condition characterized by fragile bones, has been widely publicized in the United States and rightfully so. It has assumed near epidemic proportions. Primarily it afflicts postmenopausal women. However, 20 percent of osteoporotic fractures occur in men. It is estimated that nearly 20 million American women over fifty years of age have thinning bones and that 40 percent of women over 60 have osteoporosis, that is, pathologically low bone density. Unfortunately, without measurement of bone density, the condition usually goes unrecognized. The first manifestation may be a fall with resultant bone breakage. There are about 340,000 broken hips each year among the elderly of America. Many of these patients die within a year, and many more go on walkers or are bed-ridden for the rest of their lives.

The growth and maintenance of bone is a complex equilibrium involving bone building and bone thinning. In a sense, the bones serve as a bank for minerals, especially calcium, in meeting body needs. As long as we keep plenty of calcium flowing to the bank, there is no problem. But when we cut corners on the amount of dietary calcium we need, the bank is called on to release some of its stores. The latest findings in this increasingly sophisticated area of research have been reviewed recently.[63] According to present estimates, nearly fifty substances (hormones, enzymes, receptor and signaling molecules, mineral elements) are involved in these processes. Of these, calcium is singularly important because it is the principal element giving bone its structure and strength. It is widely agreed by all manner of authorities if one does not take in adequate calcium, ones bone health will suffer; and in older women this is manifest as osteoporosis. The current hypothesis is that the female hormone, estrogen, protects against bone loss of calcium until menopause at which time production of the hormone drops rather precipitously. However, if a woman has been habitually neglecting calcium intake, there may not be much bone structure to protect.

Since milk and milk products account for 76 percent of the calcium in the diet of Americans, it is obvious that milk consumption is playing an important role in the building and maintenance of their bones. According to the USDA, milk consumption declined 25 percent between 1970 and 1997. Many nutritionists feel that we are in a dietary calcium crisis. It is forecasted that unless this trend is reversed, there will be 40 million new cases of osteoporosis over the next twenty years.

Regrettably, American girls during their teen years—by the end of which period about half of their adult bone mass will have formed —are tending to refrain from drinking milk, apparently for fear that milk will fatten them, which is not true. See the foregoing section on milk and weight control and in particular (figure 5.1).

There are many studies demonstrating the positive relationship between milk consumption and bone density. For an extensive review, see Miller et al. (suggested references). Despite this massive evidence, the anti-milk coalition persist in citing a publication[64] from the epidemiological survey known as the Nurses' Health Study, of Harvard University. In that investigation, researchers found the incidence of bone breakage (mainly hip fractures) among nurses who drank substantial milk surpassed that among their statistical counterparts who drank little or no milk. This finding certainly bears further investigation because it is completely inconsistent with much other knowledge on the subject. It has been firmly established that intake of calcium (e.g., in the form that occurs in milk and milk products) is necessary for the development and maintenance of bones, and that it is important to bone strength and preventing osteoporosis. Genetic, hormonal, motional, and/or nondietary behavioral differences may have accounted for the difference in the incidence of bone fractures between those nurses who drank milk and those who consumed little or no milk. In addition, as mentioned above, there are at least fifty known factors involved in bone maintenance. There was also a relative lack of subjects who as teenagers had consumed more than three glasses of milk daily. The researchers found the lowest rate of hip fractures in the study among such subjects, but because of the limited number of these subjects, this finding was not statistically significant. Those subjects who as teenagers had consumed more than three glasses of milk daily were the only ones in the study likely to have had a daily calcium intake approximating that which the Food and Nutrition Board of the Institute of Medicine now terms "adequate" for persons nine through eighteen years old. The lead researcher of this study has speculated that the milk intake of the milk-drinking nurses may have been "too little, too late."

Lactose Digestion Capability (LDC) About one out of every five or six Americans on average lacks the ability to digest lactose, the carbohydrate of milk. As explained in chapter 1, this is virtually a non-problem except in some people's minds. There has been a great deal of confusion generated about this subject. Some veteran milk drinkers don't even know they can't digest lactose; milk with lactose predigested is widely available; and in any event, those who can't digest lactose can easily accommodate at least one glass of milk/day if it is consumed in several small portions throughout the day. LDC is not purely a matter of race or ethnicity. Most African Americans, for example, carry some genetic contributions from Europeans and that may include the LDC gene that is dominant. They may also have inherited the gene from certain native African tribes who have a milk-drinking history.

There is no issue that has been more useful to the anti-milk coalition than lactose intolerance. There are published anecdotes that even a teaspoonful of milk in a person's tea produced incredibly painful intestinal symptoms. One gets the impression the person literally exploded. That could be, possibly for psychic or psychotic reasons, but not as a result of LDC. Stomach and intestinal complaints are sufficiently vague, uncertain as to cause, and at times emotionally driven, that they make an ideal scapegoat for the hate-milk crowd. According to recent research[65] at the University of Kansas Medical Center, ingestion of the sugar, fructose, by some people can cause the same symptoms as those of lactose intolerance including abdominal pain, diarrhea, gas, and hydrogen in the breath. Many soft drinks and fruits are rich sources of fructose. Thus, there exists another reason why lactose may not always be the problem.

The molecular cause of lactose intolerance, or adult-type lactasia as it is also known, is a very interesting problem and an active research frontier. A recent study[66] has detected genetic markers for this human limitation in a gene sequence next to (upstream) that coding for the lactase enzyme. It is possible that these polymorphic sequences somehow regulate the level of lactase expression; and in any event, they appear to provide the basis for genetic detection of lactose intolerance that could supplement several other tests now used.

Natural (genetic) selection enabled virtually the entire Northern European population, among others, to digest lactose. This made cow's milk a more valuable food than ever to those people. Because of genetics dominance of the trait, this capability is spreading all over the world. That hardly seems like something to be regretted. At the same time, for those who cannot digest lactose, many practical ways of handling the problem have been developed (chapter 1).

Allergy and Autoimmune Problems

There is no perfect food—not a single one. As with other foods, milk represents a source of foreign proteins, that is, ones we did not make ourselves. When these enter our bodies they may in rare instances promote a pattern of very unpleasant responses known as allergy. In the extreme, this involves such symptoms as vomiting, diarrhea, swelling and inflammation of tissues, nasal irritation and skin rash. The first year or two of life are often crucial with regard to development of allergies. While other substances, especially on contact with the skin, can cause allergies, proteins are by far the most important allergens in foods. It is estimated that 1 to 3 percent of young children are allergic to cow's milk proteins; however, most of those afflicted quickly out grow it. According to a recent large survey,[67] incidence of allergy in children is not growing; and the risk that a food allergic child will die of food allergy is about 1 in 800,000, a remote possibility indeed.

True allergy is due to a specific reaction of the immune system to a substance, for example, a food protein, that it cannot accommodate. People tend to confuse a variety of symptoms with those of allergy. If there is no swelling and irritation of tissues, nasal irritation or skin rash, the likelihood is something other than allergy. Many of those taking allergy prescriptions are not truly allergic. Lactose intolerance is sometimes assumed to be an allergy, which it is not.

The newborn baby has a relatively permeable intestine that allows fragments and even whole molecules of milk proteins to enter the circulation. This invasion enhances the possibility of antagonistic reaction by the immune system. As the baby grows, the gut wall becomes less permeable and the immune system becomes more mature both of which conditions facilitate normal, healthful handling of ingested food proteins. Thus, a recommendation of the American Academy of Pediatrics that breastfeeding of infants be maintained during the first year of life to encourage maturation of the gut and the immune system appears well advised. Human milk, and especially that of the baby's own mother, is thought to contain factors that promote maturation of the neonatal immune system. In addition, the chances that the baby will develop allergy to its own mother's milk is much less likely than to the proteins of infant formula. Nonetheless, allergic responses to mother's milk have been reported, for example, to cow's milk proteins or its fragments that have been ingested by the mother and traversed to her milk. The idea that food proteins are totally broken down in our stomachs can now be labeled a myth. Considering the sensitivity of some systems in our bodies, the escape of only a few molecules or parts thereof, may be all that is required at times to cause trouble.

As biomedical research further unfolds the complexities of how food proteins interact with the immune system, it appears that they can become involved in unfavorable autoimmune reactions. In such situations, the immune system that protects us from disease malfunctions and attacks us. Type 1 diabetes, which is due to insufficient production of insulin, can arise from such an attack on the pancreas. Such so-called autoimmune diseases are thought to involve genetics, viruses and other environmental factors. Among the latter, food proteins, including those in milk, may be involved *on rare occasions*. For example, epidemiological evidence has shown that both type 1 diabetes and multiple sclerosis (MS) are associated with milk consumption. In both cases, a particular milk protein has been found to induce elevated levels of antibodies against the tissue in question. In type 1 diabetes, bovine serum albumin (BSA) appears to be involved[68]; in MS, butyrophilin is implicated.[69] It develops that BSA is capable of inducing antibodies that can cross react with a cell surface protein in the pancreas. It is speculated that such binding incites an autoimmune attack that destroys the insulin-producing capability of the pancreas thus causing type 1 diabetes, a disease characterized by inability to utilize blood glucose that, if left uncorrected, produces many serious symptoms and premature death. So far, studies are divided about equally as to whether milk is involved. Butyrophilin, a protein exclusive to milk, generates antibodies that cross react with a protein in the myelin sheath of nerve cells. In this case an autoimmune attack would cause demyelination of nerves, a characteristic of MS, which renders them non-functional.

For food proteins to cause an autoimmune attack, several conditions would be required: the protein would need to be sufficiently immune-provocative to promote antibody production in the person; it would be essential that enough similarity, if not co-identity, exist between amino acid sequences of the protein receptor in the body and the foreign food protein so that antibodies generated to the latter would bind to the former; and the antibody-receptor complex thus formed would need to be capable of provoking an aggressive immune system attack at the site of the complex. Fortunately, the chances that these conditions can be met are remote. There is the fact that a properly developed and functioning immune system must learn how to deal with a huge array of foreign (food) proteins, and miraculously, it does. In addition, there is little likelihood that two different proteins will have a region of sufficient similarity in sequence, folding, and surface chemistry to enable antibody cross-reactivity.

Note that in the observed associations involving BSA and butyrophilin, no firm cause and effect relationship between these milk proteins and the particular diseases has yet been established, and the likelihood is that the numbers of individuals involved, in any event, would be few and of a specific genetic predisposition. The avoidance of cow's milk proteins during the first year of life; as prescribed by the American Association of Pediatricians may alleviate or even solve the problem. If necessary, the dairy industry can manufacture milks that are free of BSA and/or butyrophilin if there is sufficient demand.

This is a relatively new frontier in nutrition. Food proteins in addition to those in milk may be associated with autoimmune phenomena. Additional research will be required on how best to deal with these situations. It appears that part of the problem will be in detecting susceptible people regarding particular diseases, and defining who are those that require the "foreign" protein antibody as a causative factor for those diseases. It may develop that many of us carry such antibodies but that they have never caused a problem.

Bovine Growth Hormone (BGH)

For the past ten years or so, injections of BGH, also known as bovine somatotropin (bST), has been used to increase milk production of the dairy cow. This practice has been and continues to be applied effectively in many American dairy herds. What this means is that BGH is required for milk production, and that in virtually all cows, not enough of the hormone is naturally produced to achieve the maximum yield of milk. So if you give them a little more, their milk producing system is able to make more milk. It is somewhat analogous to a diabetic being able to make better use of sugars in his/her food if given a periodic shot of insulin. It was predicted in some quarters from the very beginning that BGH milk would be hazardous to human health. Some ten or fifteen years later, it seems to be a non-problem. As stated by scientists at the outset, BGH milk is fundamentally the same as any other milk, but the negativists on this issue hate to let it die. It is well established that injecting cows with BGH does not increase the BGH content of their milk or render the milk unsafe for human consumption.[70] Ironically, growth hormone therapy is being recommended for human adults in some circumstances because its production diminishes progressively in us as we age, which is one reason why older people lose muscle mass, put on weight and their skin becomes wrinkled. BGH, where is thy sting?

The Take-Away Lesson

Centuries of experience as well as extensive knowledge gained from nutritional biochemistry have established that cow's milk is an excellent human food. While current research is revealing impressive new aspects of milk's healthfulness, it is also indicating that special segments of the adult population may benefit from milks that have been suitably modified. Included in these groups are people with unique allergy, immune or genetic conditions related to milk. If there is sufficient demand for such milk products, the dairy industry should be able to produce them, as they have for reduced fat and lactose-free milks. Some dieticians and health counselors have reached near hysterical intensity in their urging of more fruits and vegetables in replacement of animal products, including milk, in the American diet. This recommendation is clearly debatable and probably ill advised for most people. While milk consumption has been falling during the past twenty-five years, being overweight has become epidemic. It is increasingly evident from research that milk can facilitate weight control. This and many other considerations suggest that the best diets include milk.

Suggested References

Bauman, D.E., B.A. Corl, L.H. Baumgard and J.M. Griinari. 2001. Conjugated linoleic acid (CLA) and the dairy cow. In: *Recent Advances in Animal Nutrition* 2001 (Eds. P.C. Garnsworthy and J. Wiseman), pp. 221-250. Nottingham University Press, Nottingham.

Picianno, M. F. Human milk: Nutritional aspects of a dynamic food. *Biology of the Neonate.* 74:84-93.1998.

Campana, W. M.; and Baumrucker, C. R. Hormones and growth factors in bovine milk. In *Handbook of Milk Composition,* edited by R. G. Jensen. San Diego: Academic, 1995.

Boirie, Y.; Dangin, M.; Gachon,P.; Vasson, M.-P.; Maubois, J.-L.; and Beaufrere, B. Slow and fast dietary proteins differently modulate postprandial protein accretion. *Proc. Natl. Acad. Sci. USA* 94:14930-35, 1997.

McCully, K. S. Homocysteine and vascular disease. *Nature Medicine* 2:386-389. 1996.

Miller, G. D., Jarvis, J. K. and Mc Bean, L. D. Handbook of Dairy Foods and Nutrition, 2nd. Ed. pp. 1-423. CRC Press, Boca Raton. 2000

Ross, R. Atherosclerosis - an inflammatory disease. *New England Journal of Medicine* 340:115-126. 1999.

Libby, P. Atherosclerosis: The New View. *Scientific American* 286:46-55. 2002

Simopoulos, A. P. Omega-3 fatty acids in health and disese and in growth and development. American *Journal of Clinical Nutrition* 54: 438-63. 1991.

Taubes, G. The soft science of dietary fat. *Science* 291: 2536-2545. 2001.

Steinberg, D. Low density lipoprotein oxidation and its patho-biological significance. *Journal of Biological Chemistry* 272:20963-66. 1997.

Notes

1. Campana, W. M.; and Baumrucker, C. R. Hormones and growth factors in bovine milk. In *Handbook of Milk Composition,* edited by R. G. Jensen. San Diego: Academic, 1995.

2. For review of casein structure, see Farrell, H. J. Jr. et al. *Journal of Dairy Science* 85: 459-71. 2002.

3. Boirie, Y. et al. Slow and fast dietary proteins differently modulate postprandial protein accretion. *Proceedings of the Natlional Academy Sciience of the USA* 94:14930-35, 1997.

4. Meister, K. Facts about "Functional Foods." *A report by the American Council on Science and Health*, New York, 2002. pp. 32.

5. For those in need of extensive information and documentation regarding dietary calcium, please consult: Miller, G. D., Jarvis, J. K. and Mc Bean, L. D. *Handbook of Dairy Foods and Nutrition, 2nd. Ed.* pp. 1-423. CRC Press, Boca Raton, FL. 2000.

6. Renner, E. *Journal of Dairy Science* 77:3498-3505. 1994.

7. Black, R. E. et al. American Journal of Clinical Nutrition 76:675-80. 2002.

8. Cadogan, J. et al. *British Medical Journal* 315:1255-70. 1997.

9. Vieth, R. *American Journal of Clinical Nutrition* 69:842-56. 1999.

10. Vieth, R. et al. *American Journal of Clinical Nutrition* 73:288-94. 2001.

11.   Jablonski, N. G. and Chapin, G. *Scientific American* 287(4):74-81. 2002.
12.   Lawson, R. E. et al. *Nutrition Research Reviews* 14:153-72. 2001.
13.   Parodi, P. W. *Journal of Dairy Science* 82:1339-49. 1999.
14.   Belury, M. A. *Annual Reviews of Nutrition* 22:505-31. 2002.
15.   Ip, C. et al. *Journal of Nutrition* 129:2135-42. 1999.
16.   Baumgard, L. H. et al. *American Journal of Physiology* 278: R179-84. 2000.
17.   Baumgard, L. H. et al. *Journal of Dairy Science* 85:2155-63. 2002.
18.   Dugan, M. E. R. et al. *Canadian Journal of Animal Science* 77: 723-5. 1997.
19.   DeLany, J. P. *American Journal of Physiology* 276: R1172- 9. 1999.
20.   Jahreis, G. et al. *European Journal of Lipid Science and Technology* 102:695-703. 2002.
21.   Kritchevsky, D. et al. *Journal of the American College of Nutrition* 19: 472S-7S. 2000.
22.   Aro, A et al. Nutrition and Cancer 38(2):151-7. 2000.
23.   National Research Council . *Carcinogens and anticarcinogens in the human diet.* 1996. National Academy Press, Washington, DC.
24.   See citations in Patton et al. note 25.
25.   Patton, S. et al. *Journal of Dairy Science* 80:264-72.1997.
26.   Kimura et al. Gastrointestinal absorption of recombinant human IGF-I in rats. *Journal of Pharmacological and Experimental Therapeutics* 283(2): 611-18. 1997.
27.   Carson et al. IGF-I increases brain growth and CNS myelination in transgenic mice. *Neuron* 10: 729-40. 1993.
28.   Kling, R. J. et al. *Pediatric Research* 43: 216-21. 1998.
29.   Campana, W. M. et al. *International Journal of Molecular Medicine* 1: 235-41. 1998.
30.   Stroynowski, I. Prions in the gut: Dietary proteins or infectious pathogens? *The Scientist* 15(15)6. 2001. See also: Prusiner, S.B. *Proceedings of the National Academy of Sciences of the USA* 95:13363-83. 1998.
31.   van Praag, H. et al. *Nature* 415:1030-4. 2002.
32.   See chapter 1 and the reviews of bactericidal activity in milk by Reiter, B. *Journal of Dairy Research* 45:131-47. 1978; and O'Toole, D. K. *Advances in Applied Microbiology.* 40: 45-94. 1995.
33.   Bellamy, W. et al. *Biochimica et Biophysica Acta* 1121: 130-6. 1992.
34.   Dionysius, D. A. and Milne, J. M. *Journal of Dairy Science* 80:667-74. 1997.
35.   Among the organisms mentioned by Bellamy et al. and Dionysius and Milne are enterotoxigenic *E. coli, P. fluorescens, P. aeruginosa, B. cereus, Salmonella salford, S. aureus, Klebsiella pneumoniae,* and *Listeria monocytogenes.*
36.   Roy, M. K. et al. Journal of Dairy Science 85:2065-74. 2002. According to the literature reviewed in that report, there is evidence that antibiotic peptides from lactoferrin combat the growth of certain malignant tumors.
37.   Barr, S. I. et al. *Journal of the American Dietetic Association* 100:810-7. 2000.
38.   Murphy, C. et al. Journal of the American Medical Association 288:2307-12. 2002.
39.   Zemel, M. B. et al. *FASEB J.* 14:1132-38. 2000.
40.   Summerbell, C. D. et al. *British Medical Journal* 317:1487-9. 1998.
41.   Pereira, M. A. et al. *JAMA* 287:2081-9. 2002.
42.   The substance of this commentary on the falling heart disease death rate is interpreted from a news service article: Kolata, G. Heart Attack Stroke Patients Live Longer. *New York Times News Service*, 1/19/03.
43.   Kris-Etherton, P. M. and Yu, S. *American Journal of Clinical Nutrition* 65: 1628s-44s. 1997.

44. Bravata, D. M. et al. *Journal of the American Medical Association* 2891837-50. 2003.
45. Note that in our concerns about cholesterol, there is quite a difference between that deposited in arterial plaques by way of the death of macrophages that came there to deal with inflammation and the cholesterol that is reputed to have gotten there from ones diet via LDLs. Further, how does one tell the difference between the two?
46. Ridker, P. M. et al. *New England Journal of Medicine* 342:836-43. 2000; ibid 344:1959-65. 2001.
47. Meister, K. Chemoprevention of Coronary Heart Disease. *A report by the American Council on Science and Health*, New York, 2002. pp. 20.
48. ASBMB Today, September 2002. p.8. This is a publication of the American Society of Biochemistry and Molecular Biology.
49. Pullinger, C. R. et al. *Journal of Clinical Investigations* 110:109-17. 2002.
50. Lucotte, G. et al. *Human Biology* 69(2);253-62. 1997.
51. Some may wish to know more precisely what is the difference between these two types of fatty acids. The terms, omega-3 and omega-6 refer to where in the carbon chain of the fatty acid the final double bond between carbons is located, that is, either 3 carbons from the CH_3- (or omega) end, CH_3-CH_2-CH=CH-; or 6 carbons from that end, CH_3-CH_2-CH_2-CH_2-CH_2-CH=CH-. Consider also our earlier discussion of fat structure in the notes for Chapter 2. From a dietary standpoint, the principal omega-6 fatty acid is the linoleate (18:2) of vegetable oils and the main omega-3's are DHA (22:6) and ECA (20:5) of fish oils and alpha-linolenate (18:3) mainly in plant lipids and at low levels there.
52. Krauss, R. N. et al. *Circulation* 102: 2284-99. 2000.
53. Ness, A. R. et al. *Journal of Eipdemiology and Community Health* 55:379-382. 2001.
54. Bostick, R. M. et al. *American Journal of Epidemiology* 149:151-61. 1999.
55. Mann, J, I., et al. *Heart* 78:450-5. 1997.
56. Abbott, R. D. et al. *Stroke* 27:813-8. 1996.
57. Meister, K. and Morgan, J. Risk factors for breast cancer. *A report of the American Council on Science and Health*, 1995 Broadway, New York, NY 10023. 2000. pp. 25.
58. Knekt, et al. *British Journal of Cancer* 73:687-91. 1996.
59. Hjartaker, A. et al. *International Journal of Cancer* 93:888-93. 2001.
60. Meister, K. Risk factors for prostate cancer: Facts, speculations and myths. *A report of American Council on Science and Health.* 2002. New York, NY. pp 21.
61. Giovannuci, E. et al. *Cancer Research* 58:442-7. 1998.
62. Veierod, M. B. et al. *International Journal of Cancer* 73:634-638. 1997.
63. De Francesco. *The Scientist* 16(5):28. 2002.
64. Feskanich, D. et al. *American Journal of Public Health* 87(6): 992-7.1997.
65. Findings by researchers of the University of Kansas Medical Center presented at the 67th Annual Scientific Meeting of the American College of Gastroenterology summarized in *Research News Companion* for Fall 2002. Published by BioSupplynet, Research Triangle, NC
66. Enattah, N. S. et al. *Nature Genetics* 30: 233-237. 2002.
67. Macdougall, C. F. et al. *Archives of Diseases in Childhood* 86:236-9. 2002.
68. Virtanen, S. et al. *Diabetes* 49:912-7. 2000.
69. Stefferl, A. et al. *Journal of Immunology* 165:2859-65. 2000.
70. Juskevich, J. C. and Guyer, C. G. *Science* 249:875-84. 1990.

Production and structure of CLA's. As a consequence of microbial action on the linoleic acid of ingested plant lipids in the rumen of the cow, a number of isomers of that acid containing conjugated double bonds are produced. These CLAs enter the animal's circulation and are incorporated into lipids of milk and body tissues. There would be nothing very unusual about such metabolism except that the two principal CLAs of milk fat, the cis 9, trans 11 and trans 10, cis 12 exhibit remarkable health-related functions.

Actually there are many CLA isomers produced in the cow, but the important ones in milk are those two. The average amount of CLA in milk fat is about 5 mg per gram of milk fat but there is considerable variation depending on the feed. Most of the total (80 – 90 percent) is normally the cis 9, trans 11 isomer. Another variable in the amount of this latter form of CLA is that there is a significant quantity of a precursor, vaccenic, or more precisely, trans 11 octadecenoic acid in milk fat. The human is capable of desaturating it to the cis 9, trans 11 CLA although the effiency of this process is not known. At times, vaccenic acid may reach a level of 5 percent in milk fat, especially when cows are on spring/summer pasture.

In order to understand CLA and its bioactive forms and properties, it may be helpful to study the structures involved. The reader may also want to consider introductory information on the structure of fatty acids (notes for chapter 2). The normal structure of linoleic acid, a common component of fats and oils, especially of vegetable origin, is that of 18 carbons with two double bonds (C18:2). Those bonds are in the 9 and 12 positions in the carbon chain:

$CH_3\text{-}CH_2\text{-}CH_2\text{-}CH_2\text{-}CH_2\text{-}CH{=}CH\text{-}CH_2\text{-}CH{=}CH\text{-}CH_2\text{-}CH_2\text{-}CH_2\text{-}CH_2\text{-}CH_2\text{-}CH_2\text{-}COOH$

The position of the double bonds in the native plant linoleate is what is known as methylene interrupted because there is a CH_2-group in between them. When such a group is missing, the arrangement is said to be conjugated, i.e., -CH=CH-CH=CH-, in which every other carbon-to-carbon union is a double bond. Conjugation of double bonds is of interest because it influences light absorption. For example, ß-carotene, the principal (yellow) pigment in milk fat, has a conjugated system of 11 double bonds.

A further consideration is that there are two possible configurations a carbon chain may have at the double bond. One is called *cis* in which case the carbon chain is bent back towards itself; and the other is called *trans* which projects the carbon chain away from itself. Thus, linoleic acid and the two CLA isomers have molecular shapes at variance with one another. This circumstance, in which two molecules have closely related size, functional groups and composition but different shapes, may help to explain their differing physiological actions. For example, linoleic acid favors the growth of cancer cells, while cis 9, trans 11 CLA suppresses growth of such cells. This may be a case of competitive inhibition in which the CLA binds to and blocks the cell growth promoting site of action used by linoleic acid.

Formation of homocysteine. Production of homocysteine, the risk factor for heart disease, involves some of the unique chemistry of our bodies. Addition and removal of chemical structures known as methyl (CH_3-) groups are very important reactions for our health and well-being. When the methyl group is removed from the essential amino acid, methionine, the resulting product is homocysteine:

$CH_3\text{-}S\text{-}CH_2\text{-}\ CH_2\text{-}CHNH_2\text{-}COOH\ <{=}>\ CH_3\text{-}\ +\ HS\text{-}CH_2\text{-}\ CH_2\text{-}CHNH_2\text{-}COOH$
(methionine)   (methyl)   (homocysteine)

As shown in the equation, the loss of the methyl group is reversible. In order to prevent this loss and the accumulation of homocysteine, it is necessary to have adequate B vitamins in the diet, particularly B_6, folic acid and B_{12}. These vitamins activate the enzymes that cause remethylation of the homocysteine. Thus too little of those vitamins in the diet can elevate the blood level of homocysteine as can certain genetic disorders.

6

Importance of the Cow
and Production of Milk

Importance of the Cow

As most people understand, the cow is a marvelous creation. It produces huge quantities of milk, a highly nutritious food, from crude plant materials, most of which are useless or unpalatable to us. The purpose of this chapter is to provide important basic information on the cow and how she accomplishes these great things.

Have a Cow?

At some point when I was little, I learned that cows make milk. That seemed pretty impressive. I pondered the idea that some day I might have a cow. As I grew up and actually had some direct experience with cows, the interest in possession remained. Except for rare moments when excited or afraid, cows are docile, friendly, and curious about people. I liked the smell of them and of barns, which are characterized by a mixture of hay, silage, and manure odors. In addition, I greatly appreciated milk. The fact that cows implied beautiful country, farming, and a family activity were also attractive aspects. One could understand how the family cow could become just as much a pet as a dog or cat because cows do something very worthwhile for people. Eventually my hope grew toward having a dairy farm but at the logical time to acquire one, I had no money. Eventually the problem was solved for me in a very unique and highly satisfactory way. I obtained a position at the Pennsylvania State University which at the time had barns full of cows, including one each for the five major dairy breeds. As we will discuss, the role of the cow in our culture goes on and for reasons of efficiency, Penn State has concentrated mainly on the Holstein breed, as has the American dairy industry as a whole. Dairying is definitely shifting to larger operations and the family farm is fading somewhat. But who knows, sometime the family cow may stage a comeback. In any event, we need to spend a few moments on how having a cow got started.

Domestication. Quite naturally, the relationships that ancient humanity developed with animals were driven by self-interest. Taming, training, and use of wild animals, where possible, could help humans to survive and to have a better life. As we do today, mankind had many basic needs including food, clothing, transportation, protection from enemies, and companionship. Domestication of cattle must have seemed a very sensible idea since it could help with a number of those needs, particularly those for food (meat), clothing (leather and hides), and beast-of-burden type operations (hauling, plowing, and transportation).

Cattle domestication must have been a daunting task when first undertaken in Europe about 8,500 years ago. One does not even need to consider the passions of wildness to understand the physical risks presented by cattle. However, a lot of wild instinctive motivation still exists in the cow. Critics talk about how some farmers crowd cows together. They like to be together because in the wild there is safety in numbers. In addition, cows are sometimes subject to mob hysteria. If one becomes frightened, somehow it is instantly communicated to those close by and then there is a stampede. When a domesticated cow decides to move, it can amount to a huge object being on a physically destructive path. In any wild foray, a cow can easily damage herself. In terms of veterinary care and milk production, this can be very costly. For the most part, cows are well behaved, but one should always be alert around them. They can suddenly get out of hand, change direction, smash things and people in their paths. Bulls are even more apt to do such things and their reputation is aptly described by "like a bull in a china shop."

Beyond this rambunctiousness, one wonders how wild cattle managed to survive against their natural enemies? They can run, trample, and gore with their horns. Water buffalo of Africa are known to be extremely tough and ferocious. However, they need to be that way because of large carnivores, such as lions, tigers, and cheetahs who can stalk or run them down, especially their calves. The ancient migration of cattle into Europe must have been highly advantageous to them in providing an escape from those carnivores. It is an interesting coincidence that this also created the basis whereby cattle would become of great value to Europeans.

Despite the risks, domestication of cattle was very worthwhile for humanity. Along with cultivation of plants, the other branch of agriculture, it helped to insure a secure food supply and to eliminate the precarious hunter-gatherer existence that had defined life for humanity and its progenitors over millions of years. A very decisive factor in cattle domestication was that they do not compete with the human for food. Under natural conditions, they graze vegetation, particularly grasses, that grow without cultivation. So all early man had to do was to manage this animal. Today some say that what I have just described, animal husbandry, is wrong. Animals have rights, and it is not fair to use them in such a way. I doubt that this idea even passed through the minds of ancient mankind. They saw animals eating each other and they had to be careful not to get eaten themselves. It must have been a pretty practical business and using animals made a lot of sense. If we bring this question down to the modern world, we find that not all that much has changed. Millions of people still lead primitive lives, starvation is still pretty widespread, and humans still haven't figured out how to treat each other. In addition our many cultural economic relationships with animals and our needs of them are deeply engrained. Most people feel our use of animals under these conditions is necessary and justified.

What's in a name? It is possible for one to become confused regarding various terms used in connection with cows. They are also called bovines, and in a collective sense, cattle. "Bovine" derives from the zoological classification of the sub-family name, *bovinae*, which includes the many breeds of dairy and beef cattle as well as water buffalo of Africa, the American and other bison, yaks, and the cattle of Southeast Asia known as zebu. All these different kinds of cattle are closely related in the way their bodies function and are structured. Except for a few modern day breeds, they all have horns, some of enormous proportions. Dairy cattle are rather massive, have cloven hoofs, multichambered stomachs and feed on grasses and other plant matter. There is a good bit of variation among them regarding size, body conformation, hairy coat, and configuration of horns. The various breeds of dairy and beef cattle are very closely related and became defined in their identities because our forbears selectively bred them to maximize either milk or meat production under a variety of climatic and geographic conditions. In fact, some breeds are used for both purposes, for example, the Shorthorn. Geographic isolation has been another important factor in evolution of the cattle breeds. For example, the Guernsey and Jersey breeds of dairy cattle evolved on islands by those names off the coast of England, the Ayrshire from a location in England, the Brown Swiss from Switzerland and the Holstein from the area of North Germany and the Low Countries.

It is not known exactly when the bovine was domesticated but there is archeological evidence that man was managing livestock 12,000 years ago in the Middle East, and that he has been milking cattle for about 8,500 years. The world of dairy is greatly indebted to Europeans who painstakingly selected animals for milk production and other desirable characteristics during hundreds of years. The major dairy breeds brought from Europe to America were Holsteins, Guernseys, Jerseys, Ayrshires, and Brown Swiss (figure 6.1). Each has unique characteristics and advantages. For example, Guernseys and Jerseys produce milk of relatively higher fat content. Their milk tastes richer than that of other breeds; and it was a better starting material for making butter in the days of home and farm butter production because one needed less milk per pound of butter. Milk fat globules of Guernsey milk are more yellow by nature than those of the other breeds and the milk is often promoted by the term "Golden Guernsey." The Holstein produces a larger volume of milk on average

Figure 6.1

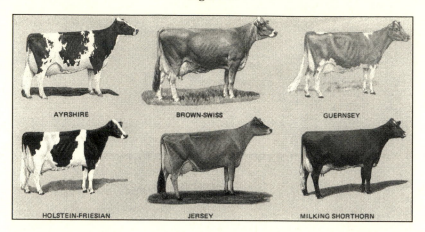

The six major dairy breeds. Photo courtesy of the Purebred Dairy Cattle Association. The classical build of the dairy cow is somewhat bony and angular with the body more or less defining a triangle from nose to udder up to topline and back to nose. Note the more rectangular and well-fleshed body of the Shorthorn which is characteristic of all beef cattle breeds.

than the other breeds. Selective breeding, particularly as aided by very careful record keeping and artificial insemination, boosted the milk production capacity and milk fat and protein output of Holsteins to the point that they have pretty much displaced the other breeds. Counting dry cows and heifers, currently there are about 20,000,000 dairy cows in the U. S., 86 percent of which are Holsteins. This is the big black and white cow. It produces 90 percent of the milk consumed in the U.S. A heifer is a female calf being retained for milk and calf production. They are first bred at about two years of age.

Regarding breeds, there are some shifts occurring. Because of its dual milk and meat use and improvement through selective breeding, the Shorthorn (see figure 6.1), is picking up in popularity, and is considered a sixth member of the major dairy breeds where there used to be five. There also is renewed interest in the Jersey because, in comparison to the Holstein, it takes heat well and produces milk of higher solids content, which in essence means the dairyman is paid more for it.

The great natural beauty and variety in breeds of cattle are brought out very impressively in the book by Rath (see selected references). In these times, there is great breast beating about how we are destroying species. It is not all negative. Humanity has achieved remarkable results through animal breeding and the world's cattle today are a great testimonial to that fact. Who knows, maybe we will get around to creating some wonderful new species.

Figure 6.2

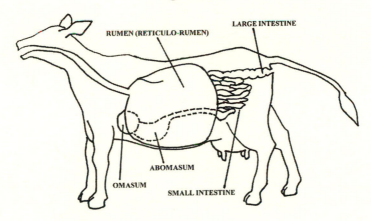

Scheme of the cow's multicompartmented digestive system.

A Cow's Unique Stomachs

A key question is how does the cow get so much more food value out of crude plant materials than we can? The simple answer is because of its unique digestive system. However, the really interesting part is in the details, which virtually defines a cow and how she functions. To begin with, a cow's stomach is unique. Where we have a short tube, known as the esophagus, connecting our mouth to our stomach, the cow has three additional component parts located in that connection route (figure 6.2).

If it were not for those additional "stomachs," the bovine digestive system would not differ in principle from our own. We are known as mono-gastric or single stomached along with cats, dogs, pigs, rodents, and many other animals. The four stomachs of the cow are the rumen, reticulum, omasum, and abomasum. The rumen is a fermentation vessel that occupies a large portion of the body cavity. The rumen and reticulum are often spoken of as one system because the reticulum is a large first pouch within the rumen. Swallowed food from the cow's esophagus first enters the reticulum pouch. While fermentation in the reticulum and the rumen are in equilibrium, the reticulum prevents large fragments of food from moving on in the digestive process. It is from the reticulum that material is regurgitated to the mouth for further chewing, the purpose of which is to mix the food with more saliva and to reduce the size of food fragments. This so-called cud chewing is one of the many familiar characteristics of the cow, just standing there peaceably with jaws in motion. It is not unlike a human chewing gum, but the cow's operation is far more essential to its well-being.

Like the reticulum, the omasum serves to separate fluid from solid matter and direct those phases for further fermentation or digestive action. Fluid is pressed out and allowed to flow on in the digestive system and the compacted solids are retained for further fermentation breakdown. What with more or less constant cud chewing and the functioning of all those stomachs, the cow does a superb job of getting what it needs out of things like grass, leaves, stems, stalks, and other crude materials. Such animals as goats, sheep, deer, antelope, moose, and elk, which also have rumens, survive in like manner. Goats are superior survivors. Left deserted on islands by humans, they have been known to consume every blade of grass and every green leaf on shrub or tree such that an island which was originally green and forested is rendered bare. Sometimes the goats are able to go on, undergoing near starvation until the next rainfall restores some plant life. As one can readily observe, sheep will graze a pasture to the point that the grass is as short as a golf putting green.

The main purpose of all those stomachs in ruminant animals is to make special improvements in the nutritive value of the relatively crude plant foods they ingest and get it ready for classical digestive action in the true stomach (abomasum) and the intestines. Note that these processes need a large amount of water. A dry cow requires about ten gallons of water a day. During lactation, twice that much or more is needed depending on the nature of the feed and the amount of milk being produced.

The rumen. The first part of the cow's digestive system, known as the rumen or reticulorumen, is a fermentation chamber with a capacity of forty to sixty gallons. A complex mixture of microorganisms comprised of bacteria and one-celled animals, called protozoa, break down the grass, leaves, stems, stalks, seeds, etc. into components usable by both the microorganisms and the cow. A piece of equipment which is designed to produce desirable products through action of living cells is known in the technology trade as a bioreactor. The rumen of the cow, and related species, is the living model of such a reactor demonstrating once again that Nature got there first. A unique aspect of the rumen fermentation is that a portion of the constantly multiplying microorganisms are moved on continuously with the digesta to become food for the cow. So these microorganisms not only break down the plant material into substances that can be used for nourishment and milk production, they multiply greatly in numbers and are themselves utilized as food further along in the digestive tract. As a result of the nutrients they make available from the ingested plant material, vitamins and other micronutrients they synthesize during the fermentation, and the nutrient content of their bodies', these microorganism are a tremendous boon to the cow and milk production.

Another unique activity of rumen bacteria is the breakdown of cellulose into products that are useful to them and to the cow. The human cannot digest cellulose. At times we may gain some minor caloric benefit from bacterial fermentation and absorption of products derived from it in the colon. Primarily, ingested foods containing cellulose contribute to the fiber and fecal bulk in human digesta. Considering the huge amount of cellulose tied up in the biomass of the world, this is unfortunate. It brings to mind things like implanting an artificial rumen in the human; or more practical, a genetic "fix" to enable us to digest cellulose. Such measures might help allay starvation in some areas of the world. It would be a sort of ultimate vegetarianism by which we could go gnaw the bark off of trees if they weren't under environmental protection.

A dividend to the cow resulting from the rumen fermentation of cellulose and other carbohydrates is the production of volatile fatty acids (VFAs). These are acetic, propionic and butyric acids. They are termed volatile because they readily evaporate into the air, and like most such substances, they have odor. Acetic acid is responsible for the pungent smell and sour taste of vinegar. Propionic acid is a principal flavor and odor component of Swiss cheese. Butyric acid contributes strongly to the odor and flavor of grating-type cheeses, such as Romano. In high concentration, its odor has an unpleasant fecal character. The cow makes very good use of the VFAs. Because they are small molecules, they readily pass from the rumen and the digestive tract into the circulation. From there they are readily used in the synthesis of milk and for the cow's own metabolic needs involving glucose, fat and energy requirements.

Yet another unique action in the rumen is the phenomenon of lipid hydrogenation. In essence this is the conversion of unsaturated fatty acids, from the consumed plant material, to saturated fatty acids (see also notes for chapter 2). Our most intimate association with this is through the labels on snacks and other processed foods which often contain hydrogenated cottonseed and/or soybean oil. Those particular hydrogenations are carried out by humans using a chemical reactor and hydrogen under pressure in the presence of a catalyst. Such commercial hydrogenation enables vegetable oil processors to convert oils into products with semisolid properties that make them more suitable as spreads (margarine) and as processed food ingredients. Whether in the cow's rumen or in a commercial hydrogenator, the principal is the same, addition of hydrogen to unsaturated fatty acids which partially or fully saturates them thus raising the temperatures at which they melt. The main product of the process in the rumen is stearic acid, a hard white solid at room temperature. Commercial hydrogentation produces the same acid in the seed oils. However, because the treatment is only partial, the yield of stearic acid is less. The cow is very well adjusted to absorbing the stearic acid into its circulation and using it. The rumen also produces a number of other unique fatty acids as a result of microbial activity and hydrogenation, see the discussion of conjugated linoleic acids (CLAs), chapter 5 and its notes.

Another facet of fat use in the cow that reflects back on the activity in the rumen is incorporation of rumen microbial fatty acids into her body and milk. That is, the fatty acids making up the structure of the bacterial and protozoal cells are released into the digesta, absorbed into the circulation and then are handled like fatty acids from the feed. For this reason, it is estimated conservatively that 10 percent of milk fat is derived from the lipids of rumen microorganisms. Because of the rumen and the complexity of its reactions and effects within the cow, bovine milk will never be easily and closely imitated. This is particularly true with respect to bioactivity of components present in milk at low concentrations. Some of them are being characterized, such as the CLAs, but many may never be defined. This is also true of milk flavor. Not only is its imitation an everlasting challenge but so are the flavors milk imparts and develops in products such as cheeses, ice cream and cultured milks (see also chapters 7 and 8). To be able to imitate the rich flavor of regular full-fat ice cream without the fat has been one of the holy grails of dairy research.

To summarize, the unique actions in the rumen on food ingested by the cow are: digestion of cellulose, production of volatile acids, hydrogenation of fatty acids and continuous production of protozoa and bacteria. All of this is going on more or less continuously and simultaneously. These capabilities render the cow very efficient in digesting plant material as food and using the products to make milk. In the broader sense, this applies also to the production of meat by both beef and dairy breeds.

Feeding Cows

In certain areas of the world, such as parts of Africa, India, and the Middle East, domestic cattle can be kept outdoors year round, and if there is plenty of good pasture, they might not require any special kinds of supplemental feeding. However, the domestication of cattle in seasonally cold climates, such as in the northern parts of Europe and the United States; and the development of dairying as a commercial endeavor presented farmers with the problems of feeding and housing cattle on a year round basis. This led to development of barns, feed preservation and supplementation of pasture grazing with additional feedstuffs to maximize milk production. A further consideration is that most cattle of European ancestry do not do well under climatic conditions of intense sun and heat. For example, Holsteins, the large black and white cow, can actually get sunburned, and their milk production suffers when summer temperatures go into the 80s and 90s. So at least shade is required and even fans under such conditions.

In the beginning there were two basic means of preserving plant materials for subsequent feeding to cattle: one was natural sun and air drying at the end of the growing period, as practiced in the production of hay and grain; and the other was making of silage, the process whereby a crop is chopped up, with or without additives and preservatives, placed in storage and allowed to ferment. Bacteria on the chopped up plant carry out a fermentation which develops acidity thereby stabilizing the material against further decomposition and preserving its food value. The situation has considerable analogy to making sauerkraut. In principle, the cabbage is shredded, layered in a jar or barrel, the layers are successively salted and then the whole is allowed to ferment. The resulting sauerkraut (sour cabbage) will keep more or less indefinitely. The most common plant for ensilage in the United States is corn but many other materials are so treated. At a proper point of maturity, the plant is cut off a few inches above the soil and the whole thing, corn ears, stalks, leaves, tassels, and all is mechanically chopped and transported into a silo, a tall cylindrical storage structure. As mentioned, there often are additives such as lactic acid or metabisulfite. In today's dairy world, hay and ensilage are massively produced and there are other varied forms such as haylage and green chop. It takes many tons of these materials to feed a large herd of cows. The production of them is still something of an art but it also requires a lot of technology. Hay needs cooperative weather for the drying. If it is bailed containing too much moisture, it can become moldy, a condition that can sicken cows. Moldy silage is also bad. Like other crops, forages for cows depend on the weather. So there is a lot to know and quite a bit of risk in growing and preparing storable feeds for cattle.

Basic requirements. Feed accounts for about 50 percent of the cost of producing milk. Thus, it is essential for dairymen to exercise good feed management. Both the health of the cows and the size of the milk check depend on it; and it is quite a complex task requiring expert knowledge of ruminant (cow) nutrition and markets for feedstuffs. Calculating a balanced ration for high-producing cows out of a large array of available feed ingredients, and at an acceptable cost, is challenging. Along with maintaining records for the individual animals in a herd, ration calculations are a computer operation.

There are a number of ways to meet the needs for human expertise in feeding cows. In these days of ever-larger dairy farm operations, some are big enough that the ownership can afford a professional manager trained in dairy science, including both the animal and economic aspects. There also are family dairy farm operations where a son or daughter went to the state university and obtained the necessary training to carry on the business. Another solution is for the farmer to lean on the university agricultural extension service for help. This can be a very constructive move in which the extension agent analyzes your problem and points you in the right direction for little or no charge. It may mean you have to take a couple of short courses at the university, buy a computer with appropriate software, and learn how to use them. However, it may save your business, make it thrive and also bring you up-to-date.

On the other hand, let's say your hands are full with demands of the farm, family, and life in general. Your are already trying to master too many things in an era of increasing specialization, and to get deep into cow nutrition, economics of ration costs and their calculations is just too much. Yet you can't afford to hire a manager. This seems to call for the dairy nutrition consultant. Such a person will develop the information you need, check in with you at regular intervals to see how things are working, and do any necessary corrections or fine-tuning. Talented consultants can easily pay for themselves in saving on feed costs, veterinary bills, management efficiencies, and new ideas. They also may enable an operator to get along with one less full-time employee and all that involves, such as wages plus medical coverage, retirement program, income tax withholding, workmen's compensation, and so on.

The menu. Cattle feeding involves special terms, some of which one must master in order to better understand the cow and how it lives. There is first of all *forage*, which in its primitive sense refers to what cattle ate when they were wandering around in the wild, primarily grass. The current usage usually means *forage crops.* These are plants specially grown to feed cattle, such as, grasses, legumes, grains, corn, sorghum, and so on. They can be fed standing, harvested or preserved in various ways. *Concentrates* are grains and other high-energy feedstuffs. *Roughages* are mainly dried structural plant materials of relatively high cellulose and low energy content. Examples are corn stalks, corncobs, wheat straw and seed hulls. *Legumes* are a large family of flowering plants which have specialized nodules on their roots. These nodules contain bacteria that "fix" atmospheric nitrogen in the soil, which is in essence a fertilization process. This helps plants to grow. Thus, many crop rotation programs on the farm attempt to have a period in which a legume is grown because it will fertilize the soil for a non-leguminous plant grown there subsequently. Legumes used as forage crops for cattle include alfalfa, clover, and soybeans. Generally a cow's total ration will contain each of these major feedstuffs in some proportion because it is well established they all play a constructive role in bovine nutrition and milk production.

Alfalfa. A crop that is a great food for animals and an improver of the soil is almost too good to be true. This is the forage crop for cattle known as alfalfa or lucerne. It is of very great importance in the United States and throughout the world. Introduced into America during colonial days, both George Washington and Thomas Jefferson grew it on their plantations but not very successfully. Until soil chemistry and plant nutrition were better established, it was not clear why crops would succeed for one farmer but not for others. Eventually it was shown that to thrive, alfalfa needs calcium in the soil to reduce the acidity. In some locations, the calcium was present naturally as limestone; in other locations, it needed to be added. In a good growing year or with irrigation, alfalfa yields a number of cuttings. As explained above, it is a legume, a plant that enriches the soil by depositing nitrogen in it. A typical stand of alfalfa is three to five years old before it is rotated to some other crop.

Other items. Beyond what cows consume by grazing pastures, the variety of materials they can use as food is quite amazing. In the not too distant past, it was simply hay, corn silage and grain concentrate. Table 6.1 presents major categories of feed ingredients currently utilized by cows and other ruminants. Remember that any single category may involve many specific items; for example, grains and seeds would include corn, wheat, oats, barley, hominy, soybeans, cottonseeds and others. In addition, items in these various categories can be fractionated and processed in many ways to facilitate their incorporation into feed mixtures and to enhance their palatability and utilization by the animals. These include: milling, chopping, rolling, heating, steaming, drying, fermenting, and other means of preservation. All in all, it turns out to be quite a menu. One thing making this possible is that cows are not particularly picky eaters.[1] Even in the case of unpalatable materials, cows can be encouraged to eat by mixing or covering the problematic ingredient with things that they like, such as molasses, silage or grain. Thinking about the menu from the dairyman's standpoint, he has the problem of feeding a balanced ration all year long that will keep the cows healthy and producing milk at a profit. This is quite a demanding project. Some crops are seasonal, the availability of many ingredients he could use fluctuate; and on top of everything else is the need to consider feed costs. Thus, it is fortunate that the potential menu is large.

Table 6.1

Forage crops	Crop wastes	Food-processing wastes	Fiber-processing wastes	Protein substitutes	Animal wastes
Legumes	Straw	Corn factory	Wood fines	Urea	Blood meal
Grasses	Corn-stalks	Apple pomace	Paper	Anhydrous-ammonia	Meat meal
Corn silage	Pea vines	Beet pulp	Cardboard		Bone meal
Grain	Bean vines	Brewers grain	Cottonseed hulls		Fish meal
Sorghum		Distillers grain			Feather meal
		Soyhulls			
		Oil meals			
		Bakery waste			
		Milling by-products			

Ingredient sources that are utilized in preparing feedstuffs for cows and other ruminants. Reproduced with permission from *From Feed to Milk....* by Ishler et al. (see Selected references at end of chapter).

The Cow as a Cultural Icon—Or Love that Cow

In America, the cow has been thoroughly absorbed and enjoyed in the culture. There are cow trinkets, gadgets, toys, and jewelry. Lots of cow art is displayed in pictures, murals, and on clothing. A cow was used as a trademark/promo by one of the big computer companies until recently. There is plenty of outlandish cow humor in the form of newspaper columns,[2] greeting cards, and cartoons about them. One of our neighbors has several life-size cow statues posing in his front yard. This is something of a joke here in La Jolla, California where most of the lots are like postage stamps but there is some irony in it, too. Early in the last century (1906), there were dairy farms in La Jolla Shores and the cows enjoyed wading in the ocean just like the natives and tourists do to day. Gary Larson, the famous humor artist, has produced many wonderful cartoons involving cows. One favorite of mine shows a group of cows in a pasture standing upright together on their hind legs socializing and one of them, pointing to a car approaching in the distance, yells, "Car!" In the next panel, the cows are down on all fours munching pasture grass. Another of his many great contributions is in figure 6.3.

A great appreciation of the cow exists in many of us. This seems to have reached an ultimate in India where the Hindu religion dictates that cows are sacred. However, the recent cow cultural event in Chicago demonstrates that the American also has a strong capacity to identify with this animal. Cows on Parade™ ran in Chicago from June 15 to October 31, 1999. Three hundred plastic, life-sized, and life-like cows were creatively decorated as objects of art and displayed for the enjoyment of residents and visitors to the city. Of course, a major purpose of the event was to promote the enterprises and artists sponsoring the individual cows. The overall response was unexpectedly large and very positive. We searched for what about the cow made this event so successful. It seems that cows are viewed as large, friendly and maternal. Somehow they seem to make it easier for us to connect with each other. Chicagoans apparently went crazy over their cows. This was an astutely promoted event but the cows sure made it a success.

Don't Have a Cow?

Despite the immense practical importance of cattle to humanity and the enjoyment they provide us, there are those who want to break up that relationship. As previously mentioned, the attacks are at many levels and often indirect. Shouldn't we have a cow if we want one? Let's look at some of the issues.

Against the grain. A favorite ploy of the animal rights/vegetarian activists is: feeding grain to animals is wasteful because it is needed by starving humans. Of course, as animal rights defenders, they could as logically protest that the animals have just as much right to the grain as humans do, but that one isn't

Figure 6.3

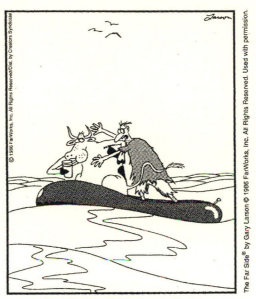

"Hey! That's milk! And you said you
were all empty, you stinkin' liar!"

Gary Larson cartoon.

convenient for them here. Appealing as it may sound, the "starving humans" argument doesn't have much substance. Foremost, there already is enough food for everyone, the real problem being to get it to those who need it. Especially vicious are political leaders in various parts of the world who use donated food, and money gained by selling it, as a weapon to reward their friends and control or eliminate their enemies—children be damned.

Perhaps the most incredible action of this type is the current rejection of food donations to starving peoples of Africa by some of the political leaders there.[3] This summer (2002) has been especially unfavorable to agriculture in many parts of Africa. The basis of the rejections is that GM (genetically modified) foods are involved and that they will poison the people. Food crops, such as corn, soybeans, and rice, have been genetically modified to enhance yields, resistance to insects and weed killers, and to improve nutritional qualities. A modification of rice to increase its vitamin A (carotene) potential is a particularly impressive improvement. This change alone should help to prevent blindness in millions of people. GM foods have the approval of agencies in the United States and the United Nations. Americans have been eating GM foods for years without problems. Even if there were some risk involved, would you rather consign your people to starvation? Greed is another factor. Sometimes the food, earmarked as a gift to the poor and starving is sold by local intermediates to the highest bidder. With tricks like these, why blame human hunger on feeding some grain (GM?) to cows, which in any event, give back something.

Another consideration in the grain argument, as already explained, cattle do not naturally compete with humans for food. Crude plant material is good for them and of no use to us. In fact, by digesting and utilizing cellulose a major plant constituent, something we cannot do, they make milk and meat which supplement and enrich our food supply. As is common knowledge, whether or not any given farmer is going to feed grain to cattle is determined by a complex of local conditions in his area of the world which determine whether it is efficient and profitable to do so. Grassland farming, which utilizes little or no grain feeding, is practiced in many areas of the world, including parts of the United States. Because of rainfall and soil conditions in New Zealand, a grassland farming country, much of the pastureland is lush and ideal for milk, lamb, and wool production, extremely important items in the country's economy. There is a great deal of flexibility in what can be fed to animals used for meat and milk production; but what actually is fed at any given time and location depends on market factors, particularly what feed ingredients are available, their prices, what will make a nutritionally balanced ration, and consumer expectations. For example, at the moment, American consumers are asking for leaner beef and leaner meat in general, which means less feeding of grain used to fatten animals for market. Grain feeding produces greater "marbling" of the meat with fat. This has favorable effects on flavor and texture. No doubt it will always be preferred by some customers.

In any case, focusing on grain feeding is misleading, cows can consume and utilize a wide array of agricultural byproducts that are unusable as human food. Spent grain left from the making of alcoholic beverages has been fed to cows for over 150 years. The needs of cattle for protein can be met in substantial degree by including simple forms of nitrogen, such as urea and ammonia in their feed. This works because the rumen organisms are able to make proteins using those raw materials. By coincidence, urea and ammonia are used as fertilizers to make plants grow. So fertilizing the cow with them could be considered a short cut that reduces the necessity in some circumstances of feeding them grain or protein concentrates.

Don't read it. Eat it or sleep on it. Regarding the feeding of industrial byproducts to cattle, there is a rather sensational research story involving one of my colleagues, Earl Kesler, at Penn State. He and his students fed cows and growing heifers chopped up newspapers mixed with molasses, a byproduct of the refined sugar industry. Both milk production of the cows and growth of the heifers were satisfactorily supported and the animals had no visible health problems.[4] Further to the point that cows are flexible in what they can eat, Arturi Virtanen, Nobel laureate of Finland, maintained a herd of cows on a completely synthetic diet comprised of cellulose, simple forms of nitrogen, minerals and vitamins.[5] Thus, the "grain-eating cow is starving humans" argument is simplistic, misleading, and, at the moment, literally not true. Another thing which Professor Kesler and his associates discovered is that cut-up newspapers also make good bedding for cows. Don't save a tree. You could be robbing some cow of her food and bedding. Hug a cow instead.

A waste of land. Another of the anti-cattle arguments is that the cow and animal agriculture in general is an inefficient and inappropriate use of the land. On that one, they are joined by some environmentalists. However, it doesn't hold up any better than the grain complaint. It is an oversimplification to state that dairy farming wastes land. Generally, supply and demand determine what happens to land in the U.S., and many different kinds of land are used here for dairy farming. Cattle can be grown and well maintained on very limited land as is clearly evident from many large milk production units in California on very limited acreage. What big modern dairy herds require are a few acres for some exercise and fresh air. The feed is often grown in other areas where it is economical to do so and the rainfall or irrigation is supportive. It is then shipped where needed. Actually the total land use situation in California is pretty unusual. It is a big state and in comparison to other countries, is said to have the sixth or seventh biggest economy in the world. It has 25 million people with about three-fourths of its total population living within five or ten miles of the ocean. What about the rest of the state? It is relatively empty. Grassland farming of dairy cows is practiced in many areas of the world today, including parts of the U.S. Such farming enables less grain feeding especially where pastures are lush year around. There are very large land areas in the United States and throughout the world for which the best use is animal grazing, in fact, some locations aren't fit for much else. How much of it will be used for that purpose, depends on the return to the investor of doing so, just as in any other business activity. For some families in the third world, it could be a good return if they only had the money for even a small investment.

The challenge. Twenty-seven years ago, we wrote, "Because the rumen is able to utilize crude cellulosic and fibrous plant materials and simple forms of nitrogen such as urea in generating high-quality nutrients in it rumen, the ruminant does not need to compete with man because man's digestive system cannot derive food value from such materials. So there is a challenge to put ruminant agriculture on an equivalent economic basis throughout the world. Meat and milk from the ruminants are an important basis of the good life in Western culture and these commodities could go a long way in fighting malnutrition and starvation in the rest of the world."[6] There have been signs of progress. For example, Japan has a thriving dairy industry[7] and China is making a major effort to establish a beef industry. However, considering the world as a whole, there is a long way to go yet in meeting the challenge.

One trouble with discussions about the world food supply problem, is the assumption that humanity will just continue to stand there and get run over. Our rise from hunting and gathering is a testimonial to human ingenuity, resourcefulness, and creativity. Further, even the best efforts to predict what lies ahead are fraught with uncertainties. We don't hear quite so much about the population explosion lately as birthrates are coming down all over the world. We should be thankful for our great capacities to contrive and adapt.

Agriculture and the environment. Despite efforts to paint American agriculture as backward on environmental issues, it is not. There is a concerted effort toward the "sustainable/renewable" approach. In other words, all practices that are using are also, at the same time, aimed at retaining and restoring. Agricultural extension services of the state universities have developed and are promoting such programs. One example out of many is the statewide Environmental Stewardship Program centered at the University of California, Davis. Another is LEAP, the Livestock Environmental Assurance Program involving Ohio State University and various other agencies in Ohio.

Ongoing constructive efforts not withstanding, the anti-cow environmentalists are heard to complain: manure stinks, is filthy and pollutes. Anyone who has walked across a pasture in the spring knows that manure is a good fertilizer. The grass and weeds that grow up next to a "cow pie" are greener and bigger than those a short distance away. So there is some good in manure. When one talks about organic farming and using "natural" as opposed to "chemical" fertilizers, then the environmentalists say manure is ok. The fact that it puts fecal and possibly pathogenic bacteria next to plants used for human food may not be ok. And on the other hand, environmentalists claim that manure washes into streams thereby polluting them, and that dairy farming produces soil erosion and contamination of the atmosphere (methane, hydrogen, and CO_2. Don't even breathe!).

Others have been thinking more positively about the manure. In a forward-looking plan to optimize the cattle/environment interaction, interest groups in South Dakota have banded together and are seeking federal and other support to create what they call a "Green Machine."[8] The organization, known as ValCap for Dakota Value Capture Cooperative, proposes to use the waste from some 28,000 beef cattle to prime a biorefining complex that will generate methane (natural gas), which will be used to heat boilers in an ethanol plant. Corn will be used to make the ethanol which will go into gasoline. Residue from the corn-to-ethanol step will be supplied to the cattle as a protein-rich feed supplement. The steps in this biocycling, which would be just as applicable to dairy cattle, are shown in figure 6.4. This ambitious and creative idea will bear watching. It could provide an excellent model of good environmental practice for widespread adoption if it works. Even if it doesn't, it illustrates the point that environmental dilemmas are also opportunities, not insoluble problems.

Figure 6.4

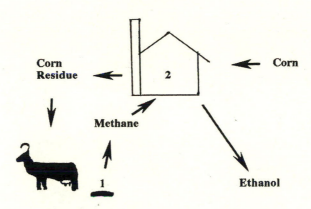

The South Dakota cattle waste biocycle. Manure from cattle (1) goes to a bioreactor where bacteria produce biogas (methane) from it. This gas is used to provide energy in a plant (2) that converts corn to ethanol by fermentation. The ethanol is used to fuel automobiles, and corn residue from the fermentation is fed to the cattle which produce more manure.

Trying to keep up with all the one-liners and non-sequiturs against animal agriculture is quite impossible and hardly necessary. However, it is a reasonable expectation in this country that any complaint will be listened to and acted on if it has real merit and is in the best interests of most people. No doubt there are infractions on land use and zoning laws by individual farm operations. Our system of government is well designed to settle such issues if the parties themselves cannot. Further, like most other large and diverse human enterprises, dairy farming is capable of being improved in some ways and in certain locations, but that isn't what many activists want. They would like nothing less than complete failure and eradication of the dairy industry.

The family cow? In all likelihood, the cow/human relationship was quite simple in the beginning. The indications are that most owners of cows in Ireland had just one or two animals and this practice probably went back for hundreds if not thousands of years. In seventeenth- and eighteenth-century America, families had a cow or two. It is hard to know whether a culture involving a pet family cow as a source of milk would pass inspection with the anti-milk activists, or whether the sacredness and religious respect accorded cows used for milk in India would suffice. Probably not. There are those that believe animals are just as important as humans and nothing should be done to interfere with an animal's life. Where does that leave the millions of pets that humans keep and control? Animal rights activists are against people having pets.

Cow philosophy. When one considers how tremendously beneficial the cow is and has been to humanity, it is hard to understand why some people try to discredit all that. It is evident that many people have intense feelings and have done a great deal of thinking about animals. Obviously there must be differences among us regarding basic assumptions about the cow's purposes in this life. While such differences can't be bridged by discussion or debate, the reader may be interested in some pertinent considerations. Many people are guided by the Bible which has this to say in the Old Testament about our care and use of animals:

> Then God said, Let us make humankind in our image, according to our likeness; and let them have dominion over the fish of the sea, and over the birds of the air, and over cattle, and over all the wild animals of the earth, and over every creeping thing that creeps upon the earth. (Genesis 1:26)

That seems pretty clear. According to it, we are put in charge of the animals. Coupled with the accepted use of animals for their milk in other contexts (see, chapter 1), the Bible is supportive of using livestock for their milk.

There is also the broadly based principle of being helpful to others that is embraced across lines of many beliefs and philosophies. From that standpoint, humanity looks with particular favor on vocations involving service to others, such as, teaching, legal and medical services, the military, the Peace Corps, and so on. At least in that sense, the life of a cow is a great and admirable thing. They aren't known as "the foster mothers of the human race" for nothing.

Perhaps we need to ponder what higher, better purpose the cow could have in this life. In my view, the existing cow/human situation is win/win. Living with them is a distinct cultural plus in many ways; they provide us with milk, meat and an industry that makes a living for millions of people. We give them plenty of food, barns with music, fresh air, exercise, health care and, where possible, nice pastures. All of them do not live perfect lives. Who does? The cows I've known have been contented. Ironically, the old profit motive works to the cow's benefit. If they aren't treated right and maintained in good health, they don't give much milk. So it pays to be nice to cows. True, we don't provide them with retirement villages for seniors but even the environmentalists don't want them around if all they are going to do is eat, poop and take up space. One thing is certain, we haven't seen anything yet. The bovine mammary gland is a fabulous producer of proteins. Among other things, it is being customized by gene manipulation to mass produce human proteins of all kinds including those needed for infant formula and in the field of human medicine.

* * *

The cow is a profound gift to humanity. A capacity to convert a large quantity and array of crude vegetation into milk makes her of unique value. Not only is bovine milk at one and the same time a nutritious food and a refreshing beverage, it has also served as a source of other greatly appreciated foods, such as, cheese, ice cream, and butter. Like other changing aspects of our culture, the management of the millions of cows making up the modern dairy industry presents some problems. In the main, these have been acknowledged and are being dealt with constructively.

Production of Milk

In the first part of this section, we extend the subject of milk secretion, discussed at the cellular/molecular level in chapter 2, to include the cow's udder. From a practical standpoint, it is a most awesome set of secretory glands.

The Udder. In the normal udder, there are four separate glands of approximately equal size. For expression of milk, each gland is served by a separate teat. For purposes of identity, the four glands are designated front or rear, left or right. On rare occasions cows will be born with a non-functional quarter or teat. More frequently there may be a noticeable variations in size of the quarters. All four quarters function in the same way. As explained in chapter 2, the number of glands is a variable among the species of mammals. The reason for four in the cow is to assure an adequate supply of milk for the maximum number of offspring. There appears to be a substantial insurance factor because cows almost never have quadruplets. However, they do have twins and in the wild, extra outlets may be needed to foster nurse other calves or to compensate for wounds to the udder.

The alveolar cells that make and secrete milk are arranged around a central lumen (open space) into which the milk is secreted. The lumens are connected by tube-like structures known as ducts. Thus, the milk can flow out of the alveolar lumens into the ducts and the smaller ducts lead to larger ones which eventually lead to the nipple, or teat as it is called in the cow. The actual mechanisms involved in milk secretion from the cell are described in greater detail in chapter 2.

Bovine mammary tissue at relatively low microscope magnification has the appearance shown in figure 6.5 (right). The alveoli which produce and secrete milk are connected by a duct system through which the milk flows to the teat and they are supported structurally by a matrix of collagen. In figure 6.5 (left), a cross-sectional scheme of a bovine udder quarter including its teat is shown. In comparison to the human mammary gland, which has fifteen or twenty relatively small ducts separately bringing milk to the nipple, the bovine gland has much larger ducts bringing milk to an accumulation area. The lower end of this region forms a hollow cistern in the center of the teat. Milk in the cistern can be withdrawn through a channel at the end of the teat either by suckling of the calf or by mechanical expression, that is, milking. The channel, known as the streak canal, is normally kept closed by sphincter muscles. This is the same kind of muscle control that keeps the anus and urinary bladder closed. On rare occasions there will be a cow, approaching milking time, that leaks milk. Serious

Figure 6.5

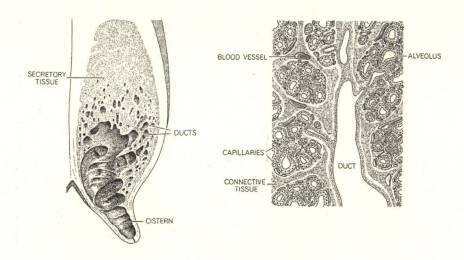

An artist's rendition of the structure of lactating bovine mammary tissue as seen under low magnification in the microscope, right; and of an intact bovine mammary gland (udder quarter), left. Milk synthesized in cells of alveoli is secreted into central lumens of the alveoli from whence it flows through the duct system into the teat cistern, lower left, where is can be removed by nursing or milking. (Reproduced from Patton, S. Scientific American 221(1):58-68. 1969.) For an actual micrograph of bovine lactating tissue, (see fig. 2.2 in chapter 2).

leakers are usually culled from the herd.

The bovine teat, which varies from about two to four inches in length, is an interesting species variation. Unlike the infant human, which has a flat face, the calf has an elongated mouth structure. The evolved teat of the cow not only fits the calf's mouth but it is so designed to deliver a lot of milk relatively quickly which meets the substantial energy and growth needs of a baby weighing close to a hundred pounds at birth. The human situation is entirely different. The breast is relatively small, it delivers milk quite slowly through a short nipple. The newborn baby is small, slow growing and relatively inactive compared to a calf. Not surprisingly both systems work well. However, fortunately for humanity, the cow's teat lends itself well to hand or machine milking.

Milking

It can be seen from the scheme of the udder, figure 6.6, that constriction of the teat at the point where it joins the udder (arrows) traps milk in the teat. Then, if the teat is compressed, milk has nowhere to go except out through the streak canal at the bottom of the teat. It is this precise combination of mechanical

Figure 6.6

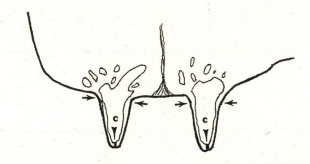

Scheme of the front and rear quarters on one side of a cow's udder showing where constriction is needed (arrows) in order to trap milk in the cisterns (C) so that it can be squeezed out through the streak canals (arrowheads).

effects that is brought about by the hand of the person doing the milking. In hand milking, the constriction at the top of the teat is accomplished by encircling and squeezing at that point with the thumb and forefinger. Then progressive pressure can be exerted down the teat with the other fingers forcing out the trapped milk. The primary problem encountered by the uninitiated is that they think all one needs to do is squeeze the teat. Without any constriction at the top of the teat, that just forces the milk up into the udder. Before the invention of the milking machine in 1903 and its gradual adoption, the only way to obtain milk from a cow was by hand. In the United States there is no longer any hand milking on commercial dairy farms. However, in many other areas of the world, hand milking of cows, goats, sheep, horses and camels continues as it has for thousands of years.

Milking machines. In essence, a milking machine is a device that delivers pulses of suction to the four teats of a cow in order to remove milk from the udder. It functions mechanically very much as does a nursing calf. The difference is that the machine acts on all four quarters of the udder at once, whereas the calf does one-at-a-time, two if there are twins. The essential parts of the machine are four cups that fit onto the teats and four hoses which connect the cups to a receiving bucket for collecting the milk. This system is connected through a pulsator to a vacuum line maintaining a suitable vacuum by means of a pump which is usually remote from the milking operation. The timing of the pulsator allows removal of all the milk that has accumulated in the teat and closely associated larger ducts and then an interruption of the vacuum for a period of time sufficient to allow additional milk in the udder to drain down into the region of the teat. This pulsating vacuum system continues pumping milk from the udder until there is no practical amount of milk becoming available for removal. At that point the milk (machine) is weighed, credited to the particular cow and transferred to a holding tank. The machine is then readied for attachment to the next cow. The washing and sterilizing of the teat cups after each individual milking is very important.

In more recent barn installations and milking parlors, milking machines are more or less built into the permanent structure. Each milking, the quantity of which is weighed and recorded electronically, is pumped to a holding tank. Any milk collecting flasks and all pipelines are cleaned in place. However, the teat cups and their connecting lines remain detachable. For further information on care use and research findings regarding milking machines, see Schmidt et al.[9]

The Rotolactor. Henry W. Jeffers, one of the greatest dairymen of all times, contributed in many ways to the advancement of the industry. He developed certified milk, that is, raw (unpasteurized) milk produced under the utmost standards of sanitation and cleanliness. He made many contributions to improved breeding, feeding, and management of cows. Perhaps most prominently, he invented the Rotolactor, a merry-go-round on which cows could be milked. The cow stepped onto a round rotating floor where she was washed and machine milked in one revolution. About ten cows could be accommodated at one time on this moving system. The Rotolactor and many of the advanced ideas of Jeffers were put into practice by him at the Walker-Gordon Farm near Princeton, N.J. Among other things, the cow manure was dried, bagged and sold as a lawn and garden fertilizer under the name of Bovung. He developed this farm into a showplace operation. His facility for imaginative public relations produced a truly great accomplishment at the New York World's Fair in 1939. The Borden Company, a major processor of milk and milk products at that time, had decided to participate with an exhibit at the Fair. Jeffers convinced Borden's management and others involved, that this shouldn't be the conventional milking of a few cows, but a grand display of 150 top-quality animals from the five major breeds being housed on-site and milked on a Rotolactor. This turned out to be an extremely successful exhibit. Jeffers' and Borden's grandiose dream entertained and informed millions of people in a very constructive way about the dairy world.

In many respects, the Rotolactor with its progressing and simultaneous (machine) milking of cows was the forerunner of the modern milking parlor. On the other hand, it was quite an investment at the time and well beyond the financial reach of most dairy farmers. Further, it was not sufficiently flexible and practical for widespread adoption. The physical limits on how many cows could be accommodated at one time were bound to limit its usefulness in the rapidly growing herd sizes in the United States. There is no question that Jeffers had a great idea for an impressive exhibition of cows being milked. Further, his vision is embodied in some modern dairies with as many as eighty cows on one giant rotating circular floor

Milking parlors. When most people hear the term "milking parlor," they probably wonder what that means? It conjures up possibilities for a Gary Larson cartoon with cows sitting around in comfortable chairs in a sunlit room visiting with each other while they are being milked. Actually that may not be too far from the truth in some instances. In essence, a milking parlor is any structure that allows cows to enter and leave an area specially equipped for their milking. It can be simply a situation in which cows in a line pass through a location in a barn where their udders can be sanitized and milked; or it can be a gleaming modern facility fully equipped to milk ninety cows simultaneously.

In order to obtain some fresh raw cow's milk for research a few years ago, on several occasions I visited a more rudimentary but nonetheless effective milking operation. It was a family owned business in coastal southern California that produced, processed and distributed milk. There were 800 cows being milked around the clock by three shifts of workers. This pretty much amounted to a never-ending stream of animals to be milked. Because of the relatively favorable year round weather at this location barns could be quite open and simple, being needed only to provide periodic shelter or shade. From a milk production standpoint this was what is known as a "dry lot" operation on fifteen or twenty acres and quite characteristic of southern California. In that region, expensive real estate, lack of rain to sustain pastures, and the high cost of transporting milk all encourage maintaining large numbers of cows on limited acres close to the masses of milk consumers along the coast. Whether or not such an enterprise fulfills ones notion of an ideal dairy farm, it can and does produce a lot of excellent milk.

Against the preceding story of down-to-earth dairying, we need to bear in mind that there are many other versions. Figure 6.7 presents an image of a more up-to-date milking parlor located in the Dairy Center at the Pennsylvania State University. It conveys the impression of modern cleanness and efficiency including computer measurement of yield for milk from each cow and stainless steel sanitary pipe for conveying the milk to storage. While this relatively new milking parlor tends to minimize labor, it is by no means an ultimate. The latest trend is to robotic milking. In such a parlor, the cow is identified electronically by a tag she is wearing. She is mechanistcally positioned, her udder is automatically washed and then robotic milk extractors attach and efficiently remove the milk. The milk yield is measured and recorded by computer and the cow is sent on to be replaced by another. In 2002, Toronto, Canada was the site of the first large international conference on robotic milking. While such a system requires minimal human oversight to make sure that everything is operating properly and that the milk is of good quality, it is a far cry from the hand milking of every animal less than a century ago.

Figure 6.7

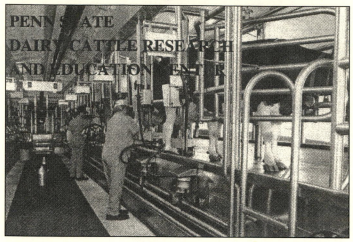

Cows being milked in the milking parlor at the Penn State Dairy Research and Education Center.

Housing and Management of Cows

Because dairy farmers have been their own bosses, the ways they have housed, fed, milked and managed their cows has been highly varied and continues to be so. There is always the search for a better, easier, more profitable way of producing milk. Anyone who worked on a dairy farm in the bygone era of the last century can readily understand the need for change. It was back-breaking labor during long days and seven days a week. There was always feeding, milking, changing bedding, and removing manure, all hand operations. So every dairy farmer under his particular set of conditions has been looking for a better way. Thus, it is not possible to say simply and precisely this is the way milk is produced. There is constant change and the two biggest driving forces are automation to reduce labor costs and growth in size, that is, numbers of milking animals, to increase an operation's competitiveness and profitability.

There are some general considerations about how and where cows live that are factors in their housing. In each of the United States there are thousands of cows and this involves them and their attendants in all manner of climates including drastic seasonal changes. There is heat and cold, dry and wet, pasture and no pasture in all kinds of combinations. Yet, with proper management, cows thrive and continuously produce milk under all these circumstances. This is quite a commentary on human ingenuity and the suitability of cows for the milk production mission.

Another set of factors that impact on housing for cows is defined by practical management requirements. How big an operation is contemplated in terms of numbers of cows? How important relatively will labor and feed costs be? About half the cost of producing milk is feed cost. Pasturing helps to cut that cost. How competitive will the milk market be? For example, one can envision a small, family operation with little or no hired help in a relatively uncompetitive market succeeding under quite different animal housing conditions than that for a large investor supported operation in a highly competitive market. So the upshot of all these diverse considerations is that housing and living conditions for cows vary greatly. Average herd size is constantly rising which means that large commercial ventures are increasing and smaller family operations are declining. So in a very real sense every "dairy barn" is a unique structure.

The functional aspects of a cow's life require that there be areas for feeding, resting, milking, exercise, medical care, and reproduction. Some of these can be accomplished in the same space and some require movement from one location to another.

Barns. Free stall barns are now the predominant housing design. Free stall arrangements provide individual open compartments for the cows. In a way, they represent a glorified milking parlor with the flexibility to handle feeding, some freedom and exercise for the animals, as well as manure removal, at more or less one location. They involve rows of stanchions under roof. The stanchions define approximately enough stalls for the number of cows in the herd. Various kinds of bedding are used. Cows enter and exit at will. The system accommodates feeding and milking rather efficiently, and the cows have a good bit of comfort and freedom to exercise, rest and move around.

A very standard barn design, still used in older smaller operations, is one in which the cows are in two rows facing each other across a feed access aisle (see figure 6.8). There is also an aisle in back of each row. It includes an adjacent gutter for catching manure which used to be removed by hand and more often now is mechanically scraped away. The rear aisles also provide access for cleaning udders and attaching a milking machine. In front of the cows is a manger or feeding trough into which silage, grain, hay, etc. can be placed. It may be partitioned to favor an allotment for each animal or the spacing may be such that they can't readily reach each other's allotment of food. This system requires that the cows be immobilized and this is accomplished by an elongated metal collar or yoke that allows the animal to stand up or lie down and to move their heads around. They are also confined by metal sidebars that keep them from swinging their bodies into the cows next to them. The metal framing for these stanchions include the air/vacuum lines needed to operate the milking machines, and a water line with individual water bowls which the cow can fill by just pressing down with her muzzle on a metal piece in the bottom of the bowl. Cows easily learn this and other tricks on how to live comfortably in this environment.

Figure 6.8

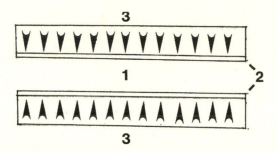

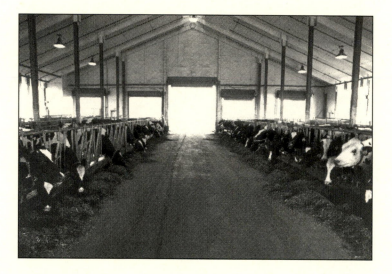

A traditional barn arrangement for housing dairy cows. Upper: the cows (arrowheads) are retained in two rows of stalls and face each other across a feed delivery aisle (1). In front of each row of cows is a feed trough (2) which may be divided into compartments, one for each animal. At the rear of the animals are aisles (3) that provide access for milking and manure removal. Lower: Photo of cows in such a barn with view down the central aisle.

In the foregoing arrangement, the cow must be brought in and out of the barn in accord with daily needs for pasturing, exercise and milking schedules. They get used to these routines and readily respond to gestures aimed at moving them in and out of the barn. Of course, herd instinct is important. They tend to move when the other cows move and in the same direction. In coming back into the barn, they also have considerable ability to remember their individual stalls. They readily come into the barn, enter their stalls and stick their heads through the open collars that can then be closed to

Figure 6.9

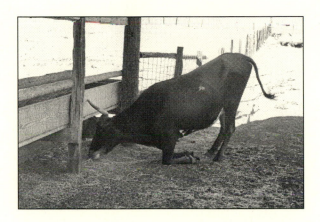

Long Horn cow scrounging for extras in and under a horse feeding manger. Photo courtesy of J and J Ranch, Big Oak Flat, CA.

facilitate feeding and milking operations. People have a tendency to think that cows are stupid and it is true in the herd they don't seem to have any mind of their own. However, left to their own devices, they can figure out a few things. The Longhorn cow in figure 6.9 learned where a horse was being fed on the ranch and came regularly to get any leftovers. Further she figured out how to get the stuff that fell under the manger.

Some people believe or imagine that cows are managed inhumanely. To the extent that one sees freedom of cattle to wander unrestrained in the wild as the ideal, that may be so. However, cattle are not necessarily safer, happier, and certainly not of greater use to us under such conditions. I've never been aware of unhappiness in a cow or of its resistance to its way of life. They don't act as though they hate being milked. True, they do complain sometimes when delivering a calf or when they have been hurt and when they are sick. But for the most part, they seem quite content, particularly if they can be with other cows and do what they do.

The round barn. In the interest of greater economy and efficiency, dairy farmers are constantly changing barn designs and arrangements. An interesting innovation was the round barn. It appears to have originated in the Midwest about 1900. Two examples of this type barn have come to the writer's attention. One, designed by a farmer named Neff and known as the Neff Barn, was constructed near Centre Hall, PA in 1910. It is a beautiful historic landmark that still stands (see figure 6.10). The other was built in 1913 near Harrisburg, Pennsylvania by the Hershey Chocolate Co. to house cows supplying milk for chocolate manufacture.

Figure 6.10

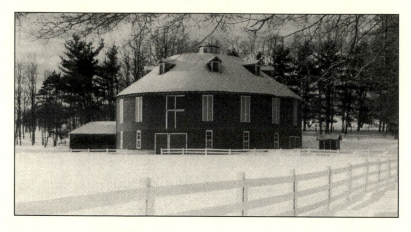

A historically famous round barn near Center Hall, PA built in 1912 for the purpose of feeding cattle more efficiently. Stalls for the cows were arranged in a circle such that all of them faced toward the center where a central shoot from the floor above could deliver their feed. Photo courtesy of Dick Brown.

The main advantage attributed to the round structure was ease of feed handling. As in most barns, hay was stored on the upper floors and the animals were housed at ground level. By arranging stalls of the round barn so that the animals faced toward the center, hay and other feed could be dropped through a central shoot to arrive right in front of all of them. Efficient construction with no waste space dictated that the barn for this feeding arrangement should be round. Another interesting explanation for the origin of the round barn, probably from the Pennsylvania Dutch, was that corners should be avoided because evil spirits liked to hide in them.

There are thousands of barns, new and old, in Pennsylvania but those are the only two round ones I ever saw or heard of. Since the size of a cow and the practical dimensions of a central feeding shoot are fixed, a round barn would only accommodate a relatively small herd. So the trend toward larger and mechanized operations was probably one factor rendering the round barn obsolete.

Other housing. Between open outdoor housing with overhead roof shelter from the elements and conventional barns with restraining stanchions, there are many arrangements directed toward keeping the animals comfortable and maximizing efficiency of feeding, milking and manure handling. For example, so-called "loose" housing allows cows to move freely in an area of a barn. Access to feed is provided at the periphery of the open space or is delivered by conveyor. Fresh bedding is spread as needed. This covers manure and helps to keep the cows clean and comfortable. Eventually the manure/bedding layer builds up and must be removed but the daily disposal problem is eliminated. Loose housing requires a milking parlor and uses a lot of bedding. The free-stall arrangement is discussed above.

Because high heat and humidity can be hard on cows and milk production, human ingenuity is creating unique housing and management to deal with the problem. Modern barns in the southern U. S. are constructed to produce a cooling updraft of air. They are equipped with fans and sprayers of water mist for individual cows. These developments have significance not only for dairying in America, but particularly for milk production in the tropics where many millions of people live. Speaking of heat stress, see figure 6.11.

Figure 6.11

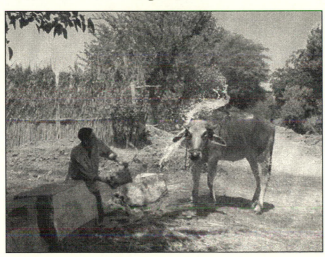

Water buffalo cow welcoming a cool shower at her home in the Nile delta. These animals are the prize possession of rural Egyptians. They are used for milk (and cheese) with male calves raised for meat.

To provide some idea of the varied structures and activities that need to be accommodated in producing milk, an aerial photograph of the facilities at the Penn State Dairy Research and Education Center is shown (figure 6.12). Although this may be a somewhat idealized and diversified version because of its teaching, research and public relations functions, it does embrace all the many necessary operations as described in the figure caption.

Milk Production

Individual animals. Early in the past century, it was considered quite acceptable for a cow to produce 5,000 pounds of milk in a lactation of nine or ten

Figure 6.12

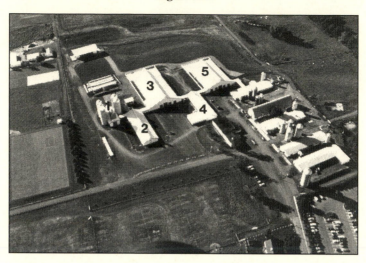

Aerial view of the Penn State Dairy Research and Education Center showing: 1. Feed center with vertical and horizontal silos, 2. Tie-stall barn, 3. Heifer barn, 4. Milking parlor and milk room, 5. Free-stall barn. The group of structures at right consist of five barns and silos formerly used for individual herds of five major breeds. They now house dry cows, calves, research facilities and animals used in experiments.

Table 6.2

State	Cows[1]	Milk /Cow[2]	Milk[3]
CA	1590	20,193	33,251
WI	1292	17,182	22,199
NY	672	17,527	11,778
PA	599	18,112	10,849
MN	510	17,278	8,812
US	9115	18,139	165, 336

Total number of cows, milk production per cow and total milk production in 2001 for the five leading milk producing states and the United States as a whole. Data from the National Agricultural Statistics Service, USDA courtesy of Marc Tosiano.
Footnotes: [1]Milking animals in thousands. [2]Pounds of milk per year. [3]Milk in millions of pounds.

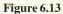

Figure 6.13

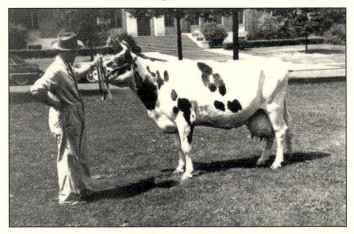

Penn State Veeman Josie, a cow that held the lifetime milk production record. For details, see text.

months. In the United States during 2001, an average cow produced 18,000 pounds of milk (table 6.2). It is not uncommon today for some cows to produce 50,000 pounds of milk during a nine- or ten- month lactation. To put it another way, that is eighty quarts a day or twenty-five tons of milk during one lactation. Such huge milk production by individual animals reveals the drive there has been for improvement and increased profitability of dairy farming. The current record for a single lactation is some 75,000 pounds of milk.

Early in my career at Penn State, someone brought to my attention a prize cow in the University herd. She was a registered Holstein by the name of Penn State Veeman Josie, (figure 6.13). She lived to be nineteen years old, and by the early 1950s, she had become the highest living lifetime producer of milk in the United States. Her final total production was 257,778 pounds of milk and 8,100 pounds of butterfat. She alone supplied humanity with close to 1,300 tons of high quality food during her lifetime. A cow like Josie gives us some idea how successful our dairy industry has been. As a result of selective breeding throughout hundreds of years, and its more recent enhancement by artificial breeding, Josie emerged as a better, more persistent milk producer than any of her forbears. In addition, she became the foundation cow of a family that numbered fifty high-producing descendants in the Penn State herd by 1954. Of course, the beneficial effects of her genes go on and on in the dairy world.

Statistics—federal and state. [10] In the last few decades numbers of smaller herds of cows and part time dairy farmers have been dwindling. There was a time when many rural Americans supplemented their incomes from non-farm jobs with a milk check derived by keeping a few cows. A herd of 100-cows is on

Figure 6.14

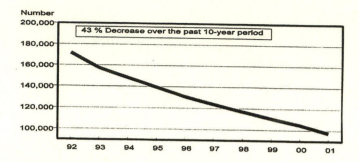

Trend in the number of dairy farms (cow operations) from 1992 through 2001. Data from the National Agricultural Statistics Service, USDA courtesy of Marc Tosiano.

Figure 6.15

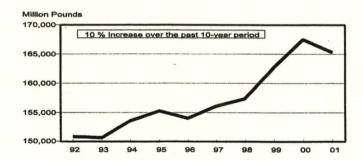

Trend in U. S. total annual milk production from 1992 through 2001. Data from the National Agricultural Statistics Service, USDA courtesy of Marc Tosiano.

the small side today. During 2001, 39 percent of all the milk produced in the United States came from operations involving 500 or more cows. These large businesses utilized 34.6 percent of the total producing animals in that year. Because of the large, sometimes factory-like nature of milk producing operations, there is less of a tendency to call them farms although many still have the traditional character of a farm. The USDA refers to them as "milk cow operations." Commensurate with the increase in average size of dairy farms, the actual numbers of them have been dropping steadily during the past decade as shown in figure 6.14. While this may involve a number of causes, increase in efficiency with greater size is a major factor. One might argue that the drop has actually been precipitous but it may be distorted somewhat by the USDA's definition of a milk cow operation as any place having one or more milk cows.

Figure 6.16

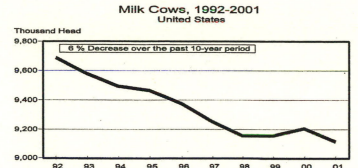

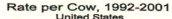

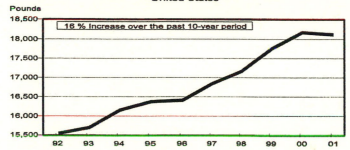

Trend in number of cows (upper) and average milk production per cow per year in the U. S. (lower) from 1992 through 2001. Data from the National Agricultural Statistics Service, USDA courtesy of Marc Tosiano.

The only category of dairy farm that actually increased in numbers during 2001 involved those with 500 or more animals, that is, the larger ones.

After falling rather steadily in the late 1970s and the 1980s, milk production in the United States picked up during the 1990s (figure 6.15). This increase was accomplished by fewer cows producing, on average, more milk (figure 6.16). Statistics for the five leading states and the U. S. as a whole for 2001 are presented in table 6.2.

Dairy farming is of major economic importance in many states of the U.S. About fifty years ago, Vermont was unique among the States for having as many cows as people. Since then, there has been a heavy swing in the direction of people, that is, 140,000 cows and 600,000 people in 2001. However, dairy farming is still a major aspect of Vermont's economy. Wisconsin, the number two milk producing state, has come to be known as America's Dairyland. Less well known is that agriculture is the number one industry of Pennsylvania and that milk is the leading agricultural commodity of the state. It has 9,700 commercial dairy farms, that is, operations with more than ten cows. They average sixty-four cows per farm. The farms produce close to 11 billion pounds of milk a year with a farm value of $1.7 billion. Major factors determining the size of a state's dairy farming economy are proximity to population centers and to cheese plants. Cheese plants are particularly important in Wisconsin, New York, and California but the milk produced in those states also is utilized by large population centers within the states or close by.

* * *

The cow is a marvelously engineered mammal. She evolved to have a digestive system (rumen) which, with the help of resident microorganisms, enables her to make a complete and nutritious diet out of crude plant materials. Incidental to this mode of life, the cow also can make relatively large volumes of milk, a highly nutritious, life-sustaining food. Human guidance of the cow's reproduction program coupled with scientific research has made her an ever more proficient producer of milk. Some people make the point that humans are the only animal that consumes the milk of another species —the idea being, it is odd of us to consume cow's milk. Humans do many unusual species specific things like smoking and flying airplanes, but the basic reason we use cow's milk as a food is simple common sense; it is nutritious, it is palatable, and the cow can make it for us cheaply and in huge amounts. Cross-nursing between species is not all that uncommon.

Destitution and starvation remain in many areas of the world today. We can be thankful here in the U.S. that from the beginning, our people took very seriously the necessity of producing food so that people would be healthy and productive in their work. Despite current criticism of it, dairy farming has made a tremendous contribution to meeting that need. Available statistics indicate that milk production is alive and well in the United States.

Suggested References

Aker, R. M. *Lactation and the Mammary Gland.* Iowa State Press, a Blackwell Publishing Company, 2002. pp. 278.

Council for Agricultural Science and Technology. *Animal Agriculture and Global Food Supply.* Task Force Report 135. Ames, IA. 1999. pp. 1-99.

Ishler, V., Heinrichs, J. and Varga, G. *From feed to milk: Understanding rumen function.* Agricultural Extension Circular 422. The Pennsylvania State University, University Park, PA 16802. pp. 27.

Rath, S. *The Complete Cow.* Voyageur Press Inc. Stillwater, MN. 1998. pp.144.

Russelle, M. P. Alfalfa. *American Scientist* 89: 252-61. 2001.

Notes

1. Suprisingly large pieces of hardware are sometimes found post mortem in the cow's reticulum. These include small tools, nails and metal objects of all kinds. Goats do a better job of feeling what's in their mouths before swallowing.
2. "We will live to rue the day that the cows ran out of gas," by Dave Barry. *San Diego Union Tribune*, Nov. 17, 2002.
3. Swarns, R. L. Food used as a political weapon in Zimbabwe (It's distributed to political supporters). *New York Times News Service*. This item, published in the *San Diego Union-Tribune* on 12/13/02, has been typical of many news reports and syndicated columns on the subject.
4. Kesler, E. M. et al. *Journal of Dairy Science* 50: 1994-6. 1967.
5. Virtanen, A. I. *Science* 153: 1603-14. 1966.
6. Patton, S. and Jensen, R. G. *Biomedical Aspects of Lactation.* Pergamon, New York. 1976. p. 12.
7. Adachi, S. *Civil Histroy of Dairy Technology Developments in the World with Special Reference to Asia* (in Japanese). Tohoku University Press, Sendai, Japan. 2002. pp. 1120.
8. Rogers, D. *Wall Street Journal.* 8/16/02. p. A4
9. Schmidt, G.H., Van Vleck, L. D. and Hutjens, M. F. *Principles of Dairy Science.* 2nd ed. 1988. Prentice Hall, Elmsford, NJ. pp. 446.
10. Statistical data in this section are courtesy of Marc Tosiano, National Agricultural Statistics Service, USDA, Harrisburg, PA; and Tammy Perkins, Dairy Alliance Program, The Pennsylvania State University.

7

Milk Processing and Products

Everyone has a need to know about cow's milk, products made from it, and the industry that provides them. Those considerations are an integral part of our culture and important for all of us. Thus, the purpose of this chapter is to provide an overview of milk processing and products and to answer questions like: Just what is homogenization? How nutritious is ice cream? What do they do with evaporated milk? What is meant by "sharp" Cheddar cheese? In addition, those bent on building and conveying a bad image of milk are counting on public ignorance and apathy on the subject to help achieve their goal. The implication that some conjured-up negativity about milk fits all its forms and products in reference to all consumers not only is untrue, it is ridiculous on the face of it. For example, there is more milk used in the U. S. to make cheese than for fluid milk purposes. Are the critics also trying to tell us that all the several hundred varieties and modifications of cheese are no good, too? What about yogurt and all the other products made from milk? As this chapter will show, milk is a remarkable raw material in dairy product manufacture; and these products are not only nutritious, they make for the good life where they are available. Thus, we pick up on our story here with the different things that can and do happen to milk after it is obtained from the cow.

Producer-Processors

Not all milk is sent from the farm to the processing plant. A small amount usually is retained for use by the farm families and hired personnel; and some farm operations are actually producer-processors, that is, the milk is kept at the farm, processed and marketed to the public. In addition to retail milk, they may also make and market other products such as cream, cottage cheese, buttermilk, ice cream and butter. Such businesses tend to be on the outskirts of fairly good-sized towns in dairy farming areas. Usually the products are offered at a roadside market on or by the farm. They may also make regular deliveries to customers by truck and sell wholesale to other markets.

One might ask why there are producer-processors? One reason is the appeal of cutting out the middlemen. Instead of making some money selling milk to a milk plant, that sells it to a store that sells it to a customer, you make more money by selling directly to the customer yourself. While in practice it isn't quite that simple, it can be true to a degree. In the case of the roadside outlet, the location must be right because people will have to make a special trip to the outskirts of town. However, seeing the cows in an adjoining pasture when one picks up milk can have a favorable impact. Even knowing that something is made locally or provides jobs for friends and neighbors can help with the image which is very important. In the end, it usually gets down to things like price, product quality and service in comparison to the supermarket, a tough outfit with which to compete. There was a newly opened dairy farm market in an area where my family and I lived at one point and we would stop to pick up milk occasionally because it was on our daily route. It developed that their skim milk, sold at a skim milk price, contained an appreciable amount of milk fat. This was before the days of 1 and 2 percent fat milks. Their "skim" milk tasted very good and sold well.

Milk Processing

Following withdrawal from the individual cow, milk is assayed for weight or volume and then delivered to a refrigerated holding tank that cools and stores the milk from all the cows until daily pickup by a tank truck. The pooled milk is cooled to and maintained at about 38° to 42 °F. Holding normal milk at this temperature will prevent spoilage for at least several days. The same temperature is maintained in the milk during its hauling to the dairy and while being held there awaiting processing. With exception of small plastic or fiberboard gaskets used to prevent leaks in pipelines, the milk comes in contact only with stainless steel. It is known to be highly inert toward foods and an exceptionally safe surface regarding food exposure. More importantly, stainless steel does not promote flavor deterioration of milk (see chapter 8). So the pipelines, pumps and bulk tank at the farm, the tank on the tank truck, plus all the milk handling systems in the plant are, almost without any exception anywhere, made of stainless steel. Consumers can take comfort in the fact that a never-ending dedicated effort is made to assure the quality and healthfulness of the milk and dairy products they buy. This extends all the way from washing the cow's udder, checking the quality of her milk, sanitizing milking machines and keeping the milk cold and clean until the additionally protective step of pasteurization is taken. The major processing steps applied to milk are clarification, separation, homogenization, pasteurization and cooling. Most if not all of these are applied to the milk used in manufacture of the various dairy products. It is not necessary to subject milk to be separated to clarification as well since separation also accomplishes clarification. A description of processing treatments follows.

Clarification. Raw milk as it comes from the cow, contains minor amounts of material that is considered extraneous. This includes tissue and cell debris, bacteria, and cells of the immune system from within the udder and the teat canal. These are consistent and normal components of all raw milk. Nursing babies would take in all this kind of material from their mothers' breasts but for reasons that will become evident, processing of cows milk includes a step to remove such substances. In addition, no matter how careful and exclusionary sanitation practices may be, traces of environmental material, "dirt" so to speak, may get into milk. This is no different in principle from the material picked up by other foods including meat, fruits, vegetables, and grains in their production and handling. Removal of these extraneous materials from milk, in so far as possible, can benefit the appearance and keeping quality of the milk. For example, unclarified milk sometimes produces a noticeable grayish sediment following homogenization. Clarification or separation of milk helps to eliminate such problems. In both instances, the extraneous material causing the problem is deposited as a sediment on the walls of the centrifuge bowls (see figure 7.1 and following regarding separator operation) as they revolve at very high speeds. Modern separators and clarifiers are both designed to be self-desludging; that is, they periodically loosen the material that has built up on the bowl wall and eject it out an exit port separate from those for the continually flowing milk, or in the case of the separator, cream or skim.

Separation. A layer of cream will form on the top of fresh milk, as it comes from the cow, if it is allowed to stand for twenty or thirty minutes. This is known as gravity creaming and it was very important prior to the invention of the cream separator. Before and during the 1800s, cream formed by gravity was skimmed off and used to make butter. This was a rather inefficient way of producing cream because a lot of the milk fat globule remained in the lower skim milk phase and, in addition, it was impossible to sharply separate the two layers. Any effort to remove the cream produces some remixing. In 1871, a device known as a cream separator was invented. It revolutionized the production of cream and skim milk that transformed the dairy industry. The all important aspect of this machine is a heavy metal bowl spinning at a very high speed which sediments the skim milk phase of incoming milk toward the wall of the bowl and displaces the cream inward along the center of the bowl. This enables the two phases to be removed separately. The amount of fat in the skim milk so produced ranges from about 0.02 to 0.06 percent. The principle of the separation process is illustrated schematically in figure 7.1. There is a good bit of similarity between a clarifier and a separator. Both involve bowls of similar design spinning at high speed (6,000 to 10,000 revolutions per minute) and both remove a very minor amount of sedimentable substances from the milk but the clarifier does not fractionate the milk into cream and skim. It simply passes on the whole milk relieved of the undesirable sediment.

The cream separator not only made a whole series of retail cream products possible, it also facilitated production of all the many no-fat, low-fat, full fat, double cream, triple cream, you name the amount of fat products that are cur-

Figure 7.1

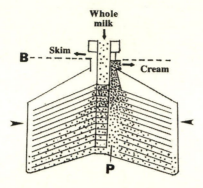

Cross-sectional view of a cream separator bowl illustrating the principle whereby it removes and concentrates the fat globules from whole milk to form cream and skim milk. The bowl has a heavy metal wall and contains a stack of closely nested metal cones. Milk continuously flows to the bottom of the bowl by means of a central tube and then rises into the cones. In operation, the bowl, spins at high speed (6,000 to 10,000 rpm). The centrifugal force thus generated sends the more dense (1.036) skim milk phase toward the bowl wall (arrowheads) thus displacing the less dense (0.930) fat globules toward the center of the bowl. Holes designed to match on the inner edge of the cones form passages, one of which is shown (P), that allow the gathering fat globules to flow upward and out a separate portal as a concentrate (cream). By the time the skim milk has moved out of the cones and upward along the walls of the bowl to its own exit, it is essentially devoid of fat. There is a barrier (B) in the separator assembly that keeps the continuously flowing skim and cream fractions from mixing.

rently available. By opening or constricting the outlet for either cream or skim from the separator, the amount of fat in the cream can be adjusted. Alternatively, the cream, as it comes from the separator, can be diluted with skim to any desired fat content. Further, skim can be used to dilute the fat content of whole milk, such as might be desirable in making 1 percent and 2 percent milks.

Homogenization. Another processing measure that has had far reaching effects in the dairy industry is homogenization. It involves pumping milk through a restricted orifice (valve) under pressures of 2,000 to 2,500 pounds per square inch with the result that the fat globules are fragmented (see figure 7.2). Homogenization was quickly and widely adopted for the manufacture of ice cream mix in the 1930s, but it took until 1950 or so for the homogenization of milk to become widespread. Fluid milk and other fluid dairy products can be homogenized either before or after pasteurization. In order for the process to be effective, the milk fat must be in a liquid state and that enzymes of the milk substantially inactivated. This means milk entering the homogenizer should be at least 140°F.

Figure 7.2

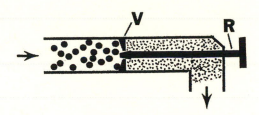

Scheme illustrating the action of a milk homogenizer. Whole milk containing intact fat globules at left is pumped under high pressure through an homogenizing valve assembly (V). This accomplishes fragmentation of the globules, the critical step in production of homogenized milk. The milk flows continuously in the direction of the arrows. Constriction of milk flow through the valve, which raises the pressure and accomplishes the homogenization, is achieved by increasing the closure of the valve via rod R.

A number of important changes take place in milk as a result of homogenization. The size of the fat particles is reduced from a mean diameter of three to four microns for the original globules to one micron or somewhat less. This greatly increases the number of fat particles, but it also increases the total amount of fat particle surface. In order to lower tension between this new fat surface and the aqueous phases, protein is bound at the interface between the two. It is estimated that 30 percent of the casein in homogenized milk is bound to the fat particles. Sometimes as a result of homogenization, the newly formed fat particles clump together. In order to breakdown these clumps, a second stage of homogenization at about 500-pound pressure may be employed. A further effect of the homogenization is an increase in the viscosity of the milk. The overall result of these new factors is that the fat will no longer rise and the composition of the milk remains the same (homogeneous) throughout its entire volume. This is true not only of the homogenized milk in your refrigerator but also of evaporated milk that often stands on the shelf at room temperature for months.

Perhaps the most important net effect of homogenization is that it makes the milk taste richer, that is, as though it had acquired more fat. In all likelihood, this is due to the increased number of fat particles and the greater viscosity. This is quite a nice dividend from a relatively inexpensive processing step. In matter of fact, 1 or 2 percent homogenized milk tastes as rich as unhomogenized whole milk. However, as a result of homogenization, it became no longer possible in the home for anyone to steal the cream off the top of the bottle, something to which I was addicted as a child. The history of homogenized milk and the research effort that went into its development at the State Universities is well presented in a book by G. M. Trout[1]

Pasteurization. When milk production and consumption was a family affair in the early years of this country, raw milk could be dealt with satisfactorily. Everyone knew it had to be used promptly or converted to something with better keeping quality, such as butter or cheese. If on rare occasions, someone got sick from drinking spoiled or disease-contaminated milk, it couldn't spread, at least not very far or via the milk. However, with the coming industrialization in the 1800s, raw milk, pooled and distributed in cities could be and sometimes was a disaster. The history of this problem in the growth of New York City during the 1800s is told very impressively by Du Puis.[2]

Pasteurization was an exceptionally beneficial development. It not only protected the public's health, it also made milk much more manageable as an industrial material. More particularly, with the ability to extend milk's keeping quality for a reasonable period of time, mass production of other milk products in which consumers would be interested became possible. The surprising thing was that pasteurization worked beautifully. It was found that a temperature treatment of 143°F for thirty minutes destroyed all pathogens and over 90 percent of the bacteria in milk. With that treatment there is little or no effect on flavor, and overall, almost no effect on nutritive value. In addition, pasteurization fits in well with homogenization which requires that the milk be heated. So in a continuous flow system, it is feasible to homogenize either immediately before or just after pasteurization. Pasteurization is known to cause slight losses of some of the vitamins: from 0 to 10 percent of the thiamine (vitamin B_1), less than 5 percent of the vitamin B_{12}, and 25 to 50 percent of the ascorbic acid (vitamin C). Even raw milk is not a good source of vitamin C, with at most, 50 percent of the recommended daily allotment in a quart. So there is some destruction of vitamin C by pasteurization. It is a small price to pay for making milk so safe from a public health standpoint. In any event, we need some fruit, a good source of vitamin C, in our diet.

Old-fashioned batch pasteurization is pretty simple. The whole process could be monitored by a recording thermometer and the record for every vat of milk kept on file. However, the need to make the process quicker and continuous led to the development of HTST (high temperature short time) treatment. Because the bacterial killing effect of heat treatment involves two variables, temperature and time, it was possible to find shorter holding times at higher temperatures that worked. Actually, there are many alternatives that work but to meet the practicalities of milk processing, 162° to 165°F for twenty to fifteen seconds is widely used. This same principle works for sterilization, the inactivation of all bacteria. As discussed following regarding evaporated milk, there is an in-can holding heat treatment of about 240°F. for fifteen minutes. However, it is possible to achieve sterilization in continuously flowing milk by heating at 275° to 300°F for two to six seconds. This milk can be aseptically filled into containers, that is, physically excluding bacteria so that there is no contamination of the sterile product during the filling operation. This heat treatment is known as UHT (ultra heat treatment).

At minimum, HTST pasteurization requires pumps to keep the milk and heating medium flowing, monitors for measuring flow rate and temperature of the milk, a section of tubing or plates in which to accomplish the required holding of the milk at pasteurizing temperature, a diversion valve for milk that did not receive adequate heating with a balance tank to hold that milk for recycling, and electronic controls for actuating and regulating the system. The heating is generally accomplished with hot water. In the interest of energy economy, heated and cooled phases are used for temperature regeneration so far as possible. For example, cold incoming raw milk could be used to cool down milk that has just been pasteurized. At the same time, the raw milk would be gaining heat for its pasteurization. Equipment needs to be specially designed to accomplish such regeneration. Generally speaking, HTST pasteurization has been very successful in meeting needs of the public and the dairy industry.

Cooling. Dairy processing is full of requirements to cool the product and keep it cold. This is because warm milk is an excellent growth medium for bacteria. The only exceptions to the keep-it-cold mandate are dried and steril-ized products. Ice cream, of course, is defined by being cold.

The basic principle of refrigeration is cooling by expansion of a gas such as ammonia or freon. When a compressed (liquified) gas is allowed to expand, it absorbs a lot of heat. So any surface that is next to the gas during this expansion will get very cold. This principle is used in the home refrigerator. It contains a small compressor driven by electricity which enables endless cycles of com-pression and expansion of a refrigerant gas that keeps the food cold and makes ice cubes. Industrial refrigeration is more or less the same. Sometimes industrial equipment will require use of an intermediate medium such as water or brine, that is, salt solution which resists freezing. These are cooled first and then pumped through the equipment that is to cool milk or milk product. However, in many commercial operations, the compressed refrigeration gas is used di-rectly in the equipment.

During my years of working in the building that housed the Penn State Creamery, once in a great while a leak would occur in the refrigeration system which used ammonia in its compressors. Ammonia gas is its own warning de-vice. The odor is readily perceived and not easily forgotten. A severe leak makes ones eyes water and may burn the skin.

In addition to the heat exchangers mentioned in connection with pasteur-ization, there are a variety of refrigerated vats and surface coolers that are used for cooling. Such vats have refrigerated walls and are equipped with agitation, which is essential. It takes a very long time to cool the center of an unstirred mass of liquid. Surface coolers are in essence stacks of fused tubes that look like corrugated sheet metal. Refrigerant circulates inside the tubes and milk flows down over the outside. Mainly these devices simply maximize exposure of warm or hot product to cold surface, and they are very important economically. Efficient use of refrigeration is essential to profitability of a dairy.

Equipment to accomplish the milk processing steps described in the foregoing is shown in a photo of the milk processing area of the Penn State Creamery (see figure 7.3). While this is a relatively small unit that meets the needs of the university community on the campus, that is, those of some 40,000 students, two hotels, a number of public dining commons, and a retail sales room; it is representative in principle of much larger operations. One thing this picture makes clear is the large amount of stainless steel sanitary pipe involved in milk processing. In the old days, this would all have had to be taken down, cleaned and put back up after each day's operations. Now it is cleaned and sanitized in place. Not all of the piping is involved in milk flow; some is used for hot and cold-water circulation in the heating and cooling of the milk. The separator (S) at left in the photo is about five feet tall at the top where the piping takes off. The centrifuge bowl which accomplishes the separation of the cream from the skim is inside the metal housing on which the S is placed. The fat content of the cream is determined by adjusting the screw (arrowheads) above the separator. The homogenizer (H) has two handles (arrowheads) which are used to adjust the resistance to the flow of milk. The resulting homogenizing pressures are regis-

Figure 7.3

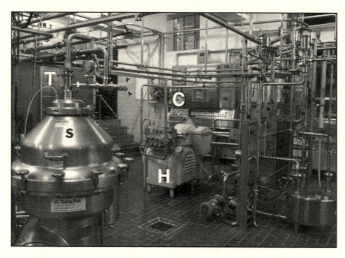

The milk processing area in the Penn State Creamery. Major equipment shown are a holding tank for pasteurized milk (T), a cream separator (S), a homogenizer (H), a plate-type heat exchanger at right (E), and a control panel (C). Also shown are a pump and a balance tank at lower right. That tank is for recirculating underpasteurized milk and to keep air out of the milk lines. Photo courtesy of Tom Palchak.

tered on the gauges attached to the stainless steel block above the H. It is in this block that homogenization of the milk takes place. The heat exchanger (E) accomplishes the heating and cooling of the milk before and after pasteurization. Between the heating up and cooling down phases, flow rate of the milk through a special length of tubing is adjusted to achieve the required fifteen seconds of holding for the HTST pasteurization. A lot of the piping in the picture is to convey milk to holding tanks and filling machines.

Packaging. For retail sales, fluid milk products are filled and sealed into many different packages ranging in size from the rather tiny cups of half and half for coffee up to gallon-sized plastic containers. There is characteristic packaging for each dairy product and for the most part this seems to be done very well. Occasionally one can note a slight burnt flavor in milk that is packaged by hot sealing the top of a coated paper carton, but it is not a devastating off-flavor. Maybe more serious, my attempts at opening these cartons by tearing and pinching the top according to instructions do not always work and I wind up having to stab them, and so far, not me. A problem that sometimes develops with gallon containers of milk, is flavor deterioration resulting from overexposure to light in the store or display cabinet. If the turnover is fairly rapid and light exposure minimal, there usually is no problem.

Milk Products

As background to aid in our consideration of the various milk products, it is of interest to know how much of the U. S. milk supply is used for the major product categories. Of the 165 billion pounds of milk produced in 2001, 33.2 percent went into fluid milk and cream, 36.7 percent for cheese, 13.3 percent for creamery butter, 8.9 percent for frozen dairy products, 0.8 percent for evaporated and condensed milk, 0.8 percent for use on farms where produced and 6.2 percent for other uses.[3] Let us focus on the cheese and fluid milk statistics for a moment. In the five-year period from 1996 to 2001, the milk supply grew by 6.5 percent and cheese production increased its use of the supply by 1.8 percent. In the process, it grew past consumption of fluid milk and cream. One may have an image of Americans as milk drinkers, they are also big cheese consumers.

We have entered an era in which food manufacturing can be extremely flexible and creative. There was a time when milk was pasteurized, cooled, bottled and distributed. Today, there are milks of varying fat content, milk with added milk solids, milk fermented by various kinds of microorganisms (buttermilk, acidophilus, yogurt), milk with its lactose hydrolyzed, flavored milks, and so on. Vitamins A and D have been added to milk for many years and it is likely that milk will continue to be utilized as a vehicle. Fortification of milk with vitamin D has been one of the most worthwhile measures ever devised to promote human well-being.

Many of the variations in milk and milk products have been developed as a result of perceived consumer health needs, especially with respect to fat content. There are low-fat and no-fat versions of milk and virtually every product made from it, even fat-free sour cream, a contradiction in terms since cream by definition is a fat-containing product. How much actual health need there is for such products is uncertain and becoming more so. The idea is that they will help consumers to contend with obesity and heart disease. However, as explained in chapter 5, milk suppresses weight gain and milk fat contains components that in experimental animals suppress accumulation of body fat and development of atherosclerosis. Perhaps the important point is that milk production and processing are now so flexible that any serious need to add something beneficial or remove detrimental components for special groups of consumers can be met. The future also holds the probability of manipulating the composition and properties of milk not only through varied feeding programs but also by genetic engineering of the cow.

One also now hears of variations in the traditional dairy products. For example, the term "frozen dessert" is used almost as often as "ice cream." This is because of the many manufactured versions of the latter including frozen yogurt, soft serve and vegetable fat ice creams. Another interesting example is diabetic ice cream, a product that looks and tastes like ice cream but by using sweeteners in the manufacture other than those containing sucrose or glucose, avoids the potential problem of blood glucose elevation in the diabetic.

Market Milk

To summarize, when milk comes into the processing plant there are two basic processing paths it can enter initially. These are to the cream separator or to the clarifier, (see figure 7.4). The milk, cream, and skim can then enter many further channels providing the multitude of products associated with the fluid milk market. The major product of this pathway is the milk millions of us drink. The main variable is the amount of fat it contains. Otherwise the processing packaging and distribution is essentially the same. Most of us know from experience that fluid milks with or without fat are palatable, reliable and consistent products.

The bulk of retail milk consumed by the public is made up of milks with varying fat content - 0, 1, and 2 percent fat and whole milk. The latter by law must contain at least 3.25 percent fat. California and some other areas of the country sell a lot of 0 percent fat milk (also known as nonfat milk or skim milk) that is fortified with a percent or so of extra nonfat milk solids. Chocolate milk, which accounts for 90 percent of the flavored milk market, continues to grow in popularity. There are a number of other specialty retail milks. These include cultured buttermilk, acidophilus milk, yogurt, and lactose hydrolyzed (lactose-free) milk. Buttermilk is produced by adding a bacterial culture to develop

Figure 7.4

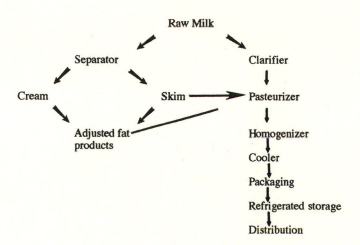

A common flow pattern for raw milk taken into a fluid milk processing plant.

flavor and acidity in the milk, a process that takes about eight to twelve hours at room temperature (72°F). Because of its resemblance to regular milk that has spoiled by turning sour, some people reject buttermilk. On the other hand, it has a loyal following and many develop a taste for it in time. Yogurt and acidophilus milk fit into the probiotic food category, that is, they are considered to have beneficial effects for their consumers beyond the conventional nutritional components. More particularly, it is held that the bacteria which are used to produce those products, and which are alive in them, benefit one through health effects in the intestinal tract. They are said to maintain a healthful population of bacteria in the lower intestine, prevent diarrhea and to aid the immune system. Acidophilus milk is indistinguishable from regular milk. Yogurt is altered from the latter in both flavor and appearance. It has the consistency of soft pudding and a flavor resembling that of buttermilk, yet distinctive to those who know it. Chocolate milk and all of the foregoing specialty milks are offered with regular and lower levels of fat.

Cream

An immediate effect of the cream separator was the creation of cream as an industrial material and a product in its own right. The main manufacturing uses of cream are in butter, ice cream, sour cream, and cream cheese and there are several standard retail creams, such as light, heavy, or whipping cream, and half and half. Many cooking and baking recipes call for cream.

Whipping cream. An important use of cream in the home is for making whipped cream. Everyone knows that a little whipped cream helps almost any dessert. The fat content of cream for whipping, which is available in any supermarket, is 30 to 35 percent fat. In the past, whether the product would whip was something of a gamble. However, in recent years the industry has made it pretty foolproof. They have added stabilizers and emulsifiers which greatly facilitates incorporation and retention of air. All one needs is for the cream, the bowl and the beaters to be cold and to whip rapidly until the product is suitably stiff. It used to be possible to easily pass the whipped stage and wind up with butter. The presence of added emulsifiers in the cream now makes this less likely.

Half and half. A mixture of half milk and half light cream began appearing widely on the American market about forty years ago. With a fat content of 12 percent and being homogenized, it has some very attractive and useful properties. Homogenization imparts viscosity and richness to the product well beyond what could be expected based on its fat content. Homogenization also gives good whitening power to half and half as a coffee additive. It is widely distributed in special small packages for the purpose. I often wonder if I am the only one who likes to drink those things, uncouth person that I am. What you do is use black coffee as a chaser. Half and half is sort of a chef's secret. It makes marvelous sauces, gravies, and soups—like lobster bisque and cream of mushroom. Because of the homogenization, there is no unsightly, possibly frightening, oiling off from half and half. In these times, there are people who become petrified when they see fat droplets on or around their food.

In the era before the fat scare, light cream was a favorite in coffee. It is hard to imagine how a teaspoonful of a product containing 18 percent fat would be that devastating but the psychological impact of these messages from the health authorities can be powerful. There used to be a product known as *creamed* cottage cheese. I can't find anything with that label anymore. What they talk about on the cottage cheese label is that the milk used in the product has been partially skimmed. One cannot blame the industry for these trends. They are simply trying to do business and satisfy customer requirements.

Buttermilk and Other Cultured Products

Milk is an excellent growth medium for bacteria. While this necessitates many sanitary precautions including pasteurization and refrigeration, it offers wonderful possibilities for production of cultured products, that is, milk products that are derived by fermentation with special varieties of non-harmful bacteria. Buttermilk, yogurt and sour cream are examples of such products. Many varieties of cheese are manufactured using treatment with a bacterial culture as an initial step. Such cultures bring about notable changes including the development of acidity, increase in viscosity, and the creation of unique flavor and aroma. The developed acidity, which is primarily lactic acid and which can reach as high as 1.0 to 1.5 percent, calculated as lactic acid, not only imparts tartness to the flavor, it also greatly aids keeping quality. With the exception of some molds, most microorganisms will not grow under such conditions.

Certain peoples of Eastern Europe are well known as consumers of fermented milks, and their notable longevity has been attributed to lifelong consumption of these products. The theory goes that bacteria in cultured milks can become dominant in the microflora of the intestinal tract, and that this is very healthy. Thus, other bacteria that produce disease as well as putrid and toxic substances are suppressed. While we know of no controlled epidemiological studies on this point, there is no question that buttermilk is an excellent food.

The term buttermilk can be a source of confusion. The practice of adding a bacterial culture to cream to be used for butter manufacture led to the naming of the by-product from the churning as buttermilk. As in other applications, the purpose of the culture was to impart desirable flavor and aroma to the butter. When butter is manufactured without benefit of culturing the cream, the by-product is called sweet cream buttermilk. Neither of these "buttermilks" is sold as beverage products at retail. Both are used in other processed foods. Used in ice cream manufacture, sweet cream buttermilk tends to promote superior body and texture in the finished product.

Because of the magnitude and importance of their use, preparation and supply of bacterial cultures is a major adjunct of the dairy industry and their care and handling is a specialty. The cultures must be carried from day to day. This means transfer periodically to fresh growth media without contamination. Another step involved in the use of cultures is the creation of starter. The making of starter is the intervening step that enables one to go from a small flask up to thousands of gallons. This involves generating a vigorously growing population of the organisms in a small quantity of the milk or cream to be inoculated. This starter can then be used to seed a much larger volume of product. Generally, incubation overnight at a suitable temperature, for buttermilk around 72° F, accomplishes the desired fermentation.

Most of the bacterial cultures employed in the dairy industry contain lactose fermentors as the dominant organism. Other special strains may be added to enhance flavor and aroma production. The culture organisms for yogurt are *Lactobacillus bulgaricus* and *Streptococcus thermophilus*. Both are lactose fermentors. Acetaldehyde is a principal aroma compound of yogurt whereas diacetyl is the more important characteristic aroma contributor to buttermilk and many other cultured dairy products. In both cases many other compounds are involved in the volatiles. Because of its powerful health food image, many people are devoted consumers of yogurt and some of them make their own at home using day-to-day transfers—not recommended here. The consumption of yogurt has increased something like sevenfold in the last twenty-five years. This gives one some understanding of the favorable health image yogurt has gained.

Sour Cream is actually a cultured buttermilk except that it is made with cream containing 18 to 20 percent fat. It has the consistency of fairly stiff pudding which results from a large increase in viscosity due to homogenization-induced clumping of its fat particles. Sour cream has a number of greatly appreciated traditional uses, such as on baked potatoes, with salsa on Mexican-American foods, and, as alternative to cream cheese, on bagels. It also has merit for improving the palatability of raw and cooked vegetables. Regarding the latter, it can be mixed in like butter or margarine but delivering more flavor and less fat than either of those. It is another one of those winners yet to be discovered by many.

Ice Cream

Regarding creativity in food preparation, it would seem that the development of ice cream was inevitable. No one seems to know just when the first ice cream was served but there are stories that it originated in Italy and stories that it was first served in America by Martha Washington while entertaining in the White House. She is supposed to have developed a special recipe whereby sweetened cream was mixed with snow and then flavored with fruit. On the theory there isn't much new under the sun, one can imagine that scenario could have happened at least a thousand years before Martha's time. Perhaps getting fruit at the same time as the snow would be limiting but the snow, cream and other interesting additives should have been no problem. As virtually everyone knows, ice cream rates at the very top of the food chart for palatability. Yes, you could refuse to eat it because of some religious or other principle, and you certainly may find flavors and brands that are not your first choice. But on the basis of how it tastes and feels in the mouth, there are no foods that can match it, at least not on a statistical basis. Many people like it best the way it comes out of the freezer, so-called soft-serve. Ice cream that is frozen hard takes a little patience and can actually be painful in the mouth because it is too cold. However, even choosy people can usually find a flavor that suits them and can condition the ice cream to the consistency they like.

There is a story that speaks pretty well to the matter of ice cream's palatability. It comes from our local newspaper[4] and concerns a young man twenty-two years old. He walked into an ice cream shop one morning at 11 A.M. and tried two free samples of ice cream. He left but later returned and threatened that if he wasn't given a bowl of chocolate ice cream, he would blow the clerk's head off. The clerk ran to the back of the shop and called the police. Apparently getting tired waiting for his treat, "the customer" grabbed a waffle cone as he departed and was greeted by the police out in front of the store. We are left to put whatever spin we want on this crazy story, but the man did make clear that he likes ice cream. Young males can have enormous appetites for ice cream. As a teenager I lived in the Philadelphia area. That city was and still is an ice cream

Mecca. The major manufacturers of those days, such as Breyers, Abbotts, Supplees, and Philadelphia Dairy Products, were in substantial degree responsible for developing the standards and quality of the outstanding product we are familiar with today. At that time, a smaller company in the area made good ice cream for $0.15 a pint, a low price even in those (mid-1930s) days. The containers were brick shaped and my friends and I would share these by cutting them in half. The cleaved container served as the dish; so all one needed was a wooden spoon. It was a great between meal treat for $0.075. Of course, sometimes one did away with the whole pint or even more depending on finances

Ice cream manufacture. What precisely is ice cream and how is it made? One way to approach these questions is to define how it differs from milk. In table 7.1, the composition of ice cream mix is compared with that of homogenized milk, mix being the product before freezing, addition of flavors (other than sugar) or the injection of fruits, nuts, cookies, and so on. Ice cream is made from milk so that the fat, and serum solids in both are qualitatively the same. Serum solids refers to the water-free part of skim milk. It includes the milk proteins, lactose and other water-soluble constituents less the water. It is evident from the table that ice cream contains several times as much fat and somewhat more serum solids than milk. The sugar added in making ice cream along with the higher fat content make it quite a bit higher in calories than milk but for an appraisal of this calorie situation, see nutritive value, following. In addition to cane sugar, a number of other sweeteners also may be included, particularly various kinds of corn syrup solids. These later also are considered to have favorable effects on the body and texture of the finished ice cream. Because of their beneficial effect on flavor and texture, eggs are used in some mix formulations.

Table 7.1
Gross Composition of Milk and Ice Cream

Component	Milk	Ice cream
Fat	3 - 4	10 -14
Serum solids	9	10 - 12
Added Sugar	0	15
stabilizer/emulsifier	0	0.1- 0.5
Water	87	62

Manufacture of ice cream mix usually utilizes cream and concentrated skim milk as primary ingredients. Cream and skim milk can be obtained by separation of milk as described in the section on separation. Condensed (concentrated) skim milk is produced by removing water from skim milk under vacuum or by using dried skim milk also known as non-fat dry milk. Actually a lot of different dairy products can be used in making mix of suitable composition. These include butter, butter oil, dried buttermilk from uncultured butter production, dried whey, dry whole milk, and various other milk fractions. If large amounts of dried ingredients are used, water will also be required. In addition to achieving the desired concentration of milk fat and serum solids, the important requirement is that all the ingredients make for a high quality finished ice cream.

When the proper formulation of milk solids has been achieved, the sugar, stabilizer and emulsifier are added under agitation to disperse and dissolve them. This is usually accomplished in a large stainless steel vat equipped with heating and agitation. It is best to premix the stabilizer and emulsifier with some sugar so that they do not irreversibly lump up during addition to the mix. The heating is continued until pasteurization is accomplished, and before cooling, the mix is passed through a homogenizer which gives the needed final dispersion of all ingredients. The homogenizer and homogenizing action is the same as that used for milk and other dairy product, as discussed earlier in this chapter. There is greater tendency for fat particles to clump as a result of homogenization in ice cream than in milk. To counteract this, an additional (second) stage of homogenization at lower pressure is usually applied to ice cream mix. After cooling (35° to 45° F.), the mix is ready for manufacture into various flavored ice creams or for storage.

Homogenization of ice cream mix was a standard practice quite a few years before it was adopted for milk in the 1940s and 1950s. If not homogenized, the fat in ice cream mix tends to churn during the freezing process which involves whipping not unlike the action and conditions for producing butter from cream. The presence of fat granules in ice cream is considered a serious defect.

Stabilizers and emulsifiers. These ingredients are added to the mix because they improve the quality of the resulting frozen product. Stabilizers are primarily vegetable gums with high water binding capability. They usually, but not always increase the viscosity (thickness) of the mix. Their main function is to organize the water structure of the product so that ice crystals in it remain small during frozen storage. Without stabilizers, commercial ice cream simply would not be able to maintain its smooth texture during distribution and storage. Gelatin is sometimes used as a stabilizer. Emulsifiers are substances that facilitate air incorporation into the mix during its freezing. They also create a very fine and stable dispersion of the resulting air cells. The wonderful palatability of ice cream results in part from its resemblance to whipped cream. It has a rich smooth somewhat fluffy feeling in the mouth. Emulsifiers are important contributors to this condition. They are so-called surface active agents and as such are related in structure and functional properties to the laundry and dishwashing detergents. Like them, emulsifiers tend to create stable foams and fine non-clinging dispersions of fat.

The incorporation of air into ice cream during freezing produces what is called overrun. If ice cream contains 100 percent overrun, half its volume is then due to incorporated air. To state it another way, the volume of a given amount of mix is doubled at 100 percent overrun. If no overrun were incorporated, frozen ice cream would have a character pretty much like an ice cube. There is no question that overrun is essential to the wonderful palatability of the product. It makes the frozen product feel softer and less cold in the mouth. Most commercial ice creams contain about 90 percent overrun although some premium brands have less.

Freezing and hardening. In the interest of keeping costs down, modern processing of ice cream is as large scale and automated as possible. Freezing, packaging and hardening in large ice cream operations are all done continuously. The mix flows continuously through the freezer which is a stainless steel cylinder that has a refrigerated jacket around it and revolving dashers and scrapers within. This equipment lowers the temperature of the mix below its freezing point, scrapes the forming ice crystals off the wall of the cylinder and whips air into the product as it freezes. Emerging from the exit end of the freezer is a semi-solid product that is ready for the various additives that will change it into the many different flavors we can buy in the stores. Feeders and injectors exist for this purpose, the most important objective being to get uniform distribution of the additive in the ice cream. The additives include an unimaginable variety of things: thickened syrups, fudges and chips, fruits and nuts of all kinds, suitably conditioned candy and cookie pieces, and so on. The Japanese, who have a great taste for fish, are now even putting it in their ice cream. Packaging machines rapidly produce pint, quart, half gallon and two and a half gallon units of product, among other sizes, which move on quickly into what is known as a hardening tunnel. This is a point on the conveyer that passes through a below 0° F. space that converts the semi-soft ice cream to a firm condition. The final and further hardening occurs in a so-called hardening room where the ice cream is stored below 0°F before distribution.

The body and texture of ice cream are very important in the way it feels in the mouth. They are not just determined and maintained by the temperature at which the ice cream is stored but also by the stability of that temperature. If the temperature fluctuates, the smaller ice crystals will melt and disappear when the temperature goes up. When it comes back down ice will selectively build on the remaining crystals making them larger. This process goes on until the ice crystal structure becomes noticeably coarse feeling in the mouth. Another thing which may happen is that growth of the ice crystals may puncture air cells thereby contributing to a condition known as shrinkage in which the actual structure of the frozen ice cream collapses, pulling away from the sides and the top of the container. That is why stabilizers and emulsifiers, which stabilize and strengthen the structure of the frozen ice cream are such useful ingredients and why a stable uniform storage temperature helps to maintain the quality of ice cream.

Varieties of ice cream. Generally, the garden variety of regular ice cream available in stores throughout the U. S. is of excellent quality, and it is rather amazing how consistent that quality is. Beyond the many variations in flavor, ice cream is sold in upscale versions with higher fat content, such as, 16 to 20 percent compared with the normal 10 to 12 percent. There are also lower- and no-fat versions; lower overrun products usually in the 60 to 70 percent range; frozen yogurt and soft-serve ice creams. The latter are very pleasant to consume. They go down so easily and are free of the mouth-numbing cold and hardness of some ice creams from the freezer. This soft condition is the same as that in commercial ice cream before it goes to the hardening room, and don't think the plant workers are unaware of that. There is a contemporary treatment for a dish or an à la mode of ice cream that is too hard, that is, about 5 to 10 seconds in the microwave.

Nutritive value. In the minds of some people, including a few nutritionists, ice cream is a no-no. "It's too rich, too calorific. It will make you fat. Anything that tastes that good, can't be good for you." A look at table 7.1 reveals that ice cream has the same nutritive components in it as does milk, a very good food. True, ice cream has added sugar and the picture may be modified somewhat by fruits, nuts, and other ingredients, but generally, it has the nutrition of milk with some additional calories. That's not so bad if one is an active person and confines the intake to a reasonable sized serving. There are possible health issues, both plus and minus, connected with the additional milk fat (see chapter 5). Remember also that ice cream is half air, so the calories per volume of it is not all that bad. The pleasure of eating ice cream also has to be taken into account. People all over the world crave it and their lives are made more tolerable when they can have it. For morale purposes among others, ice cream is a food that the U. S. makes available to its service personnel almost anywhere in the world. One way this is handled outside the U. S. is in the form of dried ice cream mix which can be reconstituted with water and frozen in soft serve machines on location. Unfortunately, ice cream is so readily available in the U. S. that it is often taken for granted.

Mr. Ice Cream. There are many people who have been involved in the development of ice cream and the advancement of the industry. As is true of the dairy field as a whole, much of the basic research and development of ice cream occurred at the state universities and was supported by tax dollars. Pennsylvania is and has been a major producer of ice cream and Penn State always has had

Figure 7.5

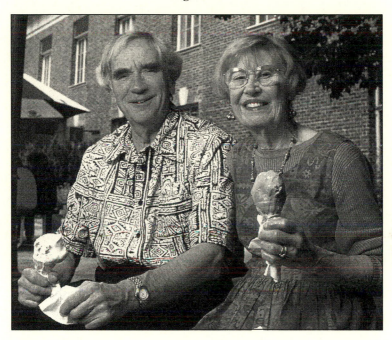

Professor Philip G. Keeney and his wife, Elsie, enjoying ice cream cones outside the sales room of the Penn State University Creamery. For Phil who is known widely as Mr. Ice Cream, this is not like the postman taking a walk on his holiday. He loves ice cream like most of the rest of us.

a strong education and research program in that area. For example, its annual Ice Cream Short Course has been taught for over 100 years and attracts students from around the world. A key person, not only in that course but in the ice cream field, is Prof. Philip G. Keeney, who is known widely as Mr. Ice Cream (figure 7.5). I have been privileged to know Phil for many years. In addition to his teaching, research by him and his students has improved the formulation and processing of ice cream. He is an ice cream consultant worldwide and has been featured in *People* magazine.[5] Europe, China, and Brazil, among other regions of the world, have received assistance from him in design and construction of ice cream plants.

It isn't surprising that Phil is an outstanding dairy scientist; he comes from that kind of family. His father, Mark Keeney, Sr., was the manager of a high-producing Holstein herd at the Essex County Hospital near Cedar Grove, NJ. Mr. Keeney developed a Holstein bull with the world's highest index at that time. The index concerns ability to genetically transfer milk-producing ability to one's offspring. He also proved that seaweed is a very nutritious food for cows.[6]

Phil had two older brothers Mark, Jr. and David who were classmates of mine. Mark became a professor and highly productive research scholar with broad interests in milk at the University of Maryland. Dave developed liquid Similac™ a substitute for breast milk and went on to become executive vice president of M and M Mars, the candy company. Phil's son, Phil, Jr., is manager of a large milk and ice cream plant in Harrisburg, PA. The Keeney family is by far the most illustrious I have ever known in the dairy field.

Cheese

Cheese is one of those very important foods that arose out of human antiquity. It is mentioned in the Old Testament[7] and appears to have been a basic food of the Israelites. Cheese is made all over the world and from the milk of many different animal species. Milk has natural tendencies to become cheese and it is entirely possible that we didn't have to invent it. First of all, milk is a good growth medium for bacteria and bacteria are important in converting milk into cheese. In addition, the sugar of milk, lactose, normally directs the bacterial fermentation of milk along lines that are healthy and non-toxic for humans. Very often these bacteria are natural contaminants of unpasteurized milk; and if milk is allowed to stand at room temperature, after a while the milk is said to have gone sour. This sourness is due to lactic acid which the bacteria have produced from the lactose. On further standing, such milk separates into a more or less clear yellowish green liquid and a semi-solid phase. The separation of milk into whey and curd in this instance is induced by the lactic acid.[8] If the whey is drained off and the curd collected and stored somewhere, the product which develops is cheese. Its character will depend a good bit on just how this curd is stored, that is, how it is packed, the temperature, the humidity, the length of time, and so on. The fact that this food turned out to be something one could store for a while and it would keep was another thing in its favor. So such very natural phenomenon could have started man on the path of cheese as food.

Another version of the cheese origin story is that it was discovered thousands of years ago when someone stored milk in an animal skin pouch, possibly a stomach, and came back to find that curd and whey had formed. Curd is what is said to result when the protein of milk, more particularly the casein, coagulates into a soft gel. It resembles the physical condition of a custard, which is normally made by heating a mixture of milk, eggs, sugar, and vanilla. Some confusion can arise about the term curd because an essential step in cheese making is to cut the curd to form pieces. (So whey and curd can form by two mechanisms; one, as explained above concerns the action of acid on milk [casein] and the other depends on the effect of enzymes on the casein of milk.) These isolated pieces of coagulated milk protein are also referred to as curd and they are the basic components used in manufacture of nearly all varieties of cheese. Our most frequent opportunity to observe curd is when we see the small cube-shaped pieces of cottage cheese. This is an instance where curd is consumed as such. Most cheese manufacture involves extensive processing of curd as discussed following.

Anyone who has been to a supermarket lately knows that there is an incredible variety of cheeses. In fact, the displays are kind of overwhelming. Some of them include an information section where one can look up in a booklet[9] the particular cheese(s) of interest and its characteristics and origin. Such help is very much needed these days because new varieties and modifications of cheese are coming out at a rapid rate. One that I like very much is a hybrid of Brie and Blue. It is soft, spreadable and contains about 40 percent fat. It sure makes a great bread and cracker spread.

Obviously, with as much milk going into cheese production as in to fluid milk in the U. S., cheese must be very popular. There is a cheese consumer culture, not unlike the wine-drinking culture. These cheese lovers take pride in their expert knowledge and firsthand experience. My hope is not to tread on anyone's toes here. It seems almost like being on sacred ground thinking and talking about a food so steeped in culture and ancient know-how. What I wish to do is briefly present principles of cheese making and to explain how so many recognizably different varieties of a food can be obtained from the same raw material, milk. Frank Kosikowski of Cornell University, a lifelong expert on cheese, wrote the definitive book on the subject. For those looking for detailed information, the modern version of Professor Kosikowski's book is the place to go, see suggested references.

Making cheese. To begin with, we might ask why would curd form from milk stored in a pouch made of skin. The answer is that the skin could have been the source of an agent(s), known as an enzyme(s), which promote formation of curd. Modern cheese making is based on adding an enzyme called rennin to milk. Originally this enzyme was extracted from calf stomach but now it is obtained more conveniently from molds. An enzyme is a protein that has the ability to repeatedly promote and greatly hasten a chemical reaction. The chemical reaction that rennin promotes is the cleavage of one big fragment, known as a glycomacropeptide, from the casein particle in milk. Removal of this peptide destroys the tendency of casein micelles in milk to repel each other. So ten or fifteen minutes after adding a suitable amount of rennin to milk, the casein micelles, which make up the white protein suspension in the skim milk phase, cross-link with each other to form a gel, or curd, as it is known.[10] This curd, when thoroughly set, is cut with special designed curd knives, ones that cut vertically and the others horizontally. The result is cube-shaped pieces. There is a natural tendency for a watery greenish yellow fluid, whey, to drain out of these pieces of curd. The whey contains all the water-soluble components of milk including the lactose, salts and water-soluble (whey) proteins. Regarding the identities of the latter, see p. 34 . The curd, on the other hand, is a concentrate of casein and the calcium and phosphate conjugated in its structure. The fat globules of the milk also become physically entrapped in the curd, so most cheeses are a concentrate of milk protein and milk fat. Since the expulsion of the whey is never 100 percent, there is always some whey with all its constituents left in the starting pieces of curd used to make cheese.

Heating the suspension of curd pieces in the whey promotes further expulsion of whey. This is one of the variables in cheese making that can promote a difference in the resulting cheese. How long was the curd heated and at what temperature? The less time and lower temperature used in the whey-expelling step, the more moisture (whey) retained in the curd and the cheese made from it, and generally, the softer the cheese.

A further step in cheese making involves placing the curd into suitable containers. The curd pieces in contact with each other during the whey drainage step have a tendency to knit together. This is further promoted by stacking cylindrical curd holders, which will eventually define the size and shape of the cheeses, and placing them under pressure. This not only expels more whey but it also closes up fissures between the curd pieces. After several days to a week or so, the individual cheeses will have assumed the proper physical condition. They are then removed from the forms and prepared for ripening. This is another key variable point in determining the character of the finished cheese. For example, at this time the surface of the cheese might be sprinkled with penicillium mold and punctured with long thin metal rods to promote air access favoring mold growth. In that case we would be off in the direction of blue-type cheeses. This would also be the time to treat the cheese surface with something to induce surface ripening with special culture of bacteria, yeasts, or molds, or to seal it with a wax dip. Finally, the cheeses are placed in a curing room where the temperature, humidity, and length of storage are further variables influencing what the cheese will be like.

Some of the other variables that are used to control what happens in the curd and thus to determine the ultimate nature of the cheese are addition of special bacterial cultures to the milk, treatment of the curd pieces with salt and washing them with water. Controlling the bacterial flora in cheese during ripening is crucial to the nature of the final product, particularly its flavor and texture. All three of these measures provide preferred bacteria with selective advantage over competitors. For example, a lactose fermenting culture that develops desirable flavor and aroma is added to the milk in cheddar cheese production. Another unique culture, added in the manufacture of Swiss cheese, contains the organism, *Propionibacterium shermanii* which helps to produce the characteristic holes and unique flavor of that cheese. Extensive whey expulsion from the curd is also an important step in Swiss cheese making.

A vital step in making soft ripened cheeses is to thoroughly wash and soak the curd in water to remove residual lactose. Lactose is a powerful fermentation controlling agent. It supports the growth of the lactic acid-producing bacteria and the resulting acidity can suppress many other strains of bacteria as well as the action of ripening enzymes. When lactose is removed by washing and soaking the curd, growth and action of bacteria and enzymes that hydrolyze proteins are favored. This condition tends to develop a soft body and the strong, stinky flavor characteristic of Liederkranz, Brick, Trappist, and Limburger-type cheeses, which many people love. The Penn State Creamery prepares and sells a Christmas gift box containing a number of their products, primarily different kinds of cheeses. It is very attractive and the Creamery personnel also do the mailing. However, a problem developed some years ago. The U. S. Postal Service was returning the boxes claiming that they contained spoiled merchandise. There was no spoilage but Penn State had to eliminate their Trappist and Brick cheeses from the gift boxes to appease the Postal Service.

Nutritive value. Cheeses generally are considered to be highly nutritious. While they are quite varied in flavor, body, and appearance, there are some aspects of their nutrition that apply across the board. Most of them contain essentially no carbohydrate, therefore they are not a source of calories from that standpoint. Some of the cheeses made from whey, such as Primost, may contain residual lactose; but in most cheeses, it is completely fermented away if not washed and soaked out of the curd. Most cheeses are primarily concentrates of casein and milk fat that vary in total food solids with moisture content. For example, a good rule of thumb for cheddar and Swiss is one-third protein, one-third fat and one-third water. Cheese making carries a substantial part of milk's calcium into the curd; thus, most cheese is a good source of calcium. Cottage cheese is a very popular un-aged cheese. It can be obtained either plain or creamed. Of course, the nutritive value of the creamed product will depend on the fat content and amount of cream. Plain cottage cheese is pretty much a pure protein food although some whey (primarily water and lactose) is retained in the curd pieces. Over all, cheeses are quality food. They definitely fit low carbohydrate diet requirements. As we acquire more and better understanding of bioactive food components, it will be interesting to reappraise cheeses, which undergo a lot of unique microbial and aging changes, the chemistry of which have received little attention.

Some varieties. Cheese can be classified in many different ways, such as by relative firmness of body, ripening agents, use, and so on. Table 7.2 classifies some of the popular varieties found in the American market. Romano and Parmesan are very popular as grating cheeses. Camembert and brie lend themselves very well to the cocktail hour because they are nicely spreadable, with wonderful flavor but not so stinky as to drive away the faint hearted and dismay the hosts. On the other hand, if there is a happy home for raunchy smells, certain revered cheeses provide it. Some of these are listed under the classification, odorous, in the table. Basically, the strong aroma of these cheeses involves sulfur compounds which are produced by decomposi-

Table 7.2
Some Popular Ripened Cheeses Classified by Several Important Attributes.

Soft	Firm	Hard	Blue Mold	Odorous
Camembert	Cheddar	Parmesan	Rocquefort	Limburger
Brie	Swiss	Romano	Gorgonzola	Liederkranz
	Colby		Stilton	Trappist
	Edam		Danish Blue	Brick
	Gouda		Iowa Blue	

tion of the protein. The odors are reminiscent of that produced during the ripening of sauerkraut.

It is interesting that long before America made blue cheese, there were popular varieties of that type made in several countries of Europe (table 7.2), Rocquefort made from sheep's milk in France, Stilton of England, Gorgonzola of Italy, and Danish Blue. About fifty years ago, researchers at Iowa State University devised a method of making blue cheese which has been widely adopted in the U. S. Mostly the penicillium mold that makes these cheeses what they are is green-looking, not blue, but in any case, these cheeses are popular. They are especially good when allowed to ripen to the point that they get at least somewhat softened and less crumbly. This has been recognized in recent years by the offering of a cheese called Cambazola™ which appears to be a cross between the soft body of Camembert and the unique flavor of Gorgonzola (blue) cheese.[11] Another close relative of that cheese is a brie with added chopped mushrooms. The two flavors go together beautifully. Of course, all kinds of other foods and flavors are added to commercial cheeses.

Cheddar and process cheese are greatly appreciated in the U. S. cheddar, originally developed in England, is firm in body, and depending on how long it is ripened, the flavor varies from mild to a condition described as "sharp." As with many sensory perceptions, precisely what sharp is evades many of us. Nonetheless, sharpness has created a cult and the term sells a lot of cheddar whether one knows what it means or can recognize it. My understanding is that sharpness increases with age: and that it is a combination of tartness with a unique flavor (aroma) that in my opinion is faintly on the skunky side.[12]

On the other hand, there is process cheese, which Americans also love. Bland and pleasant tasting, it is odds and ends of cheddar melted down, mixed with an emulsifying agent and hot-packed into plastic lined rectangular packaging. One can buy it by the box, the chunk or a pack of slices. If made out of all aged cheddar, which wouldn't make much economic sense, it could even be sharp tasting. It is good in sandwiches and for baking and cooking.

Process cheese is a marvelous example of Yankee ingenuity. Curing is a gamble with cheese just as it is with wine. Even the old-line producers with great experience have batches of cheddar that do not turn out too well. Sampling during curing can sometimes indicate there may be trouble ahead. Such cheese is not inedible; and converted into processed cheese, it is quite palatable. Being much cheaper than aged cheddar and bland in flavor, many prefer it. Thus, process cheese is a real plus in cheese manufacture and marketing. Among the problems that can derail cheddar during curing are the flavor going off, the body becoming crumbly or full of gas holes, and the appearance of mold contamination. Moldy cheddar simply isn't any more acceptable than moldy bread. For some years the Penn State Creamery made both blue and cheddar, as well as other cheeses. The mold contamination problem in the cheddar became so severe they had to give up manufacturing blue cheese.

Cheese economics in brief. For a typical semi-hard cheese such as cheddar, it takes about eleven pounds (five quarts) of milk to make one pound of cheese. Knowing this relationship can help when one is pondering whether a particular piece of cheese is a good buy. Compare the price per pound of the cheese with that for five quarts of milk. In addition, cheese is a value-added commodity in that there is capital and labor invested in its production from milk. Further, cheese requires a ripening period of months when it is an investment sitting on the shelf. It should be earning some interest, and aged cheddar should bring a better price than the green cheese for that reason alone. There are quite a few other factors that figure in. Milk going into cheese costs less than milk to be processed for the retail market. There is some return to the cheese maker for whey as a byproduct. Milk fat is the expensive component of cheeses, and it makes a difference whether the cheese is half-, full-, double- or triple-cream. Imported cheeses may involve tariffs that add to the price. So the price of a piece of cheese involves quite a few factors.

In summary, there are many variables in the manufacture and ripening of cheese that can dramatically affect its character and this is the main reason for the great variety of cheeses. A further factor is the species of animal providing the milk. Rocquefort from sheep's milk enjoys a longstanding acceptance. The popularity of goat milk cheeses seems to be growing. Innovation is ever possible. Cheeses are nutritious, highly satisfying foods. Enjoyment of them will always be a treasured part of life for many people throughout the world.

Condensed Milks

Concentration of milk, that is, the removal of water, is a primary step in many dairy operations. Many well-known dairy products, such as dried milk, evaporated milk and sweetened condensed milk involve an initial concentration.

Sometimes this step is taken with raw milk using membrane filtration to remove the water, and thus reduce the volume and the shipping cost to the processing plant, but most concentrating of milk is done at the plant in connection with some further manufacturing. The removal of water is ordinarily carried out by one of two methods, either in falling film evaporators or in what is known as a vacuum pan. The falling film systems capitalize on maximizing surface exposure and heat transfer properties of milk in a thin film. They are complex multistage systems that vary in design and operation depending on the end product being made.[13] A vacuum pan is simply a large sealed chamber for boiling away the water of milk under vacuum. Such units achieve water removal at temperatures of 120° to 140°F. These conditions are non-injurious to color or flavor of the product. Because of their greater energy efficiency and continuous product flow characteristics, falling film systems have mostly replaced vacuum pans. Either of these means of removing water from milk are the preferred initial step in producing dried milk products because the final step to total dryness, accomplished in a dryer, is the most expensive. Condensed milk, especially condensed skim milk, is also used to increase milk solids in products which require higher concentrations than are normally present in milk, for example, ice cream mix and retail skim milk with added milk solids.

Evaporated milk. Humanity must have cast around for endless years in efforts to find ways of preserving milk. Real progress required some precise understanding of the role of bacteria in food spoilage and that didn't come until the mid 1800s when the germ theory of disease was embraced and Pasteur devised pasteurization as a means of destroying bacteria. The product that really solved this problem was evaporated milk, the invention of which is generally credited to Gail Borden. In 1856, he was granted a patent on condensed milk and shortly thereafter the first condensed milk plant went into operation. In this case the terms, condensed and evaporated refer to the evaporation of water from milk which makes it more condensed or concentrated. However, in the retail trade, evaporated milk refers strictly to the canned concentrated milk that contains no added sugar. Sweetened condensed milk is the term applied to the canned milk with added sugar. Both of these products have remained pretty much unchanged in the 150 years or so since their development. Evaporated milk is concentrated 2:1 by removing water from the milk. Thus, if you wish to use it as normal milk, it should be diluted with an equal volume of water. It and sweetened condensed milk can be found in any supermarket.

From the standpoint of microbiological spoilage, evaporated milk keeps indefinitely, although extremely rare cases of spoilage show up. A real danger signal is when the can is bulged. This means something, more than likely bacteria, has been producing gas inside the can after it was sealed as the final step in manufacture. Take any such can back to where you purchased it. The producer needs to know about it and you should get your money back. Evaporated milk has a slight tan color, which intensifies during room temperature

Figure 7.6

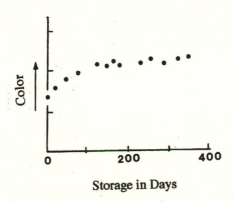

Storage in Days

Development of tan color in evaporated milk samples stored at 72°F for one year. Data points are averages for 11 commercial products used in the study (Patton, S. Journal of Dairy Science 35:1053-66. 1952).

storage. This is due to the sterilizing heat treatment it receives. Most of the change in color occurs during the first couple of months of storage and is relatively limited after six months (figure 7.6). The development of brown color is linked to an increase in caramelized flavor. While a primary benefit of evaporated milk is that it will keep without refrigeration, such storage strongly suppresses change in its color and flavor.

The processing of evaporated milk is accomplished under the exceptionally high sanitary standards of the dairy industry. In order to prevent fat separation the product is homogenized either before or after condensing 2:1. Prior to condensing, the milk is usually forewarmed to a relatively high temperature (190° to 200°F.). This treatment either reduces or eliminates the need to apply heat during condensing and it also tends to stabilize the milk against coagulation during the subsequent heat sterilization. As an additional precaution against such coagulation, a small amount of a stabilizing salt, such as dipotassium phosphate or sodium citrate, may be added to the concentrated milk prior to sterilization. Because the susceptibility of the milk to heat coagulation varies with such factors as feed and season of the year, it is common practice to conduct a pilot scale experiment using graded levels of stabilizing salt to determine how much, if any stabilizer addition is needed. The cans of milk are then sealed and subjected to sterilizing heat treatment on the order of 240°F. for fifteen minutes with continuous agitation. The cans of milk are then cooled labeled and boxed for storage or shipment to market.

With exception of minor variable losses in a few of the vitamins and the amino acid, lysine, evaporated milk appears to be fully comparable nutritionally to pasteurized whole milk. Some of the lysine is changed irreversibly by a heat-induced reaction with lactose[14] but the magnitude of this destruction during manufacture and storage of evaporated milk has not been defined. Millions of babies have been raised using diluted evaporated milk as an infant formula. This has worked quite well but it requires supplementation with vitamins and iron. Pediatricians recommend breastfeeding for infants during the first year of life. For further discussion of this matter, see chapter 3.

In addition to its nutritive value, evaporated milk has a number of other merits. On a milk solids basis, it is invariably cheaper than regular pasteurized whole milk. For example, a comparison of the two products offered in two San Diego supermarkets recently revealed a quart of reconstituted evaporated milk would have cost from $0.79 to $1.13, range for five brands, compared to $1.68 for a quart of fresh whole milk. This difference, which has existed for many years, is due to the fact that milk for product manufacture is cheaper than that for retail fluid milk as defined by milk marketing plans of the state and federal governments. Evaporated milk is sterile as purchased and thus is no problem with respect to communicable diseases or proliferating bacteria. It is a handy storable ingredient for supplying milk in cooking and baking recipes and one usually finds it in the baking materials section of the super market. Of course, once the can is opened, things can happen. From then on, it is perishable, and if not promptly used, should be refrigerated.

The primary limitation of evaporated milk is its flavor in comparison to fresh pasteurized milk which is the beverage milk flavor standard in the U. S. and other areas of the world. Once adapted to that standard, one finds it difficult if not impossible to drink evaporated milk. However, served cold, the reconstituted product to which a little sweetener and flavor has been added can be quite refreshing as well as nutritious. A few drops of vanilla or almond extract per glass seem to fit well with the normal mild caramelized flavor of this milk.

Sweetened condensed milk. In the production of evaporated milk, if at the outset we had added about eighteen pounds of sugar per 100 pounds of milk, we would have been on the way to making sweetened condensed milk. Actually both products are roughly a 2:1 concentrate of whole milk. However, sweetened condensed milk is canned without being sterilized. It does not spoil, not only because of good manufacturing sanitation, but primarily because of its high sugar (sucrose plus lactose) content which runs about 67 percent in the water phase of the product. This is analogous to jams and jellies which rely on 60 to 65 percent sugar for their keeping quality. Because it has received much less heat treatment than evaporated milk, sweetened condensed milk has less of a tendency to undergo color and flavor change.

Sweetened condensed milk should be refrigerated once opened. It is used in recipes for desserts, frostings, and other toppings, candies and ice cream. It represents sort of a shortcut for getting both sugar and milk into a recipe in one product, and with the advantage that the sugar is already dissolved. Regarding ice cream formulation, adding one part of sweetened condensed to two parts of half and half comes very close to the composition of a regular commercial ice cream mix with about 10.5 percent fat. One would also need to dissolve about 0.4 percent gelatin and add some vanilla to have a product that is ready for the ice cream freezer.

Dried Products

Because milk is a liquid of about 87 percent water and subject to microbial spoilage as well as flavor change, drying as a means of preserving milk has received a lot of attention. Other major reasons for drying milk are to reduce shipping cost, refrigeration, storage facilities, and space requirements. The dairy industry is a foremost authority on large-scale drying operations. The major dried products include whole milk, skim milk, buttermilk, whey, whey protein concentrate, and ice cream mix. Significant amounts of many other milk fractions and milk-containing products are dried.

Certain areas of the world accept dry whole milk for reconstitution as a beverage and for other uses. However, the American consumer is adapted to the very mild and consistent flavor of fresh milk. Characteristic flavor changes develop in the fat phase of dry whole milk, particularly during storage. The use of anti-oxidants and inert gas (nitrogen) packing of the dry whole milk provides only a partial solution to the problem. The particular changes are well accepted in dried ice cream mix because the additional flavoring of the product, for example, sugar, vanilla, chocolate, etc., are strong, pleasant, and overwhelming of any minor defects. Dried skim milk, also known as nonfat dry milk (NFDM), does not have the flavor problems contributed by the milk fat. As a consequence it enjoys good consumer acceptance and the product, when reconstituted with water of good quality is generally indistinguishable from fresh skim. NFDM is marketed all over the world. In addition to use in beverages, large amounts are incorporated into dry mix types of commercial foods including cake, pudding, frostings, hot chocolate, and gravy mixes. The baking industry is also a large user. The problem of flavor deterioration in dry whole milk has been substantially solved by handling the fat phase separately. At the time and place of consumption, this fat is homogenized into reconstituted NFDM. Pure milk fat is known in the trade as anhydrous milk fat or butter oil. It keeps well, particularly under refrigerated storage, and can be recombined with the skim milk phase. This innovation makes it possible now to supply the ingredients and technology for palatable milk anywhere in the world.

Milk and milk products are usually concentrated to at least 35 to 40 percent solids before drying. That is a practical and economic way of removing a lot of

Figure 7.7

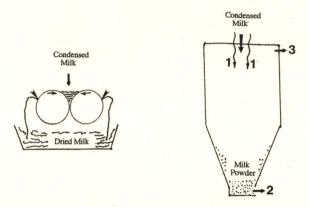

Left: Schematic representation of the process for roller drying milk. Condensed milk is deposited in the trough formed by two closely apposed steam-heated metal cylinders. As the cylinders continuously rotate, films of the milk deposited on them in the trough dry en route to knife blades which scrape the dried milk films free. Right: A scheme for the spray drying of milk. Condensed milk is atomized into the drying chamber through a spray nozzle. Hot (drying) air (1) enters the drier flowing concurrently with the liquid condensed milk particles. Dehydrated particles of milk fall to the bottom of the drier cone and are removed by conveyer and fines collection systems starting at 2. Moisture laden air exits at 3.

the water and it makes for a more dense and manageable particle in the final drying step. Both roller and spray dryers are used, but the latter much more widely today. Roller dryers are constructed of cylindrical metal drums which revolve, either a single drum or two drums in close contact rolling counter to each other. In the latter case, the drums form a trough into which the product to be dried is deposited. The rollers are steam heated and the thin film of product deposited on them is quickly dried, scraped off into a collecting system by a knife blade bearing against the roller surface. Spray dryers operate on the principle of atomizing the concentrated milk into a current of hot air. By the time the milk particles fall to the bottom of the collecting cone or floor of the drier, they are dry, that is, 1 to 3 percent water, and as they collect, can be removed at intervals by a conveyor. Compared to roller-dried products, those by spray drying are usually more soluble, uniform, and free of heat damage. The processing principles involved in these two drier systems are shown in figure 7.7. For good keeping quality, it is desirable to get the moisture content of dried milk products in the 2 to 4 percent range. One pound of NFDM is equivalent to eleven pounds of fresh skim.

Whey

There are two basic forms of whey, sweet and acid. The principal source of acid whey is from cottage cheese manufacture which employs an acid-generating bacterial culture, along with an enzyme such as rennin, to coagulate the casein and generate flavor. When only rennin or a related enzyme is used, such as in cheddar or Swiss cheese production, the whey remains sweet and essentially as it is in the original milk. On a volume basis there is a lot more sweet than acid whey produced. Both forms represent milk from which all of the fat and casein have been removed. However, a very important part of the nutrients of milk partition into the whey. This includes the whey proteins, lactose, water-soluble vitamins and most of the minerals, with the exceptions of considerable calcium and phosphorus which go with the casein into the cheese curd.

As the dairy industry advanced during the past 150 years, what to do with whey arising from the cheese industry became an enduring problem. It could be had for the hauling and was frequently returned to the farm for use as pig feed and to dump on fields. Much of it was run down drains at the cheese plants severely challenging sewage systems. The value of whey has been increasingly recognized in recent years. Versatile practical methods of fractionating and processing whey have enhanced its value. It is dried in the manner of skim milk and is used widely as an ingredient in many processed foods. Examination of labels on food products from the supermarket reveals whey as an ingredient in a surprisingly large number of foods. One important use is in frozen desserts. In oversupply and at low price, it is used as animal feed.

Membrane filtration has provided another dimension to whey processing making it possible to isolate the whey proteins and dry them as a protein concentrate of special nutritive value and utility in processed foods. Selective isolation of bioactive components from whey has opened up the possibility of producing items having very high profitability as pharmaceuticals and food supplements. This line of development is also supported by the huge amount of raw material (whey) available. Actual progress in this area of research and development is obscured by the proprietary nature of the work. However, it is a very worthwhile research frontier.

Butter

No doubt butter was discovered by humans thousands of years ago. If milk is sloshed around in a partly filled container for a while, the milk fat globules will eventually cluster together to form visible fatty particles. This could have occurred during travel when the milk was being transported. The particles may have been collected by the observer and worked into a mass which we know as butter. Such butter would not have very long shelf life, but another useful observation was probably soon in coming. When the butter was heated, such as in cooking processes, it could have been noted that an oil formed and that the oil had much longer keeping quality than the original butter. This is because the aqueous phase of the butter, which would have promoted spoilage by bacteria and/or molds would have been left behind or boiled away. We refer to this product as butter oil. It is known as *ghee* in India and *samna* in Egypt: and it is a much more important consumer product in those countries as compared to the U. S. Of course, modern day butter has relatively good keeping quality and that is a result of excellent industrial sanitation and the use of pasteurized cream in its manufacture. Even so, it is always handled under refrigeration in retail channels. Most cultures, including the American, have rather precise standards for butter and butter oil.

To elaborate for a bit on the reason that our ancestors' heating of butter could have improved its keeping quality: if the process were carried to the point where the moisture of the butter was boiled away and the remaining milk solids were caramelized (browned) in the oil, anti-oxidants that protect the flavor of the oil for a protracted period would have been developed. This fact was discovered in a study[15] conducted many years ago. The generation of anti-oxidant activity as a result of browning and roasting is a relatively neglected area of food research. Seemingly, roasted nuts, chocolate, and coffee may have health benefits that stem from anti-oxidants produced during the high temperatures employed in their production. When food systems such as milk undergo browning, they generate protein associated reducing substances with antioxidant potencies similar to those of vitamin C.[14, 16]

Manufacture. The invention of the cream separator was absolutely essential to industrial butter production, the raw material for which is cream of about 30 to 35 percent fat. The separator assured regular, large scale and efficient production of cream of the proper fat content. Commercial butter is made both in batches using a churn and by continuous butter-making equipment of which there are a number of designs and manufacturers. In either case, the churning principles are the same, the main difference being that the continuous process accomplishes the various steps more quickly which makes continuous output of product possible.

There is a choice as to whether butter will be made from sweet or cultured cream. If the latter, a culture of bacteria that will develop the desired flavor and aroma is added and the cream is allowed to incubate overnight usually at about 70° F. The organisms are generally lactose-fermenting types and the flavor/aroma is of the same type as produced in the making of buttermilk, cottage cheese and sour cream. The cream or cultured cream is temperature conditioned to make plasticity of the fat optimum for churning and then churned at about 55°F. A semi-solid condition of the fat, that is, not completely liquid and not totally hardened, seems to be very important because it will enable the fat globules to stick to each other. If they resist adhering to each other, the butter particles will be slow to form and churning will take a long time.

Figure 7.8

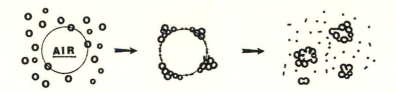

A scheme illustrating principal stages in the churning of cream to butter. Left: Agitation produces air cells amidst many small spherical milk fat globules in cream. Center: To gain structural stability as a suspension in the cream, air cells share and rob fat globules of their surface membrane. Right: This leads to clumping and merging of fat globules at membrane denuded points on their surfaces and to release of liquid fat which destabilizes the air cells. Their collapse releases minute butter granules and disperses large amounts of membrane fragments into the resulting buttermilk. Continued agitation induces merging of butter granules with consequent increase in their size.

The next phase of butter making involves incorporation of air. For the sake of simplicity, we will discuss this in terms of producing butter in a churn, a large barrel-shaped container that can be rotated. The cream is placed in the churn which is then closed and set in motion. Because of various baffles in the inner structure of the churn, vigorous agitation with incorporation of air into the cream occurs. The change going on at the level of the fat globules under these conditions is illustrated in figure 7.8. In essence, whipped cream is produced and in order to stabilize the structure of the growing dispersion of air in the cream, the membrane that encompasses fat globules is stolen by the increasing numbers of air cells. Eventually, the sticky surfaces of the denuded fat globules find each other and the globules gather together to form particles of butter which grow in size as churning continues. The removal of membrane from the fat globules also releases some liquid fat which seems to destabilize the air cells and leads to a collapse of the whip cream. At that point the small particles of butter are clearly evident. Anyone who has experience making whipped cream at home knows that the time to stop the beater is somewhat arbitrary. You want the cream to be sufficiently stiff and full of overrun (air) to obtain a good yield. But don't go too far and don't get distracted or you may get butter.

Generally the churning action is continued until the butter granules are about the size of a pea at which point the buttermilk can be drained off. The next steps are the washing, working, incorporation of salt, if it is to be salted butter, and possibly color. It is desirable to wash out residual milk solids to aid keeping quality of the butter. It is necessary to work the butter in order to make it a homogeneous mass and to incorporate the proper amount of water as well as salt. The color of butter will very depending on the cows diet. The lush pastures of spring and early summer make for butter that is very yellow. Some markets like greater yellowness than others. A yellow vegetable dye, annato, is often used to meet market requirements and to make butter color more uniform. Following the indicated steps, the butter is cut into units and packaged for marketing. In retail channels, butter is always stored under refrigeration. This is good practice in the home, too, but some temperature conditioning may be needed for best spreadability. One other note of caution, minimize exposure of butter to light, especially daylight, in order to prevent off-flavor development.

Nutritive values. Butter is approximately 80 to 82 percent fat, 15 to 16 percent water and about 2 percent salt, if salted. There are small amounts of protein and lactose, about 0.5 percent of each remaining after the washing. Thus, the nutritive value and healthfulness of butter is essentially that of milk fat. It supplies energy (calories), fat-soluble vitamins and essential fatty acids as given in chapter 2. As a result of the diet/fat/heart health advisories, no food has suffered greater image trashing than butter with the possible exception of eggs. However, eggs have been substantially rehabilitated since revelation that blood cholesterol levels are not elevated much, if at all, in most people as a result of ingesting cholesterol-containing foods. There are indications that butter contains components that inhibit both obesity and heart disease (see the discussion of milk fat, chapter 5 and the extensive review by Miller et al.[17]). There are a couple of things we definitely must hold against butter. It makes foods taste good and it has generated a lot of imitators. Families didn't produce their own butter for the first 250 years in America because it was an unsatisfactory product.

* * *

This chapter is an effort to inform the reader as to what retail milk and milk products are beyond the labels and the hearsay. The review of the information makes clear that cows' milk has been a tremendous gift to humanity. It's not just the refreshment and sound nutrition of a cold glass of milk, there are also the products made from it including cheese, ice cream, and many cultured items that are great foods in their own right. In addition, there is the capacity of milk products as ingredients and toppings to make other foods and recipes of all kinds truly enjoyable. It is not an accident that there are unrelenting efforts to imitate butter, ice cream, whipped cream and even beverage milk. Those products are standards of excellence in the food field and testimonials of success to their producers. Cheese is too, but in most forms and varieties it does not lend itself to imitation. Cheddar, America's favorite is a good example. Its inner being, an exceptionally complex state of affairs, may remain a mystery for some time to come. However, that will not keep us from appreciating it and the many other varieties. To sum up, milk in its many ways, is a major basis of the good life. For those needing a more in-depth technical treatment of milk processing and products than provided here, a number of appropriate texts have been listed under suggested references following.

Suggested References

Kosikowski, F.V. and Mistry, V.V. *Cheese and Fermented Milk Foods: Book I: Origins and Principles; Book II: Procedures and Analysis, 3rd Edition.* (Two-volume set) 1997. Publisher: F.V. Kosikowski LLC. pp. 1050.

Marshall, R. T, and Arbuckle, W. S. *Ice Cream*, 5th Edition, Chapman & Hall, New York, NY. 1996. pp. 349.

Tamime, A. Y. and Law, B. A. (eds.) *Mechanisation and Automation in Dairy Technology.* Sheffield Academic Press, Sheffield, U. K. and CRC Press, Boca Raton, FL, USA. pp. 348.

Webb, B. H. and Whittier, E. O. (eds.) *Byproducts from Milk.* Avi Publishing C., Westport, CN. 1970. pp. 428.

Notes

1. Trout, G. M. *Homogenized Milk.*. Michigan State University Press. East Lansing, MI. 1950.
2. Du Puis, E. M. *Nature's Perfect Food.* New York University Press, New York. 2002. pp. 310.
3. Data from *Milk Facts*, International Dairy Foods Association. Washington, DC. 2002. Reproduced with permission.
4. Repard, D. San Diego Union Tribune, August 15, 2002
5. July 4, 1983.
6. He also was an impressive bridge player. I remember one occasion when he got the contract for four spades doubled and redoubled. I held the ace, king, and queen of spades against him and he made it.
7. 1 Samuel 17:17.
8. The casein of milk, particles (micelles) of which give skim milk its whiteness, remain suspended in fresh milk because they are negatively charged electrically and thus repel each other. As acid develops in milk as a result of bacterial fermentation, the negative charge is neutralized, the casein particles no longer repel each other and they gather together to form clots or flakes of casein known as curd. As explained in the text, a similar result is produced by enzymes but by a different mechanism.
9. Anonymous. *The Art of Serving and Selecting Cheese.* Try Foods International Inc. Apopka, FL. 2002. pp. 92.
10. The fact that calf stomach was for many years a commercial source of rennin for cheese making is not illogical, it and a closely related enzyme, pepsin, bring about this same reaction as a first step in the digestion of casein in the stomachs of all mammals including the human.
11. The unique flavor of blue-type cheeses is due to a homologous group of aliphatic methyl ketones containing odd numbers of carbons. These are produced by the action of the blue (penicillium) mold on milk fat from which they release fatty acids that are in turn beta-oxidized to the ketones. The free fatty acids also contribute importantly to the flavor (Patton, S. *Journal of Dairy Science* 33:680-4. 1950).

12.   A great deal of research effort has been expended on trying to characterize the aroma of Cheddar cheese. A valid formulation of it would be very profitable to sell by the bottle. Further, knowing what it is could take some of the risk out of efforts to make good Cheddar because one could chemically measure progress of desired aroma development in a given lot of cheese. My guess is that the key compound(s) is one or more volatile mercaptans, that is, -SH-bearing compounds. These have very potent odor and are highly sensitive to oxidation which may explain why they have proven so elusive to identify. There is probably extremely little of them in the cheese, and by the time one has isolated them, they well may have been decomposed by oxygen of the air or altered by other molecules copresent. Another indication that -SH compounds are important to Cheddar is that better quality Cheddar contains hydrogen sulfide, the simplest -SH compound; and it may aid in the chemical production and stabilization of other -SH compounds in the cheese.

13.   For further description of falling film evaporation systems, see de Jong, P. and Verdurmen in: Tamime, A. Y. and Law, B. A. (eds.) *Mechanisation and Automation in Dairy Technology.* Sheffield Academic Press, Sheffield, U. K. and CRC Press, Boca Raton, FL, pp. 95-7.

14.   Patton, S. Browning and associated changes in milk. A review. *Journal of Dairy Science.* 38:457-478. 1955.

15.   Josephson, D. V. and Dahle, C. D. *Food Industries* 17(6):80-3. 1945.

16.   Doan, F. J. and Josephson, D. V. *Journal of Dairy Science* 26: 1031. 1943.

17.   Miller, G. D., Jarvis, J. K. and Mc Bean, L. D. *Handbook of Dairy Foods and Nutrition*, 2nd. Ed. pp. 1-423. CRC Press, Boca Raton, FL. 2000.

8

Flavor and Milk

The great enjoyment people have of milk and milk products results in a major way from their wonderful flavors. In this chapter, the nature of flavor is defined as a necessary basis for understanding the distinctive flavor characteristics of milk and its products. It will also help one understand flavor defects that may develop. With respect to foods and nutrition, it is hard to overestimate the importance of flavor. It is like a pied piper luring us down the path of our dietary fate. If we find that "deep-fried" character irresistible, it may mean continuing consumption of concentrated calories leading to problematic weight gain. Sweetness can have a similar effect. We all have our likes and dislikes about foods, and most of these are based on flavor. Before getting into this subject, please bear with me about some anecdotal background which follows.

Somehow the flavor of milk and milk products was to become important in my life and there were harbingers early on of things to come. I was about six or seven living with my family in East Aurora, NY, a bedroom community about twenty miles south of Buffalo. It was the mid-1920s and I was allowed to range pretty freely around our pleasant residential neighborhood. On one of my expeditions, I came upon an open freight car full of forty-quart milk cans on a siding by the milk processing plant a couple of blocks from our home. I noted that the can lids were loose and the cans had been emptied, but there was still something that looked like whipped cream sticking in some of the lids. I gave that stuff the taste test and was an instant convert. Using bare hand-to-mouth action, I quickly cleaned out a number of those lids. I later learned that the cans of milk were picked up daily from farm communities along the railroad route into East Aurora and that during holding, the cream rose to the top of the cans. As the train rolled along the vibration and swaying produced some whipped cream like froth in the lids—my newfound treat. I got there at just the right time, after the cans had been dumped but before they were washed up for the return.

And the rising of the cream was not wasted on me. This was is in the days before homogenized milk. Milk that stood undisturbed as little as half and hour would clearly show the cream layer on top. Our milk, which was delivered to the doorstep always exhibited this line which separated the cream from the skim about a third of the way down the bottle. I soon recognized that the top of the bottle tasted much better on my cereal than did what was in the bottom. So I would get up before anyone else, bring the milk in and pour the cream on my cereal. My father, who liked the cream for his coffee, was sorely provoked. "That little s-o-b has done it again." I was finally put under heavy duress and had to give up this pleasant practice. However, it taught me a lifelong appreciation of how good cream tastes.

Some years later, as an undergraduate at Penn State, I worked part time in the laboratories of the Department of Dairy Science. My job was to wash glassware, make up reagents, and help maintain order. It quickly became clear to me that some professors in the Department were spending a good bit of time on taste work. Much of their research involved flavor evaluation of milk and milk products that had been processed and stored under various conditions. They were pretty awesome to me in their white coats, tasting samples and recording results. I soon learned that flavor is fragile and very important in the consumer acceptance of foods. The bigger picture was that Penn State, a state-supported institution, was obligated to do things that would benefit Pennsylvania. There were two big and very important audiences for those efforts: the dairy industry and consumers. Pennsylvania had and still has plenty of both. Fluid milk and ice cream are major commodities there. By the time I had made my way through the undergraduate program at Penn State, I had a keen appreciation of flavor science.

The Nature of Flavor

For the sake of clarity, we need first to define some terms. There can be confusion about taste and smell, flavor and aroma. Flavor includes several considerations as follows:

The *aroma, odor,* or *smell* is that part of flavor detected up in the nose in what is called the olfactory area.

The *taste* part is the sensations of sweet, salt, sour, and bitter perceived by the taste buds on the tongue.

The *tactual* is the way a food feels in the mouth. Such terms as smooth, creamy, oily, crunchy, puckery, grainy, chalky, hot or burning, and many others are used to describe tactual flavor characteristics of foods.

These three components are what make up flavor. The basic distinctions among them become important when we are trying to understand the likes and dislikes people have about foods. Going back to the deep-fried foods, they are enjoyed for the crunchiness of the fried surfaces and the rich sensation of the cooking fat or oil in the mouth. Both of these sensations are tactual. Certain distinctive aroma compounds that derive from the high heat treatment of frying oils are another attractive aspect of the deep-fried flavor character.

One may ask how odor, or aroma as it is also known, can be detected by way of the mouth? This is because the olfactory epithelium, where we perceive odor, can be reached either through the nostrils by smelling or via the back of the mouth by keeping the mouth closed and exhaling through the nose, as one does while eating. A simple demonstration of the latter is to chew some food while holding your breath and then to exhale through the nose. Little or no aroma characteristic of the food will be detected during the chewing phase if there is no air movement, but a good strong response will be experienced on exhaling. Another evidence of this path is when one has a stuffy head cold and food simply goes flat with respect to aroma. At such a time one often hears, "I've lost my sense of taste," but actually it is the sense of smell that has been blocked in the nose by mucus and inflammation. There is a surface area at the top of each nostril cavity that is covered with millions of olfactory cells which are specialized in structure and function to recognize and discriminate among thousands of different odor molecules. For odor detection, air carrying the odor must be able to contact the surface of those cells The information as to what molecules have been detected is actually converted to the sensation of odor (smell) in the brain. The sense of smell is still not completely understood[1]. It involves very primitive and important drives in animals. They use it to find food and distinguish between friends and enemies as well as to find mates.

While the development of sex attractants remains one of the major objectives of research in the perfumery field, humans mainly use odor perception as a highly essential means to obtain information about food and the environment. It is a source of great pleasure in life and it can also provide unpleasant and even terrifying experiences; "I smell something burning. Is the place on fire!?" But on the subject of trying to help a lady friend find a perfume that suits both parties, it is tricky and difficult to accomplish at the perfume counter. Sensory fatigue from perfumes tends to overwhelm the situation quickly. Experience indicates that it is best to find a lady who is wearing a perfume that is very appealing, get her to identify it for you, and then take it from there—also a little tricky.

Individual Differences

The senses are quite astounding. We can all behold a certain sight and agree that what we are looking at is an elephant; or in the case of hearing, we all hear a loud noise and agree that it sounds like an explosion. However, when it comes to flavor and odor, a personal internal thing, we aren't sure whether anyone is perceiving quite what anyone else is experiencing. First of all, we may not all take in the same amount of the stimulus, food or perfume aroma, for example. Next, we may not all have the same sensitivities to the various aspects of the stimulus. Further, every food aroma is a complex of literally hundreds of odorant molecules. In the case of milk, a relatively mild smelling and tasting substance, there are at least 400 components present in the aroma, as discussed following. In addition, the shapes of molecules are being perceived by our smell receptors. For example, molecules that only differ in shape due to cis and trans configurations of a double bond can differ decidedly in odor. So odor perception is actually in a sense seeing at the molecular level. Adding to the complexity, there are something like 1,000 genes and their expression products involved in the process by which our olfactories recognize aromas. While we do communicate with each other about flavor and we often perceive agreement, how similar my precise flavor and aroma images are and my perception of molecular shapes are to yours or to anyone else's is somewhat uncertain.

The flavor threshold. One of the things that make it evident we do not all perceive things alike is differences in our sensitivity to flavor molecules. It is possible to determine a person's threshold for a particular flavor component, say saltiness, using salt as the stimulus. We will find that people vary considerably in how much salt is needed for their perception of saltiness. I remember well when and how this was driven home to me in a very scientific way. There was a professor, Samuel Renshaw, in the Department of Psychology when I was a graduate student at Ohio State University. He was one of the world's greatest experts on psychometric measurements of the senses.[2] In order to determine an individuals taste threshold for a particular substance, say salt for example, he would have the person sit in a dentist's chair in his laboratory and would administer salt solutions containing varying concentrations of salt to the observer's mouth by means of a pipette with a rubber bulb attached, a gadget like a very large eye dropper. The amount of the solutions presented was standardized but the salt concentrations varied from none to a readily perceived level. The observer would evaluate each presentation and simply respond yes or no after each one to indicate whether saltiness had or had not been detected. After a suitable number of repetitions, the data were plotted and the concentration at which the stimulus, in this case salt, was recognized 50 percent of the time defined the person's threshold for tasting salt. The 50 percent level is rather arbitrary but it is a good value for establishing that above the corresponding concentration, one recognizes the stimulus all the time and below that, one never perceives it. This is represented graphically in figure 8.1.

Professor Renshaw's data established that there were remarkable differences not only in people's sensitivity to salt but in many other taste stimuli. In my own subsequent research with Professor Donald Josephson, we went on to show that this was true of odor compounds of the type associated with milk and milk products. This led us to a means of establishing whether or not a particular aroma compound is significant to the flavor of a food.[3] For this it was necessary to determine two things: the concentration of the compound in the food and the average person's flavor threshold for the compound, that is, the minimum detectable concentration. When the former exceeds the latter, it is reasonable to assume that the compound is being detected by most consumers and thus con-

Figure 8.1

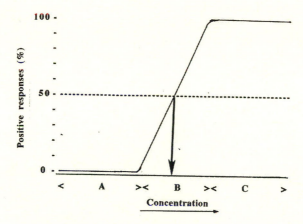

Graphic presentation of the flavor threshold concept showing the three meaningful regions of flavor concentration. A—at which it is low enough that tasters never detect it, B—the threshold region, and C—at which it is high enough that it is always detected by tasters. More or less arbitrarily, the threshold concentration is defined as that at which the tasters detect the flavor 50 percent of the time it is presented. In the figure, the arrow points from the 50 percent positive response point to the concentration of flavor or odor stimulus to which that corresponds.

tributes to the food's flavor. Such considerations are very important when one is trying to maintain or improve a product's flavor, or to devise artificial flavors that truly resemble the real things.

There is an interesting example of individual differences in odor perception involving something known as the swine sex odor. This is a urine-like aroma characteristic of the male pig. Perhaps you have purchased bacon or hot dogs on some occasion and have noticed during the cooking this very decided animal odor. When strong, it is quite unattractive. One of the functions, if not the main purpose of this aroma, which is actually due to a steroid,[4] is to attract the interest of female pigs and to facilitate interaction with them. Hence, the sex odor name. It develops that many more women (92 percent) than men (46 percent) can detect this odor.[5]

Another important principle of flavor and odor science is that the pleasantness of a particular flavor or odor may be inversely proportional to its concentration. For example, a little perfume may be fine but a lot can be quite unpleasant especially if the odor is highly persistent. If one couples this with the concept of individual differences in sensitivity, it becomes evident that what is just a nice pleasing intensity of odor or flavor to one individual may be overwhelming and unpleasant to another. This is not the only factor that may bear on whether people like or dislike a particular food but it does illustrate why we should be tolerant of each other's tastes.

One other factor about flavor that should be born in mind is the matter of fatigue. While one is eating a meal, the senses that perceive flavor and odor are under steady bombardment for an appreciable period of time. It is quite natural that at the end of the meal one is not nearly as sensitive to the various stimuli that are being presented as one was in the beginning. This is often simply stated that, "I like my first beer to be such and such a brand, after that any beer will do." This principle suggests that in meal planning, the delicately flavored courses should come first.

Eating and Flavor

Thus when one takes food into the mouth and starts chewing and swallowing it, a number of things happen more or less simultaneously. Taste buds on the tongue begin to perceive the sweet-salt-sour-bitter aspect of the food; odor or so-called aroma molecules pass out of the food into the air that is being exhaled by way of passages in the back of the mouth up into the nose where they are detected in the olfactory region; and the feel of the food in the mouth is registered simply by contact with the tissues and the teeth. As chewing, swallowing, tasting and exhaling continue, there is a heightened awareness of flavor. Chewing is particularly important because it greatly increases and constantly renews the food surfaces being exposed. This in turn provides access of more food molecules, such as sugar and salt, to the taste buds, and more opportunity for food aroma molecules to escape into the air and be detected as odor. Sometimes the warming that goes on in the mouth such as of frozen deserts and cold beverages aids that process. When we take food into the mouth, it is also the chewing that facilitates the tactual sensations, that is, whether the food is smooth, tender, chewy, gritty, crunchy, rubbery, or whatever.

While the foregoing understanding of flavor perception is not essential to the enjoyment of food, it certainly can help teach us why we like certain things, and it can be of help to food processors who have to be deeply committed to consumer acceptance of their products. Yes, they need to know whether you like or dislike their product, but it is far more helpful if you can tell them precisely why. For example, let us say you have obtained a bad-tasting half-gallon of milk from the supermarket. If you just respond that the milk "tastes bad," it is pretty vague and unhelpful. But if you say something like, "This milk tastes like the smell of sauerkraut," it is instructive in two ways: it implicates the odor aspect of flavor and suggests the cause is due to spoilage by bacteria. This indicates a number of possible origins of the problem, such as, faulty pasteurization, contamination with bacteria after pasteurization, inadequate refrigeration, or overextended storage. Despite the exceptional care given milk during production, processing and distribution, human error is always possible and any of those things could have happened. In the particular example, too long in refrigerated storage seems likely. With perishable foods, choose the freshest.

The Flavor of Milk

Milk is said to have a faint characteristic odor and to taste slightly sweet. From my own experience and from comparing notes with others, this description not only fits cows' milk but also that of human, goat, mare, camel, and alpaca. Moreover, in working with milk samples from many other species, I have never noticed much odor of any kind. That fresh milk would be bland tasting is reasonable. The mammary gland obtains the water and precursors of milk by selection and filtration from the blood which in turn, does its selection and filtration from the digestive system. However, it is possible for strongly flavored feeds to taint the flavor of milk. An interesting experiment in this regard done many years ago at Cornell University showed that if you place a bowl of chopped onions under a cow's nose, at the same time preventing her from eating the onions, the flavor of onions will show up in her milk within thirty seconds. For this reason, dairymen are very careful about what is fed to their cows. Generally, people do not want milk to have a pronounced flavor of any kind. It is suspected that babies reject the breast sometimes because of off-flavor from something the mother has eaten.

Dimethyl sulfide. In the 1950s, when I was actively engaged in flavor research, a new methodology known as gas chromatography (GC) came on the science scene. It completely revolutionized the flavor field along with many other branches of science. It enabled very efficient separation of volatile molecules and has become the basis of identifying and quantitatively measuring compounds making up complex aromas. The principle of GC concerns the sorting of molecules as they move in a carrier gas stream through a tube packed with finely divided material. The rate of movement of a volatile compound through the tube is dependent on the affinity of its molecules for the packing in the tube. In the case of an aroma, which is a mixture of volatile compounds, the sample is injected into the gas stream and, depending on their tendencies to bind to the packing phase or to remain in the gas stream, molecules of the aroma components move through the column. Each individual aroma compound is made up of identical molecules moving at the same rate but at a rate different from those for the molecules of any other aroma compound. As a consequence, a sorting out occurs and individual compounds, occasionally contaminated with another close moving component(s), exit the end of the tube. Until this innovation, there was no good way of separating complex mixtures of volatile compounds available in very limited amounts.

GC rapidly became very sophisticated. A great variety of column packings that would separate virtually any mixture were made available. For monitoring the emergence of sample components at the end of columns, instruments with extremely sensitive detecting and recording systems were developed. Individual components of aroma samples could be observed for odor, collected as they exited the column, or they could be directed into a mass spectrometer to obtain their mass spectrum for the purpose of identification.

The first GC research efforts in which I was involved had as its objective the characterization of milk aroma. We had a very primitive, pioneering gas chromatograph and we devised a way to isolate the components of interest in dry ice traps so that they could be released individually into the mass spectrometer for identification. We used an air-agitated, 1,000-gallon tank of raw milk as a source of our aroma sample. Agitation air leaving the tank was conducted through an exhaust tube packed with activated carbon to absorb odor molecules. After a trial operation of this system, we warmed a small sample of the carbon and were rewarded with a strong milk-like aroma. GC-mass spectrometry established that the principal trapped component, and the one responsible for the milk-like quality, was dimethyl sulfide (DMS), the chemical formula being, CH_3-S-CH_3, a potent odor compound which we determined had a flavor threshold of twelve parts per billion in distilled water.[6] DMS has a boiling point of 100° F. The odor of it can be observed on the breath of cows. In all likelihood, it originates in the (cow's) rumen fermentation.

The identification of DMS in milk was carried out at Penn State in collaboration with David Forss and Allen Day, two of the most gifted flavor scientists I've known. At the time, Dave Forss was a visiting research scientist from the Commonwealth Scientific and Industrial Research Organization of Australia. Al Day was a graduate student who went on to obtain his PhD and to become vice president for Research at International Flavors and Fragrances Inc. A few decades after our relatively inauspicious beginning, Dr. H. T. Badings and colleagues of the Netherlands Dairy Research Institute, in very elegant work using capillary GC-mass spectrometry, detected at least 400 compounds in the volatiles of milk.[7] They identified forty-eight of these and their results also indicated that DMS is the most important component of milk flavor. One of the components of milk volatiles identified by the Badings group was hept-4-enal, and unsaturated aldhyde with a creamy, waxy odor. This compound in its cis configuration has since been confirmed as making an extremely important contribution to the flavor of fresh homogenized milk.[8]

Not for me. For various reasons, some people do not like the flavor of milk. The problem may arise from the way it feels in the mouth, some perceived odor characteristic or an unpleasant aftertaste. In the latter case, the unfavorable reaction seems to develop after the milk has been consumed. Since this is not a problem for most regular milk drinkers, it has to do with perceptions about milk on an individual basis. If the unpleasantness is consistent at all of the individual's milk-drinking sessions, the cause may be malodorous substances produced by interaction of bacteria in the mouth and throat with residual milk. Alternatively, such substances may be produced by reaction of residual milk with unique components (enzymes?) other than bacteria in an individual's saliva. Since all these factors involve characteristics of the individual, there is not much that can be done. A possible remedy is the addition of pleasant flavor to the milk, as discussed following.

Actually, the flavor (odor) of milk is normally so mild that the individual has to be highly sensitive to find anything objectionable consistently present. There are indeed off-flavors that afflict milk, as described in the following section, and they can be readily detected. But any dairy learns how to deal with these or it is soon out of business. Nonetheless, flavor variations can always occur. Those who find the flavor of their milk objectionable can evaluate milk from several other suppliers to see if the objectionable quality varies with the source of the milk. Chocolate milk represents one solution for those who do not like the normal flavor of milk. It replaces a faint undesirable aroma with a strong pleasant (chocolate) flavor, and the faint sweet taste of milk is intensified by the addition of sugar, the most attractive of all tastes. While chocolate milk is widely distributed, making it in the home is no more complicated than stirring a teaspoonful or two of chocolate syrup into a glass of milk. There are also chocolate flavored powders that can be added to milk, either hot or cold. Another flavor enhancer for milk is about a half teaspoonful of vanilla. This can be helped with a little sugar or sugar substitute. If neither chocolate or vanilla, two of the world's most popular flavors, will do it, the situation becomes a little more challenging. Another alternative is to warm the milk. With microwaving, one can quickly and precisely produce anything from a hot sipping temperature down to just taking the chill off. For those who object to the feel of milk in the mouth, there is some latitude between skim milk, which is quite watery and normally lacking in much mouth-feel, and the relatively rich and more viscous feel of whole milk. One- and 2 percent-fat milks represent further alternatives as does buttermilk which has a completely unique flavor and feel in the mouth.

Off-Flavors

For the most part, the flavor of retail milk is excellent. One can count on the same pleasant quality from day to day and from one end of the U. S. to the other. Occasional variations and actual off-flavors are sometimes evident. Most of these are not very objectionable and some of the characteristic off-flavors are actually enjoyed by certain consumers. But because milk is so bland tasting, any off-flavors it is harboring are easily detected.

Feed and weed flavors. It is widely appreciated that what the cow eats may flavor her milk. Back in the days when dairy herds were smaller and they were pastured on large areas of land, there was a much greater possibility that they might get into feeding on weeds that could taint the milk. Wild onion, for example, was a well-known culprit. Many dairy farm operations no longer involve grazing on pasture and where they do, the maintenance of the pasture in suitable grasses with few if any weeds is the practice. The supply of feeds for dairy cows is a large-scale industrial business. Feeding things that would taint the milk is studiously avoided and, of course, a lot of experience has built up about how to avoid flavor problems.

Despite best efforts, sometimes raw milk coming into the plant just can't pass the flavor standard. Is there anything that can be done? Yes, sometimes fairly easily, and at other times drastic treatments are needed and the milk may have to be dropped down into a use classification that does not bring as good a price as that for beverage grade milk. There is equipment that is capable of evaporating a small amount of the water in the milk under vacuum and this often will strip off undesirable odor substances with the water but they have to be pretty volatile for this to work. Another approach that is more rigorous concerns diversion of the milk into condensed, evaporated or dried milks, all processes that involve heating and substantial water removal. Even if these products still carry some off-flavor, it may not be a problem if their ultimate use is in a highly flavored end product, such as, cheeses or strongly flavored ice creams (chocolate, banana, peanut butter, etc.).

Cooked flavor. Pasteurization is a minimal heat treatment of milk required by law to prevent communicable diseases from being spread by contaminated milk. At the time, early in the last century, when this processing was adopted, there were complaints that it changed the flavor of the milk. Actually the difference is almost imperceptible and, for the most part, has long since been forgotten. The heating that is employed for pasteurization is by two approved methods. One is a holder process in which the milk is brought up to a temperature of 143° F and held there for twenty minutes after which it is promptly cooled to about 38° F, a normal refrigerating temperature at which milk has good keeping quality. The other heating method is by high temperature short time treatment (HTST) in which the milk is brought to 165° F and held twelve to fifteen seconds These two methods are equivalent in heat input and HTST is more commonly used today because it facilitates large-scale continuous flow processing of the milk. Both methods are effective in killing all disease-causing organisms and in fact, they render the milk nearly sterile.

While control of the conditions of pasteurization are very rigorous, and records of the heating process for every batch of milk must be on file, some dairies choose to employ somewhat greater heat treatment as a margin of greater sanitation safety. However, any substantial holding time for milk at or above 165° F produces changes in the milk proteins that are associated with a change in flavor. In particular, the beta-lactoglobulin is involved and the change is analogous to what happens when the white of an egg is cooked. Trace amounts of volatile (odorous) sulfur compounds are produced, principally hydrogen sulfide, and this very minor chemical change from a quantitative standpoint, is readily detected as a change in flavor, the development of so-called cooked flavor.

Most consumers have no objection to cooked flavor. It is not unpleasant and it is a sign of more than adequate pasteurization. In addition, the generation of cooked flavor is usually sufficient to suppress oxidized flavor, a more objectionable change that can occur, described following.

Oxidized flavor. The lipids of milk give rise to potent flavor compounds under certain conditions, some of them desirable and others objectionable. Those causing so-called "oxidized" flavor are generally not appreciated although a notable exception is described below. The molecules that make up lipids or fats are large and in themselves not volatile so they have no odor, but if degradation occurs, the molecular fragments are often not only odorous but powerfully so. Those responsible for oxidized flavor can be easily detected at the level of a few parts in a million parts of milk. So it takes very little change in the lipids quantitatively to have a big effect on the flavor of milk. The precursors of the off-flavor in milk are polyunsaturated fatty acids, particularly linoleic (C18:2) and arachidonic (C20:4) acids. The resulting off-flavor is described as "tallowy," "oily," "waxy," or "cardboard." A very similar flavor can develop in potatoes chips that have been in an opened bag for a week or so. In fact, any food with substantial fat in it may develop this type of off-flavor.

Oxidized flavor arises from exposure of the lipids in milk to air (oxygen), light and certain trace metals, particularly cupric and ferric ions of copper and iron, respectively. Air alone is normally insufficient as a cause so no great effort is made to exclude it from milk. It is not difficult to protect milk from exposure to light. The critical period in this regard is after the milk has been put into its retail container. The best protection is to have such containers made of opaque material, a practice that is not always followed. Rust is the most common source of ferric iron and to avoid this, dairy plants utilize stainless steel for all milk-bearing surfaces. One of the biggest offenders in the past regarding oxidized flavor was the use of copper in alloys that were used up until the stainless steel era. One of these, known as white metal, was notorious for generating oxidized flavor in milk. It is a bright, silvery metal but just one piece of it in a processing line is enough to cause a problem.

In this connection, there was a community near Scranton, PA which some years ago was served by a local dairy that had white metal in some of its milk processing equipment. It had been there for years. The business was successful and no one complained about the milk. However, Penn State's College of Agriculture had dairy experts who collected samples of milk from all over the state and brought them back to the university for testing and tasting. They noted that milk from this dairy was consistently "oxidized." Eventually someone was sent from the college to the dairy to see if the trouble could not be identified and eliminated. In due course the responsible white metal components were removed from the processing lines and the problem was solved. But it wasn't. The customers did not like the new, improved flavor of the milk. This illustrates one of the classic axioms about flavor and that is: Good, bad or indifferent and irrespective of what the experts think, one can develop a taste and strong liking for a food with a certain kind of (off-) flavor.

Rancid flavor. The off-flavor of milk known as rancid is caused by the chemical cleavage of short chain fatty acids (SCFAs, fatty acids containing chains of four to ten carbon atoms) from triacyl glycerols (TGs) the basic molecules comprising fat. TGs are structurally similar in all edible fats and oils. But the TGs of milk fat are unique because they contain a group of fatty acids that are small enough when free to be volatile and odorous. In fact they are strongly and distinctively odorous. Their release from TGs is accomplished enzymatically, a process by which specially designed proteins, known as enzymes, bring about defined chemical changes. It happens that an enzyme capable of releasing the SCFAs is secreted in milk along with the TGs. So the potential to generate rancid flavor is inherent in the way milk is made. On occasions, milk is rancid as secreted and this is known as spontaneous rancidity. The name of the responsible enzyme is lipase, and the fatty acids it releases in the production of rancidity are principally butyric (C4:0), caproic (C6:0), capryllic (C8:0), and capric (C:10). All have flavor threshold concentrations at a few parts per million of milk.

Dairymen rely on two well-known facts to inhibit the development of rancid flavor in milk. One is that the milk fat globule membrane provides a barrier between the lipase enzyme, which is in the skim milk phase, and the TGs which constitute the core of milk fat globules. As long as these two remain separated, there is no problem. However, any agitation or warming and cooling that disrupt or change the membrane barrier can cause trouble because the enzyme has a strong affinity for the exposed TGs. This includes any kind of vigorous pumping, stirring or incorporation of air in the handling of the raw milk. The other control factor is heat treatment. Heating milk only momentarily to 125° F is sufficient to inactivate the milk lipase.

The term rancid may be somewhat confusing because it has other meanings than as used in connection with milk. It is also applied to the oxidized flavor of other commercial fats and oils and it is also employed generally to describe unpleasant odors. It is difficult to describe the rancid flavor of milk without implying unpleasantness., but like so many other flavors, it is at the strong end of the spectrum that most people object to it and even then, it depends on the context. A very mild degree of rancidity is enjoyed by some milk drinkers; and at the trace level, this off-flavor is probably part of the normal flavor of milk. Milk is not supposed to taste obviously rancid, but the grating cheese, Romano is characteristically rancid and that is its reason for being. People love to sprinkle it on all kinds of foods, particularly pasta and pizza. So if you have experienced this cheese, you have a good general idea of rancid flavor.

The potential of milk fat to produce unique flavor from its SCFAs has resulted in some very successful foods, particularly varieties of cheeses, and the use of these cheeses to flavor many other foods, for example, blue cheese salad dressing (for discussion, p. 210 and note 11, p. 221). One surprising application is in chocolate products. The flavor of milk solids that have developed hydrolytic rancidity in chocolate is known as the Hershey-type chocolate flavor because it was discovered and developed by the Hershey Chocolate Corp. This flavor stands out from the pleasant, mild, and more or less standard-tasting milk chocolates. The Hershey-type flavor is also present in M and M's, the popular pill-shaped bits of chocolate covered with sugar glazing of various colors. People, especially Americans, love that rancid-milk-fat chocolate flavor.

One suspects that the discovery of the Hershey chocolate flavor was one of those marvelous accidents for which science is so famous. From what we have said in the preceding, milk is teetering on the brink of rancidity as secreted, and if not properly handled, it can go over the cliff. One can imagine someone mixing a raw milk product with other ingredients in the making of milk chocolate but perhaps unintentionally delaying heat treatment. The physical mixing would be all that was needed to get the milk fat TGs next to the lipase, which otherwise would have been inactivated by the heating. By the time Mr. Hershey came back from lunch, he had a new chocolate in the making. No doubt some who tasted the product thought it was just as good if not better than the old. This then produced the challenge of generating rancidity consistently which Hershey learned how to do and managed to keep as a trade secret for many years.

The story of the sensory properties of SCFAs includes some unbelievably primitive aspects. Butyric acid in particular is strongly reminiscent of the odor of feces. Male monkeys recognize vaginal swabs of the female as "interesting" when they contain SCFAs. Humans find many putrid-tasting foods quite palatable. No doubt these are things carried forward from our earthy background of long ago. But our cultural standard for milk in this country is that it have little or no odor.

Light-activated flavor. It should be no surprise that light can produce off-flavors in milk. Light is a form of energy. It makes plants grow; it can burn or tan skin and bleach hair. In the days when milk was delivered to the door in clear glass bottles, it was necessary to use light-proof boxes for the milk. Only a few minutes of exposure of milk to direct sunlight is sufficient to develop what is known as sunlight flavor. If one has lunch at a sunny outdoor table, a glass of milk will change in flavor as it is progressively consumed. A measure developed to prevent such light-induced change in delivered milk was distribution in brown glass containers. Such glass blocks out the damaging wavelengths of light. This is the reason why beer is packaged in brown and dark green bottles. Beer in unpigmented glass containers readily develops a "skunky" flavor on exposure to sunlight. Some people actually like that flavor. The character of sunlight flavor in milk is often described as "broth-like" or like boiled cabbage.

Doorstep delivery of milk is virtually a thing of the past and the few remaining milkmen have evolved in many areas to put ones home-delivered milk in the refrigerator. However, that has not entirely solved the problem. The lighting in many supermarkets is strong enough and on long enough to affect flavor of milk held in refrigerated display cases. If the milk is in containers that are not opaque to light, off-flavor may develop, especially if turnover of the milk is slow. Gallon containers are usually of the type that lets some light through. Light-related flavor defects in milk from the super market often involve oxidized flavor as well as the broth-like quality.

Flavor defects are not the only problem resulting from the exposure of milk to light. There are detrimental nutritional effects as well. Riboflavin (vitamin B_2) is especially sensitive to destruction by light and as a result of absorbing light, it tends to photosensitize amino acids in the milk proteins to decomposition. Many years ago it was shown that the amino acid, methionine is the source of sunlight flavor in milk and that riboflavin is essential for production of the off-flavor. The flavor product from methionine, called methional, contains sulfur and is very potent.[9, 10]

Some Flavors Derived from Milk Fat

There are a number of unique and much appreciated flavors that originate from milk fat. One is the feeling of richness that is produced in the mouth, a tactual flavor response, by any milk product containing milk fat. There is the aroma that is produced by cooking or baking with butter. In chapter 7, we discussed very unique flavors of some cheeses that originate from the milk fat. Yet another unmatchable flavor contribution of milk fat is that to bisque-type soups.

Richness. Any consumer of milk and milk products knows there is a very desirable richness factor in milk that is associated with the fat content. It involves the way milk feels in the mouth. One can experience a descending intensity in this richness going from heavy cream to light cream, half-and-half, whole milk, 2 percent-fat milk, 1 percent-fat milk, and finally, skim milk, which is watery and not rich at all. The fact that richness is enhanced by homogenization suggests that it is not so much the quantity of fat as it is the number of fat particles, which are increased by such processing.

The evidence suggests that richness is due to particles or globules of fat with average diameters of 0.5 to 5 micrometers (μm) with perhaps an optimum around 1 μm. Such particles are very small, about 1/25,000 of an inch, but they still can be seen as a cloudy white suspension and they apparently can be felt in the mouth as very small ball-bearing like entities that make for a smooth sensation. From a pure numbers standpoint, skim milk has most of the fat globules that are present in whole milk, but they are too small to have any effect on mouth feel and they account for less than 5 percent of the fat in milk. Homogenization of milk, because it creates many more fat particles in the optimum size range, enhances milk richness. That this property is related to particle size is supported by other evidence that does not seem to involve fat. A treatment of skim milk which causes limited aggregation of its casein micelles clearly produces a degree of richness. Instead of the watery taste and bluish appearance, the product looks and tastes more like a 1 percent- or 2 percent-fat milk. Casein micelles normally average about 0.1 μm in diameter. So the treatment in question must produce at least a 10-fold increase in the size of the casein micelles. These special skim milks can be obtained in some supermarkets and they offer an alternative to those who want the rich taste but not the fat. However, the very limited amount of fat in milk is hardly a big dietary contributor of fat. In addition, milk fat in reasonable amount is good for one.

Heated butter flavor. Another much enjoyed flavor that derives from milk fat is due to conversion of flavorless precursors in the TGs to a series of flavorful compounds known chemically as lactones. The flavor is often described as "buttery" or "coconut-like." While these lactones are not normally detectable in the flavor of raw or pasteurized milk, the more intense heating used in cooking, frying, and baking with butter induces their formation. For those interested in the chemistry of this wonderful milk fat generated flavor, it is primarily the 10- and 12-carbon delta-aliphatic lactones that are involved. Most cooks are well aware that butter makes things taste good. In fact, this is so true that ever since its discovery, there have been concerted efforts to imitate butter, not only as a bread spread, but for its flavor potential, especially in cookies and things sauteed in the frying pan.

These lactones were first identified in connection with efforts to define the off-flavor that develops in dry whole milk during storage.[11, 12] It developed that what was an off-flavor in beverage milk was highly desirable when produced by heating butter.

Milk fat and cheese. The wonderful body, texture and mouth-feel of ripened cheeses are dependent on milk fat. In this crazy era, some people seem to want all the fat taken out of all foods; and the manufactures of cheeses and other dairy products have done their best to comply. Research and development have made available some acceptable low-fat dairy products. One thing that does not seem to work is fat-free semi-hard cheeses such as cheddar made from skim milk. I can't conceive of fat-free Camembert or Brie either. The fat content of cheddar can be halved or even reduced to one-quarter, not without sacrifice of some flavor quality, but not to zero. Without fat, it simply loses all palatability including flavor and feel in the mouth. It is like a hard tough piece of plastic and unrecognizable as cheddar. If cutting the amount of fat in the diet is all that much of a crisis, let's let cheese be the wonderful thing it is and eat a little less of it or eat something else.

* * *

A major factor in what our bodies are and will become depends on the food we eat. In turn, what we eat is greatly influenced by what tastes good to us. Thus, flavor of food and drink is no minor consideration in life. It directly involves both our health and happiness. The delightful flavor experiences that milk and milk products provide are another major reason why cow's milk is of great importance to humanity. We have to watch out that nutritionists and health care specialists don't turn eating into a daily act of self punishment—no fat, no sugar, and fill up on fiber, and so on. We have already touched on what a joy of life ice cream, with all its flavor ramifications, can be (chapter 7). Cheeses are beloved the world over. French cuisine would be nothing without butter. Fortunately, milk and milk products taste good and are good for us.

Suggested References

Badings, H. T. Flavors and off-flavors. in *Dairy Chemistry and Physics* by P. Walstra and R. Jenness. John Wiley and Sons, New York, 1984. pp. 336-357.

Smith, D. V. and Margolskee, R. F. Making sense out of taste. Scientific American 284; 32-39. 2001.

Notes

1.   An excellent progress report on the understanding of odor perception has appeared: Lyons, D. The Secret of Scent. *Forbes* 1/23/02. pp. 278, 280.
2.   Professor Renshaw was the developer of an aircraft recognition system used widely in World War II to aid military personnel in the identification of friendly and enemy planes.
3.   Patton, S. and Josephson, D. V. *Food Research* 22(3):316-18. 1957.
4.   The steroid is 5 alpha-androst-16-ene-3-one. Identification of this steroid as the swine sex odor and a review of the pertinent literature are provided by Beery, K. E. et al. *Journal of Food Science* 36:1086-90. 1971.
5.   Griffiths, N. M. and Patterson, R. L. S. Journal of the Science of Food and Agriculture 21:4. 1970.
6.   Patton, S., Day, E. A. and Forss, D. A. Methyl sulfide and the flavor of milk. *Journal of Dairy Science* 39(10):1469-1470. 1956.
7.   This work and other aspects of flavors and off-flavors in milk are presented by: Badings, H. T. Flavors and off-flavors. in: *Dairy Chemistry and Physics* by P. Walstra and R. Jenness. John Wiley and Sons, New York, 1984. pp. 336-357.
8.   Bendall, J. G. and Olney, S. D. *International Dairy Journal* 11:853-64. 2001.
9.   Patton, S. and Josephson, D.V. *Science* 118:211. 1953.
10.   Patton, S. *Journal of Dairy Science* 37:446-52. 1954.
11.   Keeney, P. G. and Patton, S. *Journal of Dairy Science* 39:1114-9. 1956.
12.   Patton, S. *Journal of Dairy Science* 44:207-14. 1961.

9

Research and Milk

Research to gain a more satisfying and useful understanding of milk and lactation will continue indefinitely. Every so often people come along who propose we have learned all that can be known about a certain thing. In fact, this has been stated recently with respect to scientific discovery in general—that all the important ones have been made and the only remaining research will involve minor odds and ends.[1] Most scientists I have talked to seriously doubt that. Actually, there now seems to be a sense of excitement that goes beyond anything in the past. Scientific research is bubbling over with possibilities and eager participants. The only limitation seems to be financial support.

Because of how important research has been in developing the modern human food supply including milk, this chapter is devoted to defining research and describing how it has made dairying such a productive and valuable enterprise to society. A discussion of the newer knowledge of genetics in relation to lactation is also presented in the hopes of showing that we aren't done yet so far as research on the mammary gland is concerned. A few examples of research that are part of my cherished experience are also described.

Milk has been the subject of vast research in order to define the most efficient and economic conditions for its production, processing, and conversion into many high-quality food products including ice cream, cheese, butter, concentrated and fermented milks. Healthfulness of milk and its products from the standpoints of nutritive value and freedom from disease-causing microorganisms has also been a primary research focus. The cost of this research has been born primarily by the federal government. The findings have been of broad benefit to dairy farmers, milk processors, and the consuming public. In recent years the dairy industry has initiated some support of milk-related research by collecting so many cents per hundredweight of milk to be used in investigational programs mainly at universities.

At this point, both human and bovine milks are fairly well characterized both compositionally and nutritionally. However, the task is by no means complete, especially with respect to bioactive substances that might be of benefit to consumers of those milks. The rise of molecular genetics in science and technology has put the mammary gland in an entirely new light from a research standpoint. Insertion of new genes into the milk synthesis process that define the production of proteins other than those normal to milk has been accomplished. As a result, milks with completely new protein components are a demonstrated fact. Because of the far-reaching benefits of dairy research in the past and implications of this new investigational area, this chapter is devoted to defining research and its application to milk and lactation.

Change

Older adults of this era have a sense of on-rushing change. The perception is that when they were young, things were not exactly at a standstill, but innovations were mostly surprising isolated events and were quite slowly absorbed into the culture. The term "newfangled" comes to mind, a description applied to the horseless carriage, as the automobile was first known. From its first appearance in the late 1800s, the automobile drove over and around piles of horse manure for many years. It was not until the late 1920s that Henry Ford developed the scheme for mass production of automobiles. In that same era and about at that same pace, incandescent light bulbs replaced kerosene lamps. Today, less than 100 years later, a major fraction of the Japanese population is using hand-held, wireless communications devices that enables voice, email, internet and computer operations. The computer is revolutionizing education, banking, shopping, even filing of income tax returns, among other things. New developments in medical practice are announced almost daily. One wonders what led to all this rapid rate of change and where it is taking us? The answer to the first part of that question is research and development or more simply, science. We live in a science and technology based culture. As to what the future holds, some of the handwriting is on the wall, but growing cultural complexity tends to obscure the longer-term view. For our purposes here, let's look at the main driving force of change, research, and what it may mean regarding milk and mammary gland

Research

Since we do live in a science-based culture, it behooves us to understand research, the means by which science expands our understanding of nature, the world and the universe. This expanded knowledge then enables the development of new devices and processes that change our way of living.

The Scientific Method. Research is a process of building on the knowledge and clues that already exist. A person who markedly influenced the efficiency of this process was Sir Francis Bacon, the English philosopher-statesman (1561-1626). His input seems to have made the way of doing research called the scientific method much more effective. This method involves the following:

1. Observations of nature that establish certain facts and relationships but which, at the same time, raise important questions.

2. Generation of a hypothesis which attempts to answer a question or explain a relationship.

3. Design and execution of an experiment to test whether or not the hypothesis is correct.

4. Cycling of new information from the experiment into creation and testing of new hypotheses to answer other questions or completely fresh questions that are raised by results from the experiment.

It is very important to note step 2. The creative generation of hypotheses, which in essence are new ideas, is something that can only start in a single human mind. It can be modified and improved by others but it starts with one person. This means that the creative individual is of paramount importance in research.

It can be seen that Bacon's system of thought and action has the properties of a chain reaction; once started, it has a natural tendency to keep going. All that is needed is human interest and ingenuity, and more particularly in these days, financing. Since man is naturally curious, and because such a system of thought can lead to profitable new products and technology, science by its very nature seems to readily generate the interest and support that it needs. And that, more or less, is how things snowballed into our current, fast-paced, information-packed age. As new information accumulates, the basis for more questions, hypotheses, and experiments is provided.

Bacon insisted upon a dispassionate approach. As a researcher, one should try not to fall in love with ones own ideas. One should take into account all of the available facts in generating a hypothesis and experiment to test it. Alternate explanations should be entertained and tested. Unfortunately as humans, scientists wrestle unsuccessfully with these requirements. One's hypothesis becomes like ones baby. There is powerful pride of ownership. It is human to detest anyone who is trying to kill your baby. And after all, nobody likes being shown wrong, especially one smart scientist by another. Even with such human limitations, science has a self-purification characteristic by which error in important matters sooner or later is revealed and rooted out of the working information base. What happens in essence is that the findings or conclusions simply cannot be repeated or do not hold in subsequent experiments by other investigators. So eventually they are rejected. The truth will out, but it is important to realize that it may not be immediately forthcoming in the unpredictable progress of science. Refining the truth to make it precise also can take a while. We often develop a pretty good rough idea of things, but knowing exactly is what truly satisfies the mind.

One thing that is shaking up Bacon's tidy scientific method somewhat is that creativity is not manifesting itself today just in hypotheses and experimental design. Data, that is, bits of raw information, coming out of experiments are so complex and massive in amount that there is a great opportunity for creativity in collecting, analyzing, and interpreting data. This emphasizes the importance of a new type of researcher, one who does not work in the conventional laboratory, but one who collates data from the literature or information files either to confirm hypotheses or to generate new ones. In scientific discussions the point is often made that you may not need to do that experiment, the needed data may already have been published in connection with other research. Thus it appears that a new breed of data analyzer-reviewer will be needed increasingly if we are to make good use of all the information that is being and has been generated.

There is evidence this new talent is already here and working hard. You may ask yourself why is it I am getting more and more news from studies suggesting what to eat, what exercise to perform, what medicine to take, and life-styles to pursue? Behind it all is that computers are enabling data handling like never before. When information about a large group of people is banked in a computer, what can be derived from it is only limited by the scientists doing computer analyses of the data. Usually the messages from such information are quite straightforward. However, not infrequently obscure and unsuspected relationships are revealed—some of them meaningful, some puzzling, others even preposterous. Nonetheless, it always has the potential for introducing new ideas and concepts. For example, let us say we have this data bank on diet and educational performance of 3,000 high school students, we wonder if any particular dietary component helps with their grades? Combing this data may put us on the track of a new brain food for high school students. It is because of the ease with which such analyses are made today that so many correlations and associations are emerging. Of course, if such a food association was detected, we could go on to many other high school populations and see how well the association held up.

Serendipity. In contrast to conducting research by the scientific method, new knowledge is also acquired in science by a process known as serendipity, which is in essence accidental discovery. For example, one may be conducting a planned experiment and some completely unplanned unsought and unanticipated phenomenon makes itself evident in the course of the work. An often-cited classic example is the discovery of saccharin in the late 1800s. It is several hundred times sweeter than sugar. A chemist while eating dinner one night noticed an intense sweetness. This was traced to his hand on which he had spilled a substance being prepared in the lab that day. By combing the records as to what chemicals had been worked with at the bench and tasting some of the suspects, the identity of saccharin was deduced. Another classic example of serendipity is the discovery of penicillin, the antibiotic by Sir Alexander Fleming in England. He noticed that when a mold spore, which is something like a seed, fell onto a bacterial culture dish, no bacteria would grow in the area around the developing mold. This led to isolation and identification of the antibiotic and a Nobel Prize for Fleming. It will be evident that serendipity can operate in computer sifting of data. The data may have been collected and banked to achieve an answer to question X, but lo and behold, on analysis, there is an answer to question Y, which was not even asked and is far more important.

Virtually every researcher who has been directly involved in the conduct of experiments for a number of years has had serendipitous experiences, and because these events can be at least surprisingly interesting and useful, if not earthshaking, it pays one to be on the lookout. Some sage has said, "Science rewards the prepared mind." It might also be said, "Science rewards the alert observer." One needs to be there, watching things, observing the results, studying the data, and particularly, wondering about weird or inconsistent happenings or data. Being so focused that one is only interested in the answer to the experimental question that has been asked can deprive one of delightful and rewarding experiences of discovery.

In thinking about serendipity, one of my own experiences comes to mind. I was doing research on the occurrence and nature of a mucin in human milk. Mucins are proteins that have a relatively large amount of carbohydrate chemically bound to them. In the case of this milk mucin, it contains 50 percent carbohydrate. It exists on the surface of lactating epithelial cells, as well as on the surface of other epthelial cells throughout the body. The mucin gets into milk at the time that milk fat globules are enveloped by the cell membrane in the process of their secretion, as discussed in chapter 2. In my work, I had been using the milk of our daughter, Mary. I was using a gel electrophoretic system to separate the milk proteins into individual bands. The system works such that proteins are sorted as to size. I got used to seeing the bands for the mucins in Mary's milk in a certain location in the pattern. One day, because I had run out of Mary's milk, I used some from another lady. The mucin bands from her milk were not in the same location as Mary's, and further, there appeared to be more bands. I then went to the freezer and got milk samples from other women and ran them all on the same gel so that I could compare the mucin bands of the various women's milk samples. They were all different! What a surprise! The number of bands and their positions on the gel varied significantly (see figure 9.1). This meant that the physical sizes of the mucin molecules were varying between the women.

What these findings were telling me was that these mucins are polymorphic, that is, they occurs in more than one form. In fact, it developed that the size of the mucin molecule is variable due to its genetics and that the reason for the two bands is that we inherit a gene for the mucin from each parent. If the two genes dictate a mucin of about the same size, only one band will be seen, but if they differ appreciably, two mucins of differing size are made and thus, two

Figure 9.1

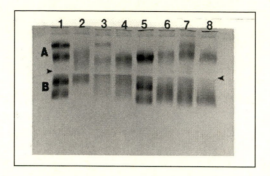

Separation and detection of two polymorphic mucins, A and B, in individual milk samples from eight women. Note that the number of bands, one or two, for each of the two mucins and position of the bands vary between samples. This demonstrates that the size of the two mucins are uniquely different (polymorphic) in milk, mammary and other tissues of the human body. Normally each milk proteins is one size and would produce only one band in the same position for all samples under the technique of separation used here. In this case, the particular method of detection only reveals bands for the mucins in the samples. For further details, see S. Patton et al. Biochimica et Biophysica Acta 980:333-8. 1989 from which this figure is adapted.

bands or one elongated band are seen. That is the take home message of figure 9.1. Dr. Sandra Gendler and colleagues at the Imperial Cancer Research Fund Laboratories in London conducted a study[2] of sixty-nine European women regarding the gene fpr the B mucin in the figure. It was found to be expressible in thirty different sizes. Most milk proteins have only one form with all of the molecules of a given protein being of the same size and structure. This mucin proved to be radically different.

Another part of my serendipitous observations was that there is a second and much larger mucin that could be detected in another location on the gel (A in figure 9.1), and it revealed this same type of genetic polymorphism. So every lactating woman's milk fat globules has a unique surface array of these two mucins which vary in size based on her genetics. It bears some analogy to fingerprint uniqueness. The individual mucin molecules appear to project from the surface of the fat globules like whiskers of various lengths. In milk, mucins may help control the kind of bacteria that inhabit the infant intestine. Mucins occurring on epithelial cells in the breast and throughout the body are thought to be a barrier against the invasion of bacteria. They also are known to bind certain kinds of bacteria that cause sickness. This may serve to present these bad bacteria to macrophages, cells of the immune system that eat and digest bacteria.

More recently, an investigation[3] has shown that one of the mucins (B in figure 9.1) occurring in the breast and milk is also found on epithelial cells of the gastric (stomach) mucosa; and that the smaller polymorphic versions of this mucin are associated with an increased risk for gastric cancer. Another risk factor for this cancer is the bacterium *Helicobacter pylori* which is also causative of stomach ulcers. It is a reasonable hypothesis that the longer form of the mucin is more effective in defending against this bacterium by holding it further away from the mucosal cell thus reducing the risk of stomach cancer. These observations define a rather specific example of how ones genes, that is, variable size of mucins on the cell surface, might influence susceptibility to disease.

Another research possibility arising from these mucins involves the question of man's place of origin on the earth. The large variety of gene sizes involved in these two mucins should make it possible to assay differences between racial, ethnic, and tribal populations throughout the world. The group of people exhibiting the greatest number of gene variations, known as alleles, should represent the earliest human gene pool within the current population. This is based on the assumption that small groups of people later leaving the earliest established population would only take a few of the total genetic variants with them and thus, would manifest less subsequent variety in the gene size of their population. Such an approach might offer another way of checking the currently held hypothesis that we all came originally from Africa.

So, serendipity can provide highly unique research experiences, but mainly what researchers need are good ideas on which to base new hypotheses and experiments. Such fresh insights can come almost any time or place. We have all heard about someone who yelled, "Eureka, I've got it!" Sometimes research is that sort of thing. One doesn't have to be burning the midnight oil at the lab. Lightning can strike during some routine task around the house, during a sleepless night, or on the golf course. It helps if one has a certain relentless and intense desire to answer some big question of the moment. So such dedication keeps the question never too far from ones ongoing conscious mental mix. This in turn seems to maximize the chances that something will make a plausible, or seemingly implausible, answer fall into place. No one knows quite where ideas come from but if the mental wheels are whirring, sometimes three bars come up, all in a line. Jackpot!

Support of Agricultural Research

Background. In its early days, dairying in the U. S. received a tremendous boost from the federal government. In 1862, legislation known as the Morrill or Land-Grant Act was passed by the Congress and signed by President Lincoln. Justin Smith Morrill, a representative from Vermont, introduced this legislation. It provided a funding arrangement, involving the sale of land, to establish and operate the state universities which were charged to educate people in the "agricultural and mechanic arts." Among other things, this meant farming, including dairy farming and milk processing. So this assured that there would be a continuing supply of trained workers for the various aspects of the growing dairy industry. Virtually every state university developed a department and educational program devoted to dairying. Subsequent acts of Congress, including a second Morrill Act (1890) and the Hatch Act (1887) provided additional funding for the land-grant universities. The Hatch Act established and funded Agricultural Experiment Stations at these institutions, and with that, a research arm in every state commenced to function in support of the dairy industry. Beyond the special consideration of dairying, this legislation establishing and supporting the land-grant universities is widely recognized to be among the most inspired actions in which the Congress ever engaged. The country continues to benefit from it immensely.

The Agricultural Experiment Station. Research in the life sciences, including agriculture and medicine, is an expensive activity and becoming more so. There are specially trained expert scientists and technicians to be paid, ever more exotic supplies and materials to be bought, laboratories to be maintained and equipped with increasingly expensive and complicated instruments; and often, costly animal and plant facilities are required. Administration and auxiliary services are other contributing costs. Our general well-being and the abundance of things in our culture are, for the most part, a testimonial that research is well worth the price. For example, Americans are the best fed and best medically cared for people on the earth. As a person involved for many years in research on milk and lactation, I sought support through the Agricultural Experiment Station program of the United States Department of Agriculture (USDA) and from grant and contract programs of the National Institutes of Health (NIH) and the National Science Foundation (NSF). While it is not my intention to make a detailed critique of these systems of support, I do want to say something in defense of the Agricultural Experiment Station program. It has been criticized despite its obvious and very great success in facilitating the U. S. food supply and in serving as a helpful model in many other areas of the world.

The principal criticism of the Experiment Station funding procedure has been its lack of peer review, a prominent characteristic of the NIH and NSF grant programs. Peer review involves having a team of experts in the field of the research proposal evaluate it and vote on whether it should be funded. In response, the USDA initiated a peer-reviewed funding program some years ago and its budget has grown steadily. So the criticism has been met. The Experiment Station program, which has grown very little in recent years, works about like this: Various acts of the Congress appropriate money, based on a formula, to the individual states, this money to be used for agricultural and home economics research at the various land-grant (state) universities. The director of the Agricultural Experiment Station at the particular university is responsible for the disbursement of the funds for his institution. Aided by assistants, department heads and consultants, the director decides what projects will be funded and for how much. Development of project proposals is in the hands of researchers just as it is for NIH/NSF grant applications. Annual reviews of projects by the director and his helpers give guidance to whether continued funding of a particular project is warranted.

One of the merits of the Experiment Station system is its relative fairness in giving people a chance. To some extent, the director is in the position of placing bets on his researchers, but when one considers the extensive sifting process that state universities go through in hiring faculty today, the director is not dealing with a bunch of losers. It was my observation at Penn State over a long period of years that everyone who wanted to be involved was given *at least a little support* which seems fair. After all, research support is something of a crapshoot no matter how it is administered. I felt privileged to watch an extremely successful research program on artificial insemination of dairy cattle blossom under support of the Pennsylvania Agricultural Experiment Station and of dairy cattle breeding organizations. Dr. John Almquist, his colleagues and students made remarkable progress in developing systems for the dilution and frozen preservation of bovine sperm. Many of their findings and innovations have become applicable in the field of human reproduction which lagged far behind in its development to that for farm animals. Of course, Penn State had its unproductive projects, too.

In some ways, the Experiment Station research system is "in house" like corporate research programs and like the intramural programs at NIH. The director gets to know his people, he can create local peer review to a degree and make educated guesses about funding research that are not as belabored and professionally threatening to the researcher as the NIH/NSF grant system. Isn't there room for both? One also wonders if the era of the research prima donna, the big shot of the lab, is not passing and that we may move on to an era of far less personal research grant competition and far more collaboration. The ever-expanding complexity and "ever-widening darkness" known as science[4] increasingly reveal the limitations of all individual researchers.

The Life Sciences Research Center. While the Experiment Station concept serves its purpose well, change is inevitable. When one looks back over the research accomplishments in dairy science, it is quite evident that the findings have not only benefited the dairy industry and the public at large, they have had an impact in many other disciplines. Further, progress in other disciplines has been essential to progress in dairy science. Recognition of this interdependence is leading to updating of research organizational arrangements. As will be evident from some of the research areas discussed following, Agriculture has a considerable interest overlap with Medicine. In fact, today there is interweaving of all the life sciences. A real pace setter in this movement is the Institute of Biosciences and Technology at Texas A and M University. To quote from a recent article about it, "The institute fosters creative research on the molecular aspects of medicine and agriculture in both its Houston location and the College Station campus. The Institute's research activities are dedicated to making a scientific impact in such important areas as cancer, heart disease, arthritis, nutrition, plant science, animal reproduction, and ethics in biotechnology.[5]"

There are pros and cons about research institutes at universities as with other campus arrangements. However, the need for this type of endeavor can only intensify with time. Research specialists are taxed severely to keep up with advancements in science, and in order to remain competent, they narrow what they are trying to cover even more. This makes collaboration with other researchers inevitable if one wants to remain professionally alive and effective. Of course, research institutes are not new, but there is a new emphasis in the life sciences including agriculture, of bringing diverse fields into an effective research focus and hopefully, using research funding more efficiently as well.

Food Supply

As noted previously, milk production per cow during the past century progressed from approximately 5,000 pounds to about 18,000 pound per lactation. One may wonder how such a remarkable increase was achieved. While many factors were involved, one was of overriding importance, that is, the system of agricultural research and extension that exists at our state universities. This system, which is administered through funds of the USDA, as discussed above, has the very practical objectives of improving agricultural productivity and efficiency thereby benefiting everyone, including farmers, consumers and the agriculture related industries. The fundamental mechanisms of this system involve research at the universities the results of which are conveyed by extension personnel to farmers who apply the findings in their farm operations. By careful record keeping, continuing education programs, and cycling farm experience back into the university research, tremendous progress has been made. In addition to milk, used here as an example, similar progress has been made with many other commodities. To repeat a cliché, which seems essential in this context, America is the best-fed nation in the world.

As a result of the knowledge base this system has established, it is reasonable to hope that, in time, the entire population of the world can be well fed. Some of the research and extension people at our state universities have been and are working hard on that very thing. In fact, experts claim that a minimum version of the goal has been achieved except for political and economic problems that stand in the way of distributing the food to the people who need it. Current conditions in India are an example. While the country produces sufficient wheat to feed all of its people, the commodity is exported at the same time that a large segment of its people are starving. For that matter, the U. S. also has its hungry and starving, though much fewer than those in India, while it sells and gives away food all over the world.

There is an astounding backlash against food research by European organizations and heads of African nations. They are in essence telling the U. S. to keep its gifts of genetically modified foods from starving African peoples. This when we have been eating such foods for years without problems. Norman Borlaug, the Nobel laureate, who, perhaps more than any other individual is helping to feed the world, has said in this connection, "Responsible biotechnology is not the enemy, starvation is.[6]" Clearly, there is more to solving the world's food problems than successful research and producing the food.

Charitable donations of food is not a long-term solution to the numerous pockets of starvation throughout the world. The countries involved must become capable of feeding their people. Until this is accomplished, the chances of achieving a decent standard of living and cultural progress in those countries will remain remote. While currently successful agricultural practices may not work in all the needy areas of the world, it is impressive how much progress has been made in some countries based on technical know-how developed in the Ag Experiment Station programs. We just need to keep trying both at the research and the geopolitical levels.

An inadequate food supply is intolerable in the U. S. Farm subsidies and price support programs are designed to prevent such situations. While there are everlasting complaints about this aspect of the federal government, it continues to achieve its objectives quite effectively. We absolutely need to encourage those who produce our food to stay in business. We may have surpluses but that is far better than going hungry. The current crisis in California regarding insufficient electric power is a classic example of what happens when no one is assuring the supply. Such things as the supply of food, water and electricity are too essential to be allowed to drift completely unattended.

One may ask what kinds of research did the Ag Experiment Stations do to make such a huge increase in milk yield per animal possible? Every conceivable variable with relevance to that objective was evaluated including: kinds of feed, nutrition supplements, feeding conditions, milking conditions, housing, length of time between lactations (dry period), age, breed, health factors of all kinds, and most importantly, genetic factors, such as selecting the best milk producers and their sires to be parents.

Speaking of sires, the perfection of bovine sperm collection, preservation, and use in artificial insemination has had a huge impact on the quantity of milk produced in the modern world. By keeping careful records not only on milk composition and production of individual cows, but also about many other attributes of the animal and the capacity of bulls to transmit desirable traits to daughters, it became possible rather quickly to select for excellence and to cull marginal and unprofitable animals.

It was this type of research which very quickly brought the Holstein to the fore. By nature a big animal, it had the body size and feed capacity to produce more milk than other breeds. However, its milk tended to be quite low in fat. Whereas Jersey and Guernsey cows produce milk of 4 to 7 percent fat, the Holstein fat test was normally 2 to 3 percent and very often below the legal minimum for fat content of market milk (3.25 percent). By selective breeding for fat content as well as for milk yield, the Holstein was soon in a position of superiority to all other breeds; and over time, milk production per cow steadily increased to reach the astounding levels being achieved today. At this writing, the record for milk production of a single animal during a 305-day lactation is 75,000 pounds.

Regarding milk yield, it was shown some years ago by Dr. Dale Bauman and his colleagues at Cornell University that administration of bovine growth hormone (BGH) to cows would enhance their milk production. The implication is that the amount of this hormone elaborated by the cow is not sufficient to sustain her maximum milk producing capacity. This is rather surprising. One would think that selection for a high level of this hormone would occur automatically in breeding for increased milk production, but apparently a well-defined physiological limit in output of growth hormone exists in the cow. Many dairy herds are now treated with growth hormone to increase their milk production. Such treatment appears to have no significant effects on the flavor, nutritive value or healthfulness of milk from those animals—a real net gain.

There are a couple of points to be made about research that yields highly useful results such as the BGH-milk yield work. Its success rested on an extensive understanding of the cow developed from many earlier investigations. That's not to take anything away from the indispensable contribution of Bauman et al.,[7] but all contemporary researchers stand on the shoulders of those who went before. In this case, those many years of effort by untold numbers of Agricultural Experiment Station and other researchers led to a worthy pay-off. For the purposes of both researchers and the research funding agencies including the Congress, it is important that such successes are duly publicized. If those handling the purse strings do not receive feedback about concrete examples of research success, further funding may dwindle and even disappear.

Milk and Conception

A big dividend of university employment is the opportunity it provides to collaborate with other faculty and students on research of mutual interest. I have benefited from many rewarding collaborations during my career. The following one seemed well worth describing here.

Being in a large Department of Dairy Science at Penn State, I had a chance to observe and wonder about research across a very broad spectrum of interests and objectives. It ranged all the way from fertility problems of cows to new uses of cheese whey. One of the major research emphases within the Department was on breeding of dairy cattle, a very important practical consideration in dairy farming. In fact, conception, the uniting of sperm and egg, is a key event because it is, or was indispensable to producing another calf and another lactation. Yes, I realize that cloning individuals is a reality and that lactation can be induced in virgin animals by hormone injections. But for the time being at least, we still need the bull and he has been essential in the evolution of the dairy industry. And remember, we wouldn't even know about these as yet unproven alternatives to the bull except for a huge amount of research.

In any event, I found the whole reproductive process intriguing and especially so the cellular and molecular events of conception. How does the individual sperm, of which there are millions in an ejaculate, find the egg? What holds this sperm to the egg? How does it then penetrate the egg so that the male and female genetic material may interact in formation of the new individual? Not being a reproductive physiologist, I wasn't very well informed in this area but that didn't subdue my wonder and interest.

An opportunity developed for me to collaborate in the research program of the Department's Dairy Breeding Research Center. The then director of the Center, Dr. John Almquist was, and still is, a world renowned scientist in the field of reproductive physiology. At the time, his research interest was artificial insemination and more particularly how to preserve sperm so that they could be stored and used at some later date or shipped for distant use. At that time there were many practical problems to be solved in order to reach those goals. Let us say you have collected sperm from a prize bull, one that has the capacity to transmit excellent genes for milk production, animal health, appearance, and fertility. You want to divide this ejaculate into many samples that can be used for future inseminations of cows. You want to preserve these samples in a manner that will retain sperm viability for months, if not years. With solutions to these problems, the fabulous genetic potential of the bull can be applied in dairy herds far and wide and well into the future.

Research by Dr. Almquist and his co-workers provided the answers. They devised materials and procedures for diluting and freezing the sperm such that on thawing, they retained substantial viability and motility and thus could be used to inseminate cows as needed. One of Dr. Almquist's graduate students at the time was Dr. Richard Saacke, who now is a renowned reproductive physiologist in his own right and a long time member of the faculty at Virginia Polytechnic Institute and State University. In his graduate work, Dr. Saacke was pursuing a clue that cow's milk would make a good material with which to dilute bovine sperm. Indeed, it makes sense using a body fluid from the same species to dilute its sperm. He was assigned by his mentor to explore the matter further and I was retained as a consultant because of my knowledge of milk. It was found that unheated milk was actually toxic to sperm. So the problem was to determine whether heating would inactivate the toxic principle, and if so define optimum heating conditions for the milk with respect to maintaining viability and conception rates with the sperm. This was accomplished and many years later, milk is still being used as a diluter for semen. It developed that heat treatment somewhat greater than pasteurization, 206°F for ten minutes, was required in order to inactivate a toxic protein in the milk.[8, 9]

From time to time, I have pondered why milk works so well in this application. Beyond keeping the sperm alive and motile, the diluter must not interfere with conception that involves sperm binding to and then penetration of the egg. There is at least one milk protein, called prosaposin,[10] which might be a facilitator of the binding process. It appears to have special functions in the reproductive system[11] including binding sperm to egg.[12] Maybe this protein might be of use in human fertility problems. Another relevant fact, soaking sperm in milk enhances their capacity to penetrate eggs.[13] So, on with the research. The latest findings about conception seem almost too romantic. It appears that the egg releases a substance(s) that is detected by an olfactory (odor) receptor on the sperm. A review of the research is entitled, "Smelling the Roses?"[14] The sperm are apparently able to home on the source (egg) and one of them wins the prize. What an exciting new research lead!

Milk and the Gene

In the 1970s it was becoming clear that foreign genes could be inserted into cells and that these so-called transfected genes could be constructed in such a way that they would be expressed by the cell so treated. In other words such cells would produce proteins that were not part of their normal inventory. That is to say also that the cell would thus become capable of doing something it was not inherently capable of doing. This technique has found a very appropriate application in relation to milk.

Germ line insertion. The fact that new genes can be placed in germ cells, that is, sperm, egg, or embryo stem cell, the ones that can give rise to a whole new individual, means that potentially, the inserted gene can be expressed throughout the body and the life of the new individual as well as passed on to progeny. While the potentialities and limitations of this technique are still being explored, we know it can be done. By using specific regulators and promoters in the construction of the gene to be inserted, it has been possible to specify expression of the gene in the lactating mammary gland so that the gene product is secreted in the milk. Human milk proteins are being produced in milks of many species of animals, including cow, goat, sheep, guinea pig, and mouse. Some of these proteins, such as growth hormone, used to overcome arrested growth, and alpha-1-antitrypsin, an agent used to treat emphysema, a lung disorder, are valuable pharmaceuticals. All manner of proteins, or functional portions of them, are candidates for custom synthesis by this technique. Research in this area indicates the feasibility of very diverse biotechnical applications.

Mammary infusion. In addition to the germ line, there is another route for manipulating the genetics of the mammary gland, and thus the milk. That is by infusion into the mammary gland by way of the teat canal. The udder of ruminants, that is, cows, goats, sheep, are constructed in such a way that liquids injected into the canal (see chapter 6 and p. 254) can diffuse via the duct system within the gland to every lactating cell. For delivery, a small tube connected to a syringe containing the material to be infused works very well. In comparison to the germ line approach, infusion has the advantage that for practical purposes, expression of the gene is limited to the infused section of the udder and to the oncoming or ongoing lactation at the time. This could be an advantage when one does not want the lifetime lactations of the animal committed to the foreign protein in the milk. In both techniques, there is the challenge of purifying the desired protein from the complex mixture of proteins in the milk. Yields of proteins in the realm of milligrams per liter of milk have been achieved, and in the case of exotic drug-type proteins such yields could be worth thousands of dollars.

A pioneering achievement by this transfection technique has been accomplished at the laboratory of Professor Ian Mather of the University of Maryland. He and his collaborators introduced the human growth hormone gene into the guinea pig mammary gland and witnessed a sustained yield of the hormone in the milk[15]. In fact, the production and secretion of it continued throughout the lactation.

It can be anticipated that genetic manipulation of the mammary gland will be used to modify milk in many ways. Such things as the many years of selective breeding to raise the fat content of Holstein milk should not be necessary. At this point, no one can anticipate all the potentialities of this approach but certainly improvements in the processing characteristics and the nutrition/ healthfulness aspects of milk will provide diverse research objectives. One frequently mentioned target is installation of the gene for the lactose-digestion protein so that lactose intolerance need no longer limit milk consumption by anyone. One can conceive of adding factors or deleting others from milk depending on needs of particular consumers. This makes the point that despite attempts of cranks and special interest advocates to defame milk, it is here to stay—now more than ever. Using the new powerful tools of molecular genetics, what few inadequacies milk may have for special subsets of our population can be modified or eliminated. For example, if it proves true that amino acid sequences of certain milk proteins incite production of antibodies in certain people that are detrimental to them, such sequences can be genetically altered or removed. A constructive attitude regarding complaints about milk, if there is any substance to them, is to see them as promoting new versions of milk to meet special needs. Of course, genetic modification (GM) of milk will have its adversaries just as currently available GM foods already do, but it seems likely that the value of these foods will eventually be widely appreciated, especially when opposing geopolitics is overcome.

The breast. From a research standpoint, it is important to realize that the new genetics also has implications for the human breast. Whether any research and development along such lines will occur remains to be seen but there are significant possibilities. The breasts are such personal attributes and are so involved in cultural taboos that they are not readily available for scientific study. They are the only glands that are greatly appreciated whether they function or not. In addition, it is not easy to use humans for any kind of invasive research let alone studies involving the breast. But if the research goals are sufficiently worthy, and potentially rewarding, things may get done.

It is now known that the resting, that is, non-lactating, breast is nonetheless engaged in some secretion. This is evident from research by Dr. Ulrich Welsch and coworkers at the Anatomy Department of the University of Munich.[16] What is being secreted and whether the product(s) have local functions or functions elsewhere in the body, as a result of release into the circulation, need to be the subjects of further investigation. It seems likely that such secretion may be more active in women who have gone through pregnancy but this point also requires study. Not that there is always a close correlation between species, but it has been observed that the cow carries about 20 percent of her lactating epithelial cells forward from one lactation to the next. Although these cells are relatively non-productive during this so-called dry period, it is always possible to hand express some fluid from the gland at that time. Normally, this fluid must somehow be reabsorbed in the body.

The interesting fact here is that during lactation, the mammary gland is pretty much shut off from cycling things back into the mother's body, the purpose being to deliver the secretion out of her body into the baby. Despite this fact, when milk over-accumulates in the breast, some milk constituents can be detected in the mother's blood stream. So there is a pathway from lactating cells into the general circulation. When lactation shuts down, this tight outward-directed system loosens up and it is then much easier for secretory products made in the breast to diffuse throughout the breast and into the circulation. If this type of post-lactational secretory activity occurs in women, they are producing and absorbing substances that would not be normal to a woman who had never lactated. Could this be a factor in the reduced incidence of breast cancer in women who have breast fed?[17]

Bearing the foregoing in mind, my colleagues and I have suggested that the breast might have endocrine functions, perhaps relatively minor in importance and as yet unidentified, but like in principle, those of the thyroid, pituitary, pancreas, and so on. The circumstances in which this could become more meaningful and demanding genetic manipulation or therapy is when the woman has an inadequacy of an important protein, for example, insulin. It might be possible to infuse the insulin gene(s) into her breast(s) by way of the nipple and achieve sufficient expression to satisfactorily control diabetes. Such infusions by way of the nipple, because of its small multiple-duct structure, would not be as simple as in the ruminant mammary gland where there is a large single channel to the surface of the gland. However, it should be possible. Infusions via the relatively tiny teats of rats and mice are done consistently with practice[18]; and remarkable intranuclear gene placements are being accomplished with the aid of current micromanipulation systems. Another consideration with respect to breast infusion is prevention and control of breast cancer. It may develop that this route is not only useful for infusion of genes that may generate cancer antagonists and metastasis inhibitors but other therapeutic agents might be delivered with improved effects and less side reactions by direct infusion into the breast.

Beyond needs of the woman herself for gene therapy, are there other reasons for gene transfer into the breast? At the moment needs of an infant for a unique and expensive therapeutic protein, enhancement of protein content of milk, and need for a therapeutic protein (drug) to be produced in a human system are among possibilities. In protein synthesis, making the backbone, that is, the chain of amino acids, is often just the first step. Adding sugars, lipids, phosphates, and other groups in the right location on the backbone, as well as achieving the proper final folded structure are challenging steps that can require very special circumstances. Thus, for some human proteins, the simplest solution to synthesis with complete and correct final structure may be synthesis in a human.

Thinking a little more broadly, one needs to remember that there are quite a few cell types in the mammary gland including not only the mammary epithelial cell that can make milk, but also fat cells (adipocytes), cell of capillary blood vessels (endothelial), connective tissue cells (fibroblasts), muscle type cells (myoepithelial), a variety of cells of the immune system, and multilayers of dermal (skin) cells. These latter could also be approached for delivery of substances by transdermal techniques. The particular objective would determine which of these many cell types might best be targeted for a particular gene transfection experiment.

Thinking a little more wildly, one might consider making the size of the breasts either larger or smaller by means of infused therapeutics. There is very extensive knowledge developing about the process of natural cell death, apoptosis as it is known. In fact, pioneering research was done on the nature of this phenomenon in the mammary gland because it is part of the normal involution and consequent shrinking of the gland at the end of lactation. Approaches to smaller or larger breasts also need to focus on fat cells, since they are the primary determinant of non-lactating breast size. This is not only a matter of how many cells but how much fat is deposited in them. Blocking or enhancing fat deposition in the breasts specifically is conceivable and, as far as augmentation is concerned, would be more natural than inserting foreign materials. Exercise or surgery are other well-known approaches to this situation.

Finally, transfecting of specific genes into the breast might represent another means of controlling aging. There is extensive evidence that one cause of aging is the loss of function in various glands and tissues in the body. Perhaps transfection of genes into breast tissue might help to maintain some functions by supplementing another fresh and continuing source of the bioactive substances that are needed. As an example, consider growth hormone (GH). Our capacity to produce this pituitary hormone declines steadily during adulthood and there is some evidence that we continue to need it in order to retain such things as muscle mass and skin tone while suppressing fat deposition. GH is by no means on completely solid ground yet for slowing the wasting, wrinkling and sagging that are so characteristic of getting old. Here again, more research is needed, but GH is a protein of the type that well might be naturally augmented for the long term via gene therapy in the breast. Further, there may be other proteinaceous products to be generated in the mammary gland with other health-producing potentialities. You ask, what about the male in this connection? At this point, there seems to be a distinct female advantage.

Dairy Research

Funding outlook. To a large extent, the future of dairy research depends on how much financial support it is given. There will always be the federal grant pathway, which is difficult, competitive and subject to funding agency budget limitations. With a few notable exceptions, dairy corporations never have played much of a direct role in dairy research. However, there is always the opportunity to obtain small grants from them and to involve them in collaborations. We also should bear in mind the new game, venture capital. This means the researcher or his partners need a sound business plan and someone who can make good oral presentations. One thing certain, the dairy markets are huge; and if one has a product or process that can obtain even a small piece of one, it is worth money. Venture capital is running lots of research operations. Just like always, researchers have to scramble for money.

Research agendas. While lack of funding is limiting the effort somewhat, dairy research is alive and well. There is great potential in applications of molecular genetics to utilize in new ways and improve milk, cows and the plants on which they feed. There will always be standard economic advancement research questions being pursued, such as: How can we feed and manage cows more efficiently? How can we reduce the expense of processing milk and milk products? Discovery of the beneficial components and properties of milk is by no means exhausted. An area in which the public is greatly interested concerns clinical and epidemiological findings on the healthfulness of milk and milk products. This is an example of an area where the relevance of research to agriculture, nutrition and medicine clearly overlaps. Even if projected dairy research were to dwindle, accidental discoveries (serendipity) would continue and liven things up.

*   *   *

Research is an incredibly important occupation. It is what has moved humanity from a primitive existence to the sophisticated modern culture and high standard of living now typical in many areas of the world. While the organization and support of research is changing with the times, it remains fundamentally an occupation of individual minds from a creative standpoint. One thing that is not widely appreciated about research is its merits as a mechanism of teaching. Young people who have become personally involved in developing an answer to a real unsolved problem in science are motivated to learn the existing relevant knowledge surrounding the problem in a way that is hard if not impossible to match in the classroom.

A tremendous amount of taxpayer-supported research is largely responsible for the vastly increased milk production capability of the cow. Such support also has made milk and milk products the outstanding and widely appreciated foods they are. Research will produce new and different possibilities for us tomorrow. Among many findings that will be coming, those via the new genetics in application to cows and milk should be quite valuable and interesting. In addition, there may be surprises, which is research at its exciting best.

Suggested References

Medawar, P. B. *Advice to a Young Scientist.* Pan Books, London and Sydney. 1979. pp. 109.

Zartman, D. L. et al. (eds.) *Milk Synthesis, Production and Nutritional Qualities. A symposium in observance of the centennial year of the Ohio Agricultural Research and Development Center in Wooster.* Ohio State University, Wooster, OH. 1992. pp. 168.

Notes

1.   Horgan, J. *The End of Science.* Addison-Wesley Publishing Co. Reading, MA. 1996. pp. 308.
2.   Gendler, S. J. et al. *Journal of Biological Chemistry* 265:15286-93. 1990. For a review of the epithelial mucins which occur in milk and on mammary and other epithelial cells, see: Patton, S. et al. *Biochimica Biophysica Acta* 1241: 407-424.1995.
3.   Carvalho, F. et al. *Glycoconjugate Journal* 14: 107-111. 1997.
4.   This profound definition of science comes to us from Hans Selye, a well-known life scientist.
5.   Thompson, J. D. *ASBMB Today* 1(5):12-15. 2002.
6.   Borlaug, N. E. Science vs. Hysteria. *Wall Street Journal.* 1/23/03.
7.   For an extensive review of the research and development regarding BHT and milk yield, see Bauman, D. E. *Journal of Dairy Science* 75:3432-51. 1992.
8.   Saacke, R. G. et al. *Journal of Dairy Science* 38:1046-7. 1955.
9.   Flipse, R. J. et al. *Journal of Dairy Science* 37:1205-11. 1954.
10.   Patton, S. et al. *Journal of Dairy Science* 80:265-72. 1997.
11.   Sylvester, D. R. et al. *Biology of Reproduction* 41:941-8. 1989.
12.   Hammerstedt, R. H. et al. *Journal of Andrology* 18:29. 1997.
13.   Barisic, D. et al. *Fertility and Sterility* 62: 172-175. 1994.
14.   Babcock, D. F. Smelling the Roses? *Science* 299:1993-4. 2003; a review of research by Spehr, M. et al. in the same issue, pp. 2054-8.

15. Hens, J. R. et al. *Biochimica et Biophysica Acta* 1523: 161-171. 2000.
16. Schinko, I. H. et al. (in English) *Zeitschrift fur mikroskopisch-anatatomische Forschung* 104: S578-92. 1990.
17. Beral, V. et al. Breast cancer and breast feeding: collaborative analysis of individual data from 47 epidemiological studies in thirty countries, including 50,302 women with breast cancer and 96,973 women without the disease. *Lancet* 360:187-95. 2002.
18. Patton, S. et al. *Journal of Dairy Science* 67:1323-1326. 1984.

Index

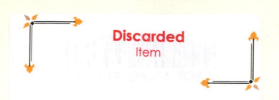